1997
YEAR BOOK OF
DIGESTIVE DISEASES®

Statement of Purpose

The YEAR BOOK Service

The YEAR BOOK series was devised in 1901 by practicing health professionals who observed that the literature of medicine and related disciplines had become so voluminous that no one individual could read and place in perspective every potential advance in a major specialty. In the final decade of the 20th century, this recognition is more acutely true than it was in 1901.

More than merely a series of books, YEAR BOOK volumes are the tangible results of a unique service designed to accomplish the following:

- to *survey* a wide range of journals of proven value
- to *select* from those journals papers representing significant advances and statements of important clinical principles
- to provide *abstracts* of those articles that are readable, convenient summaries of their key points
- to provide *commentary* about those articles to place them in perspective

These publications grow out of a unique process that calls on the talents of outstanding authorities in clinical and fundamental disciplines, trained literature specialists, and professional writers, all supported by the resources of Mosby, the world's preeminent publisher for the health professions.

The Literature Base

Mosby and its editors survey more than 1,000 journals published worldwide, covering the full range of the health professions. On an annual basis, the publisher examines usage patterns and polls its expert authorities to add new journals to the literature base and to delete journals that are no longer useful as potential YEAR BOOK sources.

The Literature Survey

The publisher's team of literature specialists, all of whom are trained and experienced health professionals, examines every original, peer-reviewed article in each journal issue. More than 250,000 articles per year are scanned systematically, including title, text, illustrations, tables, and references. Each scan is compared, article by article, to the search strategies that the publisher has developed in consultation with the 270 outside experts who form the pool of YEAR BOOK editors. A given article may be reviewed by any number of editors, from one to a dozen or more, regardless of the discipline for which the paper was originally published. In turn, each editor who receives the article reviews it to determine whether or not the article should be included in the YEAR BOOK. This decision is based on the article's inherent quality, its probable usefulness to readers of that YEAR BOOK, and the editor's goal to represent a balanced picture of a given field in each volume of the YEAR BOOK. In addition, the editor indicates when to include figures and tables from the article to help the YEAR BOOK reader better understand the information.

Of the quarter million articles scanned each year, only 5% are selected for detailed analysis within the YEAR BOOK series, thereby assuring readers of the high value of every selection.

The Abstract

The publisher's abstracting staff is headed by a seasoned medical professional and includes individuals with training in the life sciences, medicine, and other areas, plus extensive experience in writing for the health professions and related industries. Each selected article is assigned to a specific writer on this abstracting staff. The abstracter, guided in many cases by notations supplied by the expert editor, writes a structured, condensed summary designed so that the reader can rapidly acquire the essential information contained in the article.

The Commentary

The YEAR BOOK editorial boards, sometimes assisted by guest commentators, write comments that place each article in perspective for the reader. This provides the reader with the equivalent of a personal consultation with a leading international authority—an opportunity to better understand the value of the article and to benefit from the authority's thought processes in assessing the article.

Additional Editorial Features

The editorial boards of each YEAR BOOK organize the abstracts and comments to provide a logical and satisfying sequence of information. To enhance the organization, editors also provide introductions to sections or individual chapters, comments linking a number of abstracts, citations to additional literature, and other features.

The published YEAR BOOK contains enhanced bibliographic citations for each selected article, including extended listings of multiple authors and identification of author affiliations. Each YEAR BOOK contains a Table of Contents specific to that year's volume. From year to year, the Table of Contents for a given YEAR BOOK will vary depending on developments within the field.

Every YEAR BOOK contains a list of the journals from which papers have been selected. This list represents a subset of the more than 1,000 journals surveyed by the publisher and occasionally reflects a particularly pertinent article from a journal that is not surveyed on a routine basis.

Finally, each volume contains a comprehensive subject index and an index to authors of each selected paper.

The 1997 Year Book Series

Year Book of Allergy, Asthma, and Clinical Immunology: Drs. Rosenwasser, Borish, Gelfand, Leung, Nelson, and Szefler

Year Book of Anesthesiology and Pain Management®: Drs. Tinker, Abram, Chestnut, Roizen, Rothenberg, and Wood

Year Book of Cardiology®: Drs. Schlant, Collins, Gersh, Graham, Kaplan, and Waldo

Year Book of Chiropractic®: Dr. Lawrence

Year Book of Critical Care Medicine®: Drs. Parrillo, Balk, Calvin, Franklin, and Shapiro

Year Book of Dentistry®: Drs. Meskin, Berry, Kennedy, Leinfelder, Roser, Summitt, and Zakariasen

Year Book of Dermatologic Surgery®: Drs. Greenway, Papadopoulos, and Whitaker

Year Book of Dermatology®: Drs. Sober and Fitzpatrick

Year Book of Diagnostic Radiology®: Drs. Federle, Gross, Dalinka, Maynard, Rebner, Smirniotopolous, and Young

Year Book of Digestive Diseases®: Drs. Greenberger and Moody

Year Book of Drug Therapy®: Drs. Lasagna and Weintraub

Year Book of Emergency Medicine®: Drs. Wagner, Dronen, Davidson, King, Niemann, and Roberts

Year Book of Endocrinology®: Drs. Bagdade, Braverman, Horton, Kannan, Landsberg, Molitch, Morley, Nathan, Odell, Poehlman, Rogol, and Ryan

Year Book of Family Practice®: Drs. Berg, Bowman, Davidson, Dexter, and Scherger

Year Book of Geriatrics and Gerontology®: Drs. Beck, Burton, Ostwald, Rabins, Reuben, Roth, Shapiro, and Whitehouse

Year Book of Hand Surgery®: Drs. Amadio and Hentz

Year Book of Hematology®: Drs. Spivak, Bell, Ness, Quesenberry, Wiernik, and Blume

Year Book of Infectious Diseases®: Drs. Keusch, Barza, Bennish, Poutsiaka, Skolnik, and Snydman

Year Book of Medicine®: Drs. Klahr, Cline, Petty, Frishman, Greenberger, Malawista, Mandell, and Utiger

Year Book of Neonatal and Perinatal Medicine®: Drs. Fanaroff, Maisels, and Stevenson

Year Book of Nephrology, Hypertension, and Mineral Metabolism: Drs. Schwab, Bennett, Emmett, Hostetter, Kumar, and Toto

Year Book of Neurology and Neurosurgery®: Drs. Bradley and Wilkins

Year Book of Nuclear Medicine®: Drs. Gottschalk, Blaufox, Neumann, Strauss, and Zubal

Year Book of Obstetrics, Gynecology, and Women's Health: Drs. Mishell, Herbst, and Kirschbaum

Year Book of Occupational and Environmental Medicine®: Drs. Emmett, Frank, Gochfeld, and Hessl

Year Book of Oncology®: Drs. Ozols, Cohen, Glatstein, Loehrer, Tallman, and Wiersma

Year Book of Ophthalmology®: Drs. Wilson, Augsburger, Cohen, Eagle, Flanagan, Grossman, Laibson, Maguire, Nelson, Penne, Rapuano, Sergott, Spaeth, Tipperman, Ms. Gosfield, and Ms. Salmon

Year Book of Orthopedics®: Drs. Sledge, Poss, Cofield, Dobyns, Griffin, Springfield, Swiontkowski, Wiesel, and Wilson

Year Book of Otolaryngology–Head and Neck Surgery®: Drs. Paparella and Holt

Year Book of Pathology and Laboratory Medicine: Drs. Mills, Bruns, Gaffey, and Stoler

Year Book of Pediatrics®: Dr. Stockman

Year Book of Plastic, Reconstructive, and Aesthetic Surgery®: Drs. Miller, Cohen, McKinney, Robson, Ruberg, Smith, and Whitaker

Year Book of Podiatric Medicine and Surgery®: Dr. Kominsky

Year Book of Psychiatry and Applied Mental Health®: Drs. Talbott, Ballenger, Breier, Frances, Meltzer, Schowalter, and Tasman

Year Book of Pulmonary Disease®: Dr. Petty

Year Book of Rheumatology®: Drs. Sergent, LeRoy, Meenan, Panush, and Reichlin

Year Book of Sports Medicine®: Drs. Shephard, Drinkwater, Eichner, George, and Torg

Year Book of Surgery®: Drs. Copeland, Bland, Deitch, Eberlein, Howard, Luce, Seeger, Souba, and Sugarbaker

Year Book of Thoracic and Cardiovascular Surgery®: Drs. Ginsberg, Wechsler, and Williams

Year Book of Urology®: Drs. Andriole and Coplen

Year Book of Vascular Surgery®: Dr. Porter

1997

The Year Book of DIGESTIVE DISEASES®

Editors

Norton J. Greenberger, M.D.
Peter T. Bohan Professor and Chairman, Department of Internal Medicine, University of Kansas Medical Center, Kansas City, Kansas

Frank G. Moody, M.D.
Denton A. Cooley Professor, Department of Surgery, The University of Texas Medical School-Houston Medical School, Houston, Texas

Editorial Assistants

To Dr. Greenberger
Shirley Sears
Ruth Stricklen
Mary Lynch

To Dr. Moody
Flora Roeder

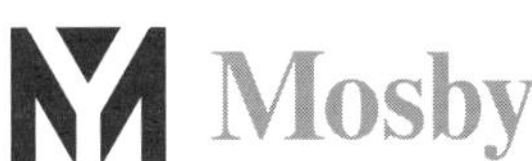

St. Louis   Baltimore   Boston   Carlsbad   Naples   New York   Philadelphia   Portland   London
Madrid   Mexico City   Singapore   Sydney   Tokyo   Toronto   Wiesbaden

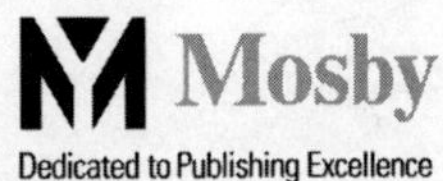

Mosby

Dedicated to Publishing Excellence

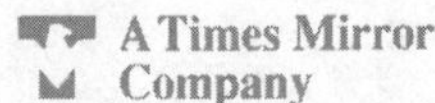

A Times Mirror
Company

Vice President and Publisher, Continuity Publishing: Kenneth H. Killion
Director, Editorial Development: Gretchen C. Murphy
Acquisitions Editor: Gina G. Byrd
Developmental Editor: Kris Horeis, R.N.
Project Specialist, Editing: Denise M. Dungey
Senior Project Manager, Production: Max F. Perez
Freelance Staff Supervisor: Barbara M. Kelly
Illustrations and Permissions Coordinator: Lois M. Ruebensam
Director, Editorial Services: Edith M. Podrazik, B.S.N., R.N.
Information Specialist: Terri Santo, R.N.
Information Specialist: Margery Marble, B.S., R.N.
Circulation Manager: Lynn D. Stevenson

1997 EDITION
Copyright © October 1997 by Mosby–Year Book, Inc.

Printed in the United States of America
Composition by Reed Technology and Information Services, Inc.
Printing/binding by Maple–Vail

Editorial Office:
Mosby–Year Book, Inc.
11830 Westline Industrial Drive
St. Louis, MO 63146
Customer Service: customer.support@mosby.com
      www.mosby.com/Mosby/CustomerSupport/index.html

International Standard Serial Number: 0739–5930
International Standard Book Number: 0-8151-9618-0

Table of Contents

Journals Represented

Mosby and its editors survey more than 1,000 journals for its abstract and commentary publications. From these journals, the editors select the articles to be abstracted. Journals represented in this YEAR BOOK are listed below.

Acta Cytologica
Acta Radiologica
Alimentary Pharmacology and Therapeutics
American Journal of Gastroenterology
American Journal of Medicine
American Journal of Physiology
American Journal of Roentgenology
American Journal of Surgery
American Journal of Surgical Pathology
American Surgeon
Annals of Internal Medicine
Annals of Oncology
Annals of Surgery
Annals of Surgical Oncology
Archives of Surgery
Artificial Organs
British Journal of Surgery
Cancer
Digestive Diseases and Sciences
Diseases of the Colon and Rectum
European Journal of Cancer
European Journal of Surgery
Gastroenterology
Gastrointestinal Endoscopy
Gut
Hepatology
Investigative Radiology
Journal of Clinical Endocrinology and Metabolism
Journal of Clinical Investigation
Journal of Computer Assisted Tomography
Journal of Pediatric Gastroenterology and Nutrition
Journal of Pediatric Surgery
Journal of Surgical Oncology
Journal of Thoracic and Cardiovascular Surgery
Journal of the American College of Surgeons
Journal of the American Medical Association
Lancet
Mayo Clinic Proceedings
Medicine
New England Journal of Medicine
Science
Surgery
Transplantation
Transplantation Proceedings
World Journal of Surgery

Standard Abbreviations

The following terms are abbreviated in this edition: acquired immunodeficiency syndrome (AIDS), cardiopulmonary resuscitation (CPR), central nervous system (CNS), cerebrospinal fluid (CSF), computed tomography (CT), deoxyribonucleic acid (DNA), electrocardiography (ECG), health maintenance organization (HMO), human immunodeficiency virus (HIV), intensive care unit (ICU), intramuscular (IM), intravenous (IV), magnetic resonance (MR) imaging (MRI), and ribonucleic acid (RNA).

Note

The YEAR BOOK OF DIGESTIVE DISEASES is a literature survey service providing abstracts of articles published in the professional literature. Every effort is made to assure the accuracy of the information presented in these pages. Neither the editors nor the publisher of the YEAR BOOK OF DIGESTIVE DISEASES can be responsible for errors in the original materials. The editors' comments are their own opinions. Mention of specific products within this publication does not constitute endorsement.

To facilitate the use of the YEAR BOOK OF DIGESTIVE DISEASES as a reference tool, all illustrations and tables included in this publication are now identified as they appear in the original article. This change is meant to help the reader recognize that any illustration or table appearing in the YEAR BOOK OF DIGESTIVE DISEASES may be only one of many in the original article. For this reason, figure and table numbers will often appear to be out of sequence within the YEAR BOOK OF DIGESTIVE DISEASES.

Introduction

The 1997 YEAR BOOK OF DIGESTIVE DISEASES follows our traditional format based on an organ system orientation but also includes various sections that cross the broad disciplines of Gastroenterology, Hepatology, and Digestive Surgery. We have reviewed more than 3,500 articles and selected 227 for inclusion with abstracts and comments. There are an additional 21 abstracts in the capsules and comments section. The selections once again include a mix of basic advances and new insights into the mechanisms of disease and clinical studies. We have emphasized the selection of papers that will be of practical value to Gastroenterologists, Hepatologists, Radiologists, Pediatricians, and Surgeons. This year, as in past years, there is an introduction in each chapter that highlights some of the key articles.

We thank Shirley Sears, Ruth Stricklen, Linda Taylor, Mary Lynch, and Flora Roeder for their continued fine efforts in the preparation of the manuscript and Miranda Jackson and Kris Horeis at Mosby–Year Book, Inc., for editorial support.

Norton J. Greenberger, M.D.

Frank G. Moody, M.D.

PART ONE

THE ESOPHAGUS

Introduction

The treatment of diseases of the esophagus continues to outpace our understanding of their pathogenesis. It is now clear, however, that patients with gastroesophageal reflux and Barrett's epithelium are at high risk for esophageal cancer developing. That laparoscopic antireflux procedures are both safe and effective offers hope for a more efficient and less intrusive way to control reflux esophagitis that is otherwise difficult to manage medically. Enough cases have now been treated and studied for a sufficient period to reveal that the results of such procedures done by experienced laparoscopic surgeons are comparable to those obtained by the open approach, and with a much shorter hospital stay.

Adenocarcinoma of the lower end of the esophagus most likely results from longstanding reflux esophagitis. If it is identified early, it can be treated by a transhiatal esophagectomy, a procedure with much less morbidity than a transthoracic approach. Laparoscopic technology offers a way to lessen the extent of the intra-abdominal portion of the procedure and, thereby, the length of stay associated with this component of the operation. I do not mean to be provocative by emphasizing the hospital side of these therapies, but, as is well known to physicians in the United States, hospital days equate to dollars and expenditure of increasingly scarce health resources. But of equal importance is patient acceptance of these less intrusive procedures.

Also in this section is a summary of a report that emphasizes the importance of the quality rather than the quantity of life in patients with esophageal carcinoma. In the course of trying to help patients with an incurable disease, we often lose sight of the reality of therapeutic outcomes and provide options that may in fact decrease the number of happy days that our patients may experience.

Frank G. Moody, M.D.

1 Medication Associated Esophagitis

Esophagitis Associated With the Use of Alendronate
de Groen PC, Lubbe DF, Hirsch LJ, et al (Mayo Clinic and Found, Rochester, Minn; Merck Research Labs, Rahway, NJ; Univ of South Florida, Tampa)
N Engl J Med 335:1016–1021, 1996   1–1

Background.—Alendronate, used to treat osteoporosis in postmenopausal women and Paget's disease of the bone, is an aminobisphosphonate and selective inhibitor of osteoclast-mediated bone resorption that can irritate the upper gastrointestinal mucosa. The adverse esophageal effects reported to Merck, the manufacturer of alendronate, were reviewed, and 3 new affected patients reported.

Methods and Findings.—A total of 1,213 reports of adverse effects had been received as of March 1996 from among an estimated 475,000 patients given the drug worldwide. In 199 patients, adverse effects were related to the esophagus. In 51 patients, including the 3 current ones, the adverse effects were considered serious or severe. Thirty-two patients needed to be hospitalized, and 2 were disabled temporarily. Findings on endoscopic examination were chemical esophagitis with erosions or ulcerations and exudative inflammation, accompanied by thickening of the esophageal wall. Bleeding was rare. Stomach and duodenal involvement were uncommon. Esophagitis appeared to be associated with swallowing alendronate with little or no water, lying down during or after ingestion, continuing alendronate use after symptom onset, and having pre-existing esophageal disorders.

Conclusions.—In some patients, alendronate can cause chemical esophagitis, including severe ulcerations. The risk of this complication may be reduced by drinking 6–8 oz of water when taking the tablet, taking it in the morning after getting up and remaining upright for at least 30 minutes afterward, and stopping medication immediately if esophageal symptoms occur.

▶ The potential for several drugs such as potassium salts, tetracycline, and quinidine to cause esophagitis is now well recognized. The report by de Groen, et al. indicates that alendronate, a drug used to treat osteoporosis in postmenopausal women, can cause chemical esophagitis, including severe ulceration, in some patients. Indeed, the severity of the esophageal lesions in de Groen's report is particularly bothersome because of the extensive degree of esophageal ulceration noted. It appears that failure of an alendronate tablet to pass promptly through a poorly lubricated esophagus may result in prolonged exposure to the drug. To reduce the risk of esophagitis, physicians prescribing alendronate should advise their patients as follows:

- Swallow alendronate with 6–8 oz of water
- Do not chew or suck the tablet
- Do not lie down for at least 30 minutes after taking the medication
- Do not take alendronate at bedtime
- Patients should stop the drug if dysphagia, odynophagia, retrosternal pain, or new and increased heartburn develops
- Do not continue or resume the medication after onset of symptoms

In addition, de Groen, et al. advise that alendronate is now contraindicated in patients with abnormal esophageal emptying because of achalasia or stricture. Finally, acid-suppressing drugs may not prevent alendronate-induced esophageal drainage.

N.J. Greenberger, M.D.

2 Reflux Esophagitis

Medical Therapy

Natural History of Reflux Oesophagitis: A 10 Year Follow Up of Its Effect on Patient Symptomatology and Quality of Life
McDougall NI, Johnston BT, Kee F, et al (Queen's Univ of Belfast, Northern Ireland; Royal Victoria Hosp, Belfast, Northern Ireland Ulster Hosp, Dundonald, Northern Ireland)
Gut 38:481–486, 1996
1–2

Background.—Gastroesophageal reflux disease affects 4% to 10% of the general population, and 50% to 68% of the patients who seek treatment are given a diagnosis of esophagitis. Esophagitis is presumed to be a chronic relapsing condition, but insufficient long-term studies have been performed to support this impression. Nor do any published studies investigate the long-term effect of gastroesophageal reflux disease on quality of life. To clarify these issues, the level of reflux symptoms, quality of life, drug consumption, and complications experienced by 152 patients with a diagnosis of esophagitis given at least 10 years previously were examined.

Methods.—Patients showed typical reflux symptoms and received a diagnosis of grade I–III esophagitis via endoscopy between 1981 and 1984. Follow-up was accomplished through postal questionnaire (including the Short Form 36 general health questionnaire for assessing quality of life) and telephone interview.

Results.—Thirty-three patients did not respond to the questionnaire and 18 had died; the 101 responses obtained allowed an average follow-up of 11 years from first diagnosis. Heartburn was still present in more than 70% of patients either daily (32%) or weekly (19%), requiring daily acid suppression treatment in 20% (Fig 2). Barrett's esophagus occurred in 1 patient and esophageal stricture in 2. Quality-of-life scores for physical function and social function were significantly lower for this population than for the Northern Ireland population at large.

Conclusion.—These data show the long-term natural history of a clearly defined subgroup of patients with gastroesophageal reflux disease: those with endoscopically confirmed esophagitis. The data indicate a worse prognosis for these patients than previously indicated, although the incidence of stricture formation was lower than previously reported. Esophagitis grade does not appear to be a useful predictor of the long-term

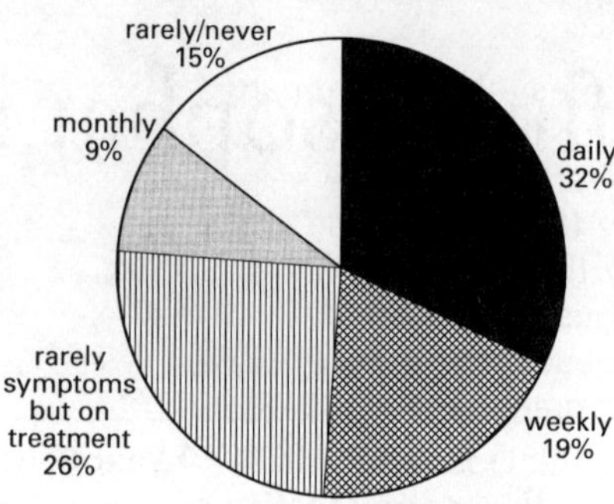

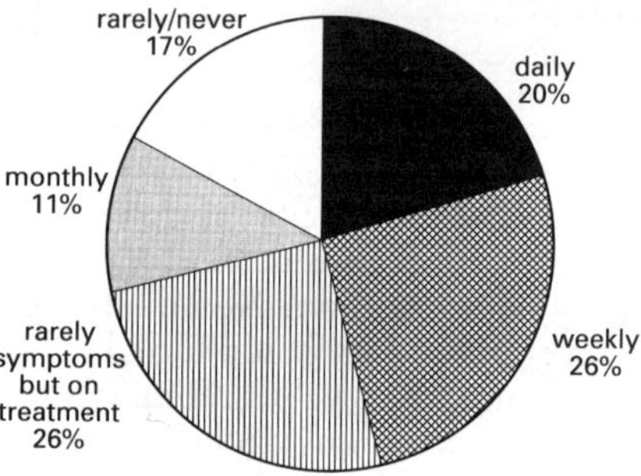

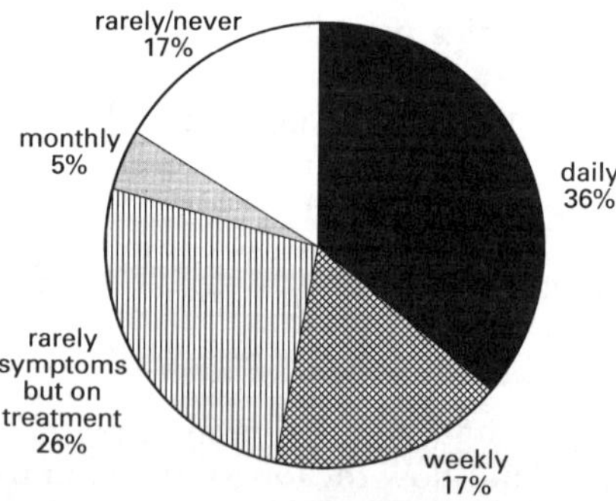

FIGURE 2.—Frequency of heartburn at follow-up. (Courtesy of McDougall NI, Johnston BT, Kee F, et al: Natural history of reflux esophagitis: A 10 year follow up of its effect on patient symptomatology and quality of life. *Gut* 38:481–486, 1996.)

outcome, but older age at the time of diagnosis did prove to be independently associated with poorer outcome.

▶ This study underscores the fact that patients with a first-time endoscopic diagnosis of grade II or III reflux esophagitis are likely to have a lifelong problem. Over a 10-year period, 70% of patients still had heartburn either daily (32%) or weekly (19%), requiring daily acid suppression treatment in 20%. I was struck by the seemingly low incidence of stricture (2 patients) and Barrett's esophagus (1 patient) in this series of 152 patients.

Patients with gastroesophageal reflux disease (GERD) and endoscopically verified esophagitis of grade II to IV are more likely to respond to long-term treatment with proton pump inhibitors (PPIs) than to histamine H_2 receptor antagonists. In approximately half the patients, the dose of omeprazole can be reduced to 20 mg every other day. I suspect that similar findings will obtain for lansoprazole.

There is no evidence to date that long term PPI therapy will reduce the likelihood of the development of Barrett's esophagus, but controlled long-term studies to clarify this issue have not yet been carried out. I am guided, in large part, by my patients with GERD and endoscopically verified esophagitis who clearly state that their symptoms are usually well controlled if they continue taking PPIs. Because the long-term safety of PPIs (10 years plus) has not been fully established, I try to taper the dosage to the lowest dose that will control symptoms.

N.J. Greenberger, M.D.

Optimal Dosing of Omeprazole 40 mg Daily: Effects on Gastric and Esophageal pH and Serum Gastrin in Healthy Controls
Kuo B, Castell DO (Graduate Hosp, Philadelphia)
Am J Gastroenterol 91:1532–1538, 1996   1–3

Background.—The optimal regimen of omeprazole 40 mg/day for suppressing gastric acid and distal esophageal acid exposure has not been established. The association of serum gastrin and gastric pH levels with this treatment also remains uncertain. The relative efficacy of a split dose of 20 mm twice a day (bid) and single-dose regimens of 40 mg every morning (qAM) or every evening (qPM) in suppressing acid was investigated.

Methods.—Nineteen healthy men volunteered for the study. Baseline fasting serum gastrin and 24-hour ambulatory combined distal esophageal and gastric pH monitoring were performed. Three regimens of omeprazole 40 mg were given for 7 days with repeated pH and gastrin determinations on day 6. The regimens were 20 mg bid, 40 mg qAM, and 40 mg qPM. The volunteers took the medication before meals.

Findings.—All dosing regimens significantly reduced acid compared with baseline values in the stomach and distal esophagus. The amount of acid exposure among the 3 dosing regimens in the esophagus and between

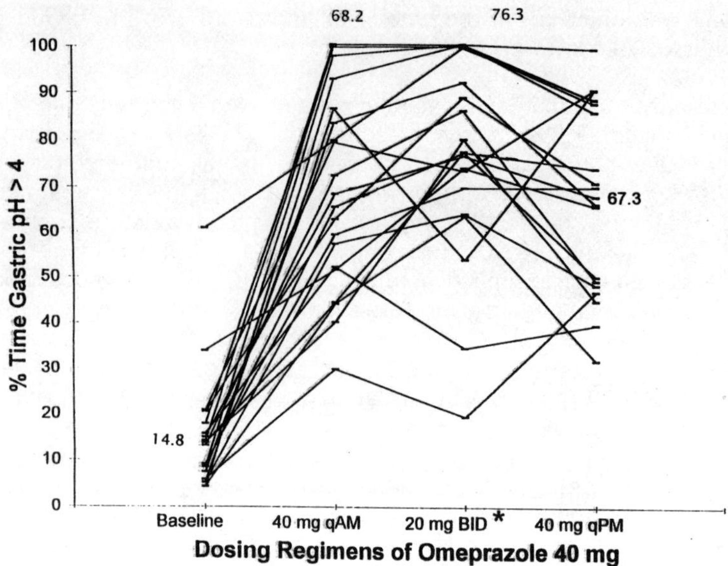

FIGURE 1.—Total percentage time gastric pH greater than 4 using different dosing regimens of omeprazole 40 mg daily. Research subjects were receiving no medications at baseline. Numerical values indicate mean for each dose. The *connecting lines* show that 15 of 19 patients had superior acid control receiving 20 mg bid dosing ($p < 0.05$) compared with once-a-day dosing qAM or qPM. (Courtesy of Kuo B, Castell DO: Optimal dosing of omeprazole 40 mg daily: Effects on gastric and esophageal pH and serum gastrin in healthy volunteers. *Am J Gastroenterol* 91:1532–1538, 1996.)

qAM and qPM dosing in the stomach did not differ significantly. However, twice-a-day dosing was more effective than the single daily dose in suppressing gastric acid in 15 of the 19 volunteers. When baseline values were compared with all regimens of omeprazole 40 mg, serum gastrin and percentage time gastric pH less than 4 differed significantly (Fig 1). There was a poor correlation between change in serum gastrin and change in percentage time gastric pH less than 4.

Conclusions.—In most individuals, gastric acid suppression is better with divided dosing of omeprazole 20 mg bid than with a once-a-day regimen of omeprazole 40 mg. Because serum gastrin levels do not correspond well to gastric pH, gastric pH monitoring is needed to determine accurately the response to gastric acid suppression.

▶ Although omeprazole at a dosage of 20 mg/day often is sufficient to control symptoms of gastroesophageal reflux disease (GERD) and other gastric acid–related disorders in most patients, many patients require high doses. This study was carried out to determine whether split dosing of omeprazole would provide superior acid suppression compared to a single-dose regimen. Note from the above figures that 15 of 19 patients had superior acid control using 20 mg of omeprazole bid.

In a companion paper, Leite and colleagues[1] studied 88 patients with GERD who had persistent symptoms while being maintained on omeprazole, 20 mg bid. Seventeen (19%) demonstrated abnormal gastric acid secretion (percentage time gastric pH less than 4 greater than 50%). Gastric pH studies resembled those of normal subjects receiving a placebo. Six of the "omeprazole failure" patients did respond to higher doses of omeprazole (i.e., 80 mg/day). Why certain patients are resistant to the acid suppression effects of proton pump inhibitors remains imcompletely defined.

N.J. Greenberger, M.D.

Reference

1. Leite LP, Johnston BT, Just RJ, et al: Persistent acid secretion during omeprazole therapy: A study of gastric acid profiles in patients demonstrating failure of omeprazole therapy. *Am J Gastroenterol* 91:1527–1531, 1996.

Effective Maintenance Treatment of Reflux Esophagitis With Low-dose Lansoprazole: A Randomized, Double-blind, Placebo-controlled Trial
Robinson M, Lanza F, Avner D, et al (Univ of Oklahoma, Oklahoma City; Baylor College of Medicine, Houston; Hahnemann Univ, Philadelphia)
Ann Intern Med 124:859–867, 1996 1–4

Background.—Erosive reflux esophagitis can usually be temporarily healed with short-term therapy with acid-suppressing agents. However, because relapse recurs within 6 months in 28% to 80% of these patients, a maintenance regimen is needed. Lansoprazole is a new proton pump inhibitor that is highly effective in the primary treatment of erosive esophagitis. Its efficacy as a maintenance treatment was evaluated in a randomized, double-blind, parallel, placebo-controlled trial.

Methods.—Patients with a recent history of erosive reflux esophagitis who had healing of erosive esophagitis after short-term treatment were randomly assigned to treatment with either placebo, 15 mg of lansoprazole, or 30 mg of lansoprazole in a single daily dose before breakfast for 1 year. Endoscopy was performed at 1, 2, 3, 6, 9, and 12 months. Any patient with an erosive recurrence was treated with 30 mg of lansoprazole daily for 8 weeks, then returned to the assigned maintenance regimen. The treatment groups were compared for the time to the first recurrence, the number of recurrences, and the maintenance of symptom relief.

Results.—There were 170 evaluable patients. Maintenance treatment with lansoprazole significantly prolonged healing, with no significant difference between the 2 doses. At 1 month, healing was maintained in 45% of the placebo group, 93% of the group receiving 15 mg of lansoprazole, and 98% of the group receiving 30 mg of lansoprazole. At 12 months, healing was maintained in 24% of the placebo group, 79% of the 15-mg lansoprazole group, and 90% of the 30-mg lansoprazole group (Fig 1). At least 2 erosive recurrences occurred in 45% of the placebo group, 8% of the 15-mg group, 5% of 30-mg group. At least 3 erosive recurrences occurred in 35% of the placebo group and 2% of the lansoprazole patients. Lansoprazole maintenance treatment also produced superior symptom relief, with a probability of remaining asymptomatic for 12 months of

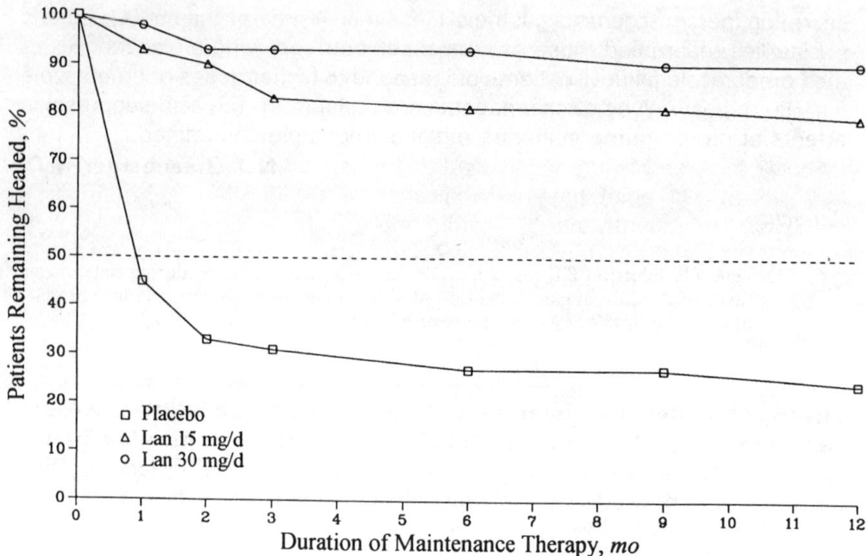

FIGURE 1.—Proportion of patients who remained healed (that is, no erosions seen on endoscopy) during the 1-year maintenance period. Lansoprazole significantly improved maintenance of healing rates compared with placebo ($P < 0.001$). Within 1 month, 45% of placebo recipients remained healed compared with 93% of patients receiving 15 mg of lansoprazole and 98% of patients receiving 30 mg of lansoprazole. (Courtesy of Robinson M, Lanza F, Avner D, et al: Effective maintenance treatment of reflux esophagitis with low-dose lansoprazole: A randomized, double-blind, placebo-controlled trial. *Ann Intern Med* 124:859–867, 1996.)

35% in the placebo group, 72% in the 15-mg lansoprazole group, and 67% in the 30-mg lansoprazole group. There were no significant differences between the placebo and lansoprazole groups in adverse events.

Conclusion.—Lansoprazole was effective in maintaining the healing of erosive esophagitis and controlling symptoms. The daily dose of 15 mg was as effective as the daily dose of 30 mg of lansoprazole. Therefore, it is suggested that 30 mg of lansoprazole daily be used as treatment of erosive esophagitis for 8 weeks, followed by a maintenance regimen of 15 mg of lansoprazole daily.

▶ The reader is referred to an excellent recent review article[1] that presents a consensus opinion on the treatment of gastroesophageal reflux disease (GERD). It bears emphasizing that there is a broad and ever-widening *spectrum* of GERD ranging from patients with endoscopy-negative GERD to patients with severe erosive esophagitis. Symptoms are poor indicators of underlying pathology. It appears that there are several subgroups of GERD and the natural history of these subgroups is not clear. For example, there are patients with classic reflux symptoms who have normal endoscopic studies as well as normal studies for 24-hour pH monitoring. Such patients are unusually sensitive to even small amounts of refluxate. It is possible and indeed likely that patients in this group do not progress to erosive esophagitis. Conversely, there are patients with erosive esophagitis who will invariably relapse if maintenance therapy is discontinued. It is generally agreed that patients who have classic symptoms of GERD without what are termed alarm or alert signals will infrequently need a confirmatory test. Such alarm or alert signals include anorexia, nausea, vomiting, dysphagia, weight loss, family history of peptic ulcer disease, anemia, and blood in the stools. To this list could be added failure to respond to intensive therapy for GERD. Again, to underscore the point, patients who have classic symptoms of intermittent GERD will infrequently need a confirmatory diagnostic test. If there is a question as to the extent of mucosal damage, endoscopy is the most appropriate test. In patients who have undergone endoscopy and who have not responded to intensive therapy, 24-hour pH monitoring may be useful to document that acid secretion has actually been reduced and to determine whether such patients are unusually sensitive to small amounts of refluxate.

Long-term studies of the natural history of GERD, especially to examine the various subgroups of GERD, are needed to define optimal therapy for these patients. It seems clear, however, that for patients with evidence of erosive esophagitis, maintenance therapy with a proton pump inhibitor provides the best current therapy available to ameliorate symptoms and maintain healing of esophagitis. The study by Robinson and colleagues provides additional support for this concept. However, long-term maintenance therapy with the proton pump inhibitors has been associated with some significant potential problems as illustrated in the following articles.

N.J. Greenberger, M.D.

Reference

1. Fennerty BM, Castall DO, Fendrick M, et al: The diagnosis and treatment of gastroesophageal reflux disease in a managed care environment. *Arch Intern Med* 156:477–484, 1996.

Predictors for Frequent Esophageal Dilations of Benign Peptic Strictures

Agnew SR, Pandya SP, Reynolds RPE, et al (Univ of Western Ontario & Lawson Research Inst, London, Canada)
Dig Dis Sci 41:931–936,1996   1–5

Background.—Many patients have recurrences of esophageal peptic stricture that necessitate repeated dilation treatments, despite optimal acid suppressive treatment. The correlated factors of frequent relapses are not well understood.

Methods.—Fifty-eight patients with benign peptic strictures and dysphagia were studied retrospectively. All had been treated by esophageal dilation. Mean follow-up was 66.5 months. The variables investigated were age, sex, heartburn, weight loss, esophagitis, Barrett's esophagus, number of dilation treatments in the first year of follow-up, frequency and number of subsequent dilation treatments, type of dilator used, and history of other concurrent treatments.

Findings.—More frequent dilations in the first year of follow-up were required in patients without heartburn and in those with a history of weight loss at their initial evaluation. Patients without heartburn had a mean of 6.2 dilations in the first year, compared with 3.2 for those with heartburn. Patients who had lost weight had a mean of 9 dilations, compared with 4.1 in those who did not. Patients who needed frequent treatment in their first year also needed frequent subsequent dilations because of stricture recurrence. There were no correlations between treatment frequency and the other variables studied.

Conclusions.—Patients who require frequent retreatment for recurrent peptic stricture are more likely to report a history of weight loss and less likely to report heartburn at the initial evaluation. The pattern of frequent repeat dilation for recurrent peptic strictures becomes evident in the first year of follow-up.

▶ The authors provide 2 self-predictive observations. Patients with benign esophageal strictures and who lose weight will require more dilatations than their counterparts who do not lose weight (but are dyspeptic). They further observed that patients who require frequent dilatations during the initial year of treatment will require frequent subsequent treatment, even in the presence of acid suppression. What they do not mention is the effectiveness of surgical therapy (fundoplication and intraoperative dilatation, if needed) for such patients. The availability and effectiveness of the laparoscopic antireflux approach should reduce the incidence of advanced strictures over the years ahead as more patients are definitively treated in the early phases of their disease.

F.G. Moody, M.D.

Surgical Therapy

Laparoscopic Nissen Fundoplication: 200 Consecutive Cases
Gotley DC, Smithers BM, Rhodes M, et al (Univ of Queensland, Australia; Royal Brisbane Hosp, Queensland, Australia)
Gut 38:487–491, 1996   1–6

Background.—The most common surgical procedure for correcting gastroesophageal reflux is the Nissen fundoplication. With the recently introduced laparoscopic approach, postoperative pain may be reduced, resulting in a shorter hospital stay and convalescent time. One experience with laparoscopic Nissen fundoplication was described.

Methods.—Two hundred patients underwent the procedure between 1991 and 1994. Preoperative evaluation included symptom score, endoscopy, manometry, and 24-hour pH monitoring of the esophagus. Assessments were performed at 3 and 12 months after surgery. Ninety-six patients also underwent 24-hour pH studies at 3 to 6 months after surgery.

Findings.—The median duration of surgery was 155 minutes in the first 100 patients. The conversion rate to laparotomy was 7%, the median hospital stay was 3 days, total morbidity was 16%. In the second hundred patients, the median operation time was 120 minutes, the conversion rate was 2%, the hospital stay was 3 days, and total morbidity was 7%. The median total symptom scores dropped from 5/9 to 0/9 after fundoplication. The median 24-hour esophageal acid exposure in 96 patients was decreased from 10% to 1%.

Conclusion.—Laparoscopic Nissen fundoplication is safe and effective in patients with gastroesophageal reflux disease. The duration of surgery and length of hospitalization decline with experience. Surgery consistently improves short-term symptomatic and pH results.

▶ This report from the Princess Alexandra and Royal Brisbane hospitals in Australia has documented, in a large number of cases, that Nissen fundoplication done laparoscopically is as effective as open fundoplication, after the learning curve has reached its asymptote. Is it less morbid? Probably. Certainly, the patients get home sooner, but are they the same patients as were referred for open surgery? The sheer number performed (200) during a 3-year period suggests not. The fact that less than 20% had significant dysphagia attests to this point of view.

F.G. Moody, M.D.

Intermediate Follow-up of Laparoscopic Antireflux Surgery
Trus TL, Laycock WS, Branum G, et al (Emory Univ, Atlanta, Ga)
Am J Surg 171:32–35, 1996   1–7

Introduction.—Laparoscopic antireflux surgery for chronic gastroesophageal reflux disease (GERD) is now viewed as an excellent alternative to lifelong medical therapy. Long-term outcome, however, is not yet available for a comparison of this procedure with open antireflux surgery. Intermediate follow-up, 1–3 years after operation, was reviewed for 35 patients who underwent laparoscopic fundoplication.

Methods.—Of the 288 patients with symptomatic GERD who underwent laparoscopic fundoplication, 100 were at least 1 year postoperative and 35 of the 100 had successfully completed 24-hour pH monitoring studies. The 23 men and 12 women in this group had a mean age of 50 years. Symptom scores and 24-hour ambulatory pH monitoring were collected before surgery and at 4–6 weeks and 1–3 years postoperatively. In most cases, laparoscopic antireflux surgery was performed through 5 trocars; some patients required a sixth trocar. The fundoplication measured approximately 2 cm in length and was fixed to the diaphragm in 2 places anteriorly.

Results.—Symptoms of reflux—heartburn, regurgitation, chest pain, and dysphagia—had improved significantly by the 6-week follow-up visit. Of the 59 patients with 24-hour ambulatory pH monitoring at 6 weeks, 51 had normal results. Five of the 8 patients with abnormal monitoring results were asymptomatic and continued to be asymptomatic at a median of 20 months later. All but 2 of the 35 patients with a second complete

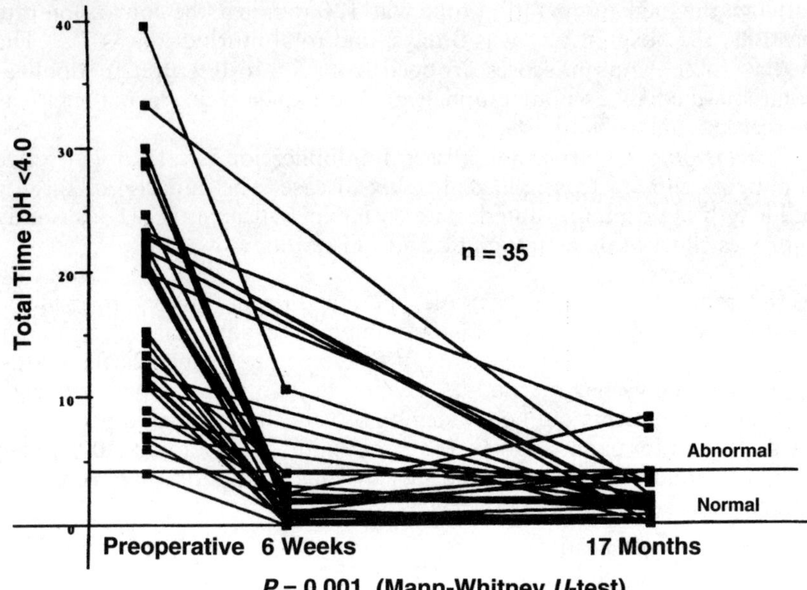

FIGURE 2.—Twenty-four-hour ambulatory pH results in laparoscopic fundoplication patients 1–3 years postoperatively. (Reprinted by permission of the publisher from Trus TL, Laycock WS, Branum G, et al: Intermediate follow-up of laparoscopic antireflux surgery. *Am J Surg* 171:32–35, 1996. Copyright 1996 by Excerpta Medica, Inc.)

24-hour ambulatory pH monitoring (median 17 months after laparoscopic surgery) had normal findings (Fig 2). There was no relationship between symptomatic or 24-hour ambulatory pH outcomes and partial versus total fundoplication.

Conclusion.—Most failures among patients who undergo open antireflux surgery for symptomatic GERD occur within the first 2 years after operation. The intermediate-term results of laparoscopic fundoplication in this series of patients suggest that the laparoscopic procedure should be as successful as open surgery. Patient satisfaction with laparoscopic antireflux surgery has been excellent.

▶ Long-term outcome studies on antireflux surgery performed laparoscopically are hard to find. The Emory group has made a valiant attempt to study patients at 1 or more years after their operations. They were able to trace 75 of 100 patients who fulfilled this criterion, and were able to perform 24-hour esophageal pH monitoring for 38 on whom the study had been performed before their operations. If you are satisfied with the sample size, and some who heard the work presented at the 36th annual meeting of the Society of Surgery of Alimentary Tract were not, then it appears that the laparoscopic approach provides results that are comparable to the open technique.

F.G. Moody, M.D.

Laparoscopic Surgery for Gastro-oesophageal Reflux: Beyond the Learning Curve
Watson DI, Jamieson GG, Baigrie RJ, et al (Royal Adelaide Hosp, South Australia)
Br J Surg 83:1284–1287, 1996   1–8

Introduction.—Laparoscopic antireflux surgery first was described in 1991, and early reports of the success of the procedure relative to open techniques indicated a 10% rate of conversion to open surgery and a significant reoperation rate. Now that surgeons have had more experience with the laparoscopic technique, it is likely that results have improved. An evaluation was performed that excluded the first 20 procedures done by each surgeon so that outcome could be judged when there was greater familiarity with laparoscopic antireflux surgery.

Methods.—Over a 4-year period, 320 patients underwent laparoscopic Nissen fundoplication at the study institution. All procedures were performed by 1 of 12 surgeons and trainees. Postoperative clinical follow-up was obtained at 3 and 12 months, then annually thereafter. Data were collected on patient satisfaction, complications, and hospital readmissions.

Results.—The study group included 174 patients (103 men and 71 women; median age 48) operated on by 5 experienced surgeons who each had performed between 27 and 102 laparoscopic Nissen fundoplications. The rate of intraoperative conversion to open surgery was 9.2%. Median operating time was 80 minutes and median postoperative hospital stay was 3 days. Within 30 days of surgery, complications occurred in 5.2% of patients and reoperations were performed in 2.3%. An additional 6 patients (3.4%) required a second procedure between 2 and 11 months after the initial surgery. All 113 patients who had a barium swallow examination 3 to 6 months after surgery were found to have an intact fundoplication, but 7 patients with postoperative dysphagia exhibited delayed emptying of barium through the fundoplication. Two years after surgery, 31 of 32 interviewed patients were satisfied with the outcome.

Discussion.—Laparoscopic Nissen fundoplication appears to have a significant learning curve because of the procedure's technical challenges. With more experienced surgeons, the rates of complication and reoperation were lower than previously reported. Although patient morbidity is greatly reduced by the laparoscopic procedure, long-term results will need to be compared with those of open surgery.

▶ This report on the outcome of laparoscopic Nissen fundoplication has the right design and numerical power to provide a benchmark for this approach to symptomatic gastroesophageal reflux. Notice that all the procedures were done in 1 hospital (the Royal Adelaide) and accessed into the study after the learning curve of the surgeons involved had been satisfied. A strict follow-up routine was adhered to and a nonclinical scientific officer kept score. The operating time (median) was 1 hour and 20 minutes, the conversion rate was less than 10%, and the hospital stay (median) was 3 days. The morbidity was low (5%), and there were no deaths. The success rate was comparable to that reported for fundoplication when performed in an open manner. This study should leave little doubt that this is the preferred therapy for patients with medically difficult-to-manage reflux esophagitis.

F.G. Moody, M.D.

3 Barrett's Esophagus

Eradication of High-grade Dysplasia in Columnar-lined (Barrett's) Oesophagus by Photodynamic Therapy With Endogenously Generated Protoporphyrin IX
Barr H, Shepherd NA, Dix A, et al (Gloustershire Royal and Cranfield Univ Inst of Medical Sciences, Gloucester, England; Univ of Leeds, England; Aintree Hosps, Liverpool, England)
Lancet 348:584–585, 1996   1–9

Background.—Dysplasia is premalignant in columnar-lined (Barrett's) esophagus, and high-grade dysplasia presents a therapeutic dilemma in choice of endoscopic surveillance for malignancy vs. esophagectomy. Photodynamic therapy has been used to destroy dysplasia and superficial esophageal adenocarcinoma. Selective mucosal ablation with little risk of perforation may be possible with the use of endogenous photosensitization with orally administered 5-aminolaevulinic acid (5-ALA).

Methods.—Participating were 5 patients with histologically confirmed high-grade dysplasia in Barrett's esophagus and no evidence of invasive carcinoma. Quantitative fluorescence microscopy was used to measure the accumulated photosensitizer protoporphyrin IX that was endogenously generated after the oral administration of 5-ALA. The photosensitizer was then activated with endoscopic photodynamic therapy with 630-nm laser light.

Results.—Protoporphyrin IX accumulated in the dysplastic epithelium, not in the adjacent stroma, and light activation resulted in selective necrosis of the dysplastic epithelium in columnar-lined esophagus. High-grade dysplasia was eradicated in all patients. Acid suppression with a proton-pump inhibitor allowed squamous regeneration. Endoscopic and histologic follow-up of 26–44 months revealed no complications or recurrences; nondysplastic Barrett's epithelium was noted underneath regenerated squamous mucosa in 2 patients.

Conclusion.—Endoscopic photodynamic therapy with endogenously generated protoporphyrin IX can eradicate high-grade dysplasia in columnar-lined esophagus, although remaining nondysplastic tissue requires surveillance. The progression of dysplasia through to carcinoma may be interrupted or delayed by this therapy, which may prevent the need for surgical excision of this lesion in some patients. Determining whether the risk of carcinoma is actually reduced requires additional long-term patient follow-up.

▶ The association of Barrett's esophagus and adenocarcinoma of the esophagus is well established, and the risk of cancer developing in such patients is 40-fold greater than that of the general population. In high-grade dysplasia, the risk of carcinoma is even higher—25% to 45%. Most authorities currently recommend esophageal resection. Photodynamic therapy involves light-induced activation of an administered photosensitizer in tissue to produce local necrosis. The exciting report by Barr et al. shows that high-grade dysplasia in Barrett's esophagus can be eradicated by endoscopic photodynamic therapy with endogenously generated protoporphyrin IX. Further, such therapy can allow regeneration of squamous epithelium. However, the presence of residual nondysplastic Barrett's mucosa contiguous to and/or under regenerative squamous epithelia indicates that close endoscopic and histologic surveillance is required.

Although photodynamic therapy offers a nonsurgical alternative to esophageal resection, long-term follow-up studies are needed to determine whether such therapy will reduce the risk of carcinoma. Similar reservations apply to laser therapy of Barrett's esophagus.

N.J. Greenberger, M.D.

4 Achalasia

Controlled Trial of Botulinum Toxin Injection Versus Placebo and Pneumatic Dilation in Achalasia

Annese V, Basciani M, Perri F, et al (Istituto di Ricovero a Cura a Carattere Scientifico, San Giovanni Rotondo, Italy; Univ of Leuven, Belgium)

Gastroenterology 111:1418–1424, 1996   1–10

Introduction.—Pharmacologic therapy, surgical myotomy, and pneumatic dilation were the traditional therapeutic options for patients with achalasia. Another alternative nonsurgical treatment modality is intrasphincteric injection of botulinum toxin. This alternative treatment should be compared with pneumatic dilation, which is considered the most effective nonsurgical treatment for achalasia, and its efficacy should be examined. Botulinum toxin injection was compared with placebo injection and with pneumatic dilation.

Methods.—Saline or botulinum toxin was injected intrasphincterally to 16 patients in a random fashion. Esophageal manometry, symptom score, and scintigraphy were used to measure the efficacy of treatment. Pneumatic dilation was performed in case of failure.

Results.—All patients treated with botulinum toxin had an improvement in symptoms 1 month after injection (symptom score, 0.9 ± 0.6 vs. 5.5 ± 1.4). Patients who were in the placebo group had no change in their symptoms. These patients subsequently had pneumatic dilation. After treatment with botulinum toxin, lower esophageal sphincter pressure decreased by 49%, and after dilation, it decreased by 72%. After treatment with botulinum toxin, esophageal retention decreased by 47%, and after dilation, it decreased by 59%. A comparison of patients treated with botulinum toxin injection and those with dilation did not reveal any significant differences in symptom score and esophageal function test results (Fig 4). Because of recurrent dysphagia, 7 of 8 patients in the botulinum toxin group required a second injection.

Conclusion.—In relieving symptoms and improving esophageal function, treatment of achalasia with botulinum toxin was as effective as pneumatic dilation. Although most patients treated with botulinum toxin needed 2 injections, the effect of the second injection lasted longer than the first one; however, it is still unknown how long the injection will last and how often they will be needed. This treatment should be restricted to clinical trials until more research is conducted on the long-term effects of

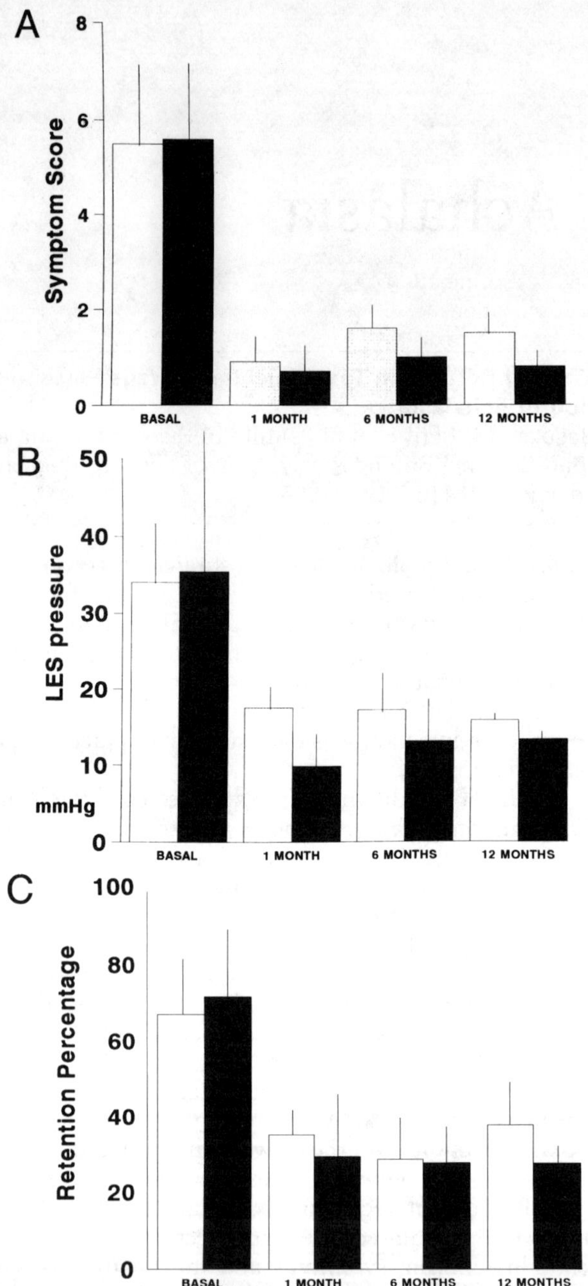

FIGURE 4.—A, symptom score; B, mean lower esophageal sphincter (*LES*) pressure; and C, esophageal retention rate during the follow-up period. All patients completed 6 months of follow-up, and 10 patients reached 12 months. Two patients were administered a second injection of toxin before the sixth month, whereas another 5 patients were administered a second injection within the first year of follow-up. *Dotted bars*, botulinum toxin; *filled bars*, dilation. (Courtesy of Annese V, Basciani M, Perri F, et al: Controlled trial of botulinum toxin injection versus placebo and pneumatic dilation in achalasia. *Gastroenterology* 111:1418–1424, 1996.)

multiple injections. Patients who are elderly or severely malnourished can have 1 or 2 injections.

▶ Although there have been several recent reports on the use of botulinum toxin injections in the treatment of achalasia, this is the first double-blind controlled trial comparing botulinum toxin with placebo injection. However, because all placebo injection recipients failed the trial, they were treated with pneumatic dilation, thus providing an additional means to assess the efficacy of botulinum toxin injections. At 6 and 12 months after treatment, no significant differences were noted in symptom score, lower esophageal sphincter pressure, and esophageal retention rate between the 2 treatment groups. However, it should be noted that 7 of 8 patients in the botulinum group required a second injection because of recurrent dysphagia. Obviously, the effect of the second injection lasted much longer. The authors caution that until more is known about the long-term effects of multiple injections, it would be appropriate to restrict this treatment to carefully designed clinical trials.

N.J. Greenberger, M.D.

Botulinum Toxin for Achalasia: Long-term Outcome and Predictors of Response

Pasricha PJ, Rai R, Ravich WJ, et al (Johns Hopkins Univ, Baltimore, Md)
Gastroenterology 110:1410–1415, 1996   1–11

Background.—Botulinum toxin (BoTx) is used to treat skeletal muscle conditions and was recently found to lower smooth muscle tone in the gastrointestinal tract. Studies with short-term follow-up report that BoTx is a safe and effective treatment for patients with achalasia, a condition leading to severe difficulty in swallowing. Thirty-one patients were followed to determine long-term effects of BoTx in achalasia and the factors predictive of response.

Patients and Methods.—The patients, 18 women and 13 men with a median age of 55 years, had taken part in 2 previously reported trials of BoTx. All were symptomatic and had the clinical, radiographic, and manometric features of achalasia. Seventeen had previously undergone esophageal dilation. Patients who did not achieve clinical remission after the first injection of BoTx received further injections, all administered through a 5-mm sclerotherapy needle into the lower esophageal sphincter region. Symptomatic response was scored according to the presence and frequency of dysphagia, regurgitation, and chest pain.

Results.—Twenty-eight patients (90%) showed an immediate clinical response with significant symptomatic improvement. Eleven of these patients, however, reported worsening of their symptoms within 2–3 months of the first injection. A second injection resulted in a sustained remission in 3 of 14 patients who either did not respond or did not have a lasting response to the first BoTx injection. Twenty patients remained in remission at 6 months. With a median follow-up of 890 days, 19 responders have relapsed. Remission periods have ranged from 5 months to 2 years and 4 months. Responders to BoTx were significantly older than nonresponders and were more likely to have vigorous achalasia rather than classic achalasia. In patients with vigorous achalasia, however, age did not affect the response to BoTx. All patients with lower esophageal sphincter pressures less than 20 mm Hg 1 week after treatment responded, whereas the response rate was only 50% for those with sphincter pressures greater than 20 mm Hg.

Conclusion.—Approximately two thirds of these patients with achalasia responded to BoTx (80 U); the average period of response was 1.3 years. The treatment was safe and side effects minimal. Both patient age and type of achalasia appeared to predict response. Intrasphinteric BoTx may be a useful alternative for patients at high risk for more invasive procedures or those unresponsive to conventional treatment.

▶ There have been several recent studies reporting the efficacy of BoTx in the treatment of achalasia.[1-4] Kozarek et al.[1] studied 23 patients with achalasia who were given either 50 or 100 units of BoTx. It was demonstrated that there was a discordance in symptom response and objective parameters of esophageal function, and that patients appeared to respond to the higher dose of 100 units of BoTx compared with the lower dose of 50 units. The failure to respond to balloon dilation or surgery were not necessarily predictors of clinical response to BoTx. Cuilliere et al.[2] studied 53 symptomatic patients with manometrically proved achalasia and demonstrated that intrasphincteric injection of BoTx is a safe procedure resulting in clinical improvement in 60% of the patients with achalasia, and that such improvement lasted more than 6 months. On the other hand, Graves et al. studied the effect of BoTx in a smaller group of 11 patients with achalasia and found no significant improvement in chest pain, regurgitation scores, and reduction in lower esophageal sphincter pressure.[3] Eaker and Gordon studied a series of high-risk patients with achalasia. Criteria included an age of 70 years and concomitant medical problems such as coronary artery disease or chronic obstructive pulmonary disease that made these patients poor surgical candidates. Eaker suggests that in high-risk patients with achalasia, intrasphincteric BoTx is an ideal alternative for providing symptomatic relief.[4]

To sum up, these studies indicate that BoTx treatment of achalasia can bring about symptomatic improvement as well as improvement in esophageal function. Such improvement can be expected to occur in approximately 60% to 65% of the patients and to last for 6 months. However, the need for additional treatment and the cost-effectiveness of this approach vs. standard therapy, i.e., pneumatic dilation or Heller myotomy, remain to be determined by comparative studies. The subset of patients with severe medical problems who are at high risk for either pneumatic dilation or surgery appear to be good candidates for BoTx.

N.J. Greenberger, M.D.

References

1. Kozarek RA, Gelfand MD, Patterson DJ, et al: Prospective trial of 50 versus 100 units of international IU of type A botulinum toxin for idiopathic achalasia. *Gastroenterology* 110:162A, 1996.
2. Cuilliere C, Ducrotte P, Zerbib F, et al: Achalasia:Outcome of patients treated by intraenteric injection of botulinum toxin. *Gastroenterology* 110:86A,1996.
3. Graves RRSH, Mulcahyi HE, Patchettse SE, et al: Botulinum toxin in the treatment of achalasia: A promise unfulfilled. *Gastroenterology* 110:123A, 1996.
4. Eaker EY, Gordon JM: Esophageal botulinum toxin injection in high-risk achalasia patients. *Gastroenterology* 110:99A, 1996.

Perendoscopic Injection of Botulinum Toxin Is Effective in Achalasia After Failure of Myotomy or Pneumatic Dilation

Annese V, Basciani M, Lombardi G, et al ("Casa Sollievo della Sofferenza" Hosp, San Giovanni Rotondo, Italy)
Gastrointest Endosc 44:461–465, 1996

1–12

Background.—Achalasia, a severe motor disorder of the esophagus, can have serious clinical sequelae. The goal of therapy is to reduce lower esophageal sphincter (LES) pressure. Surgical myotomy or pneumatic dilation achieve good to excellent results in 65% to 90% of patients, but such procedures carry a significant risk for major complications. Pharmacologic treatment has been less successful. After the injection of botulinum A toxin significantly reduced LES pressure in piglets, a double-blind, placebo-controlled trial confirmed the benefits of this treatment in patients

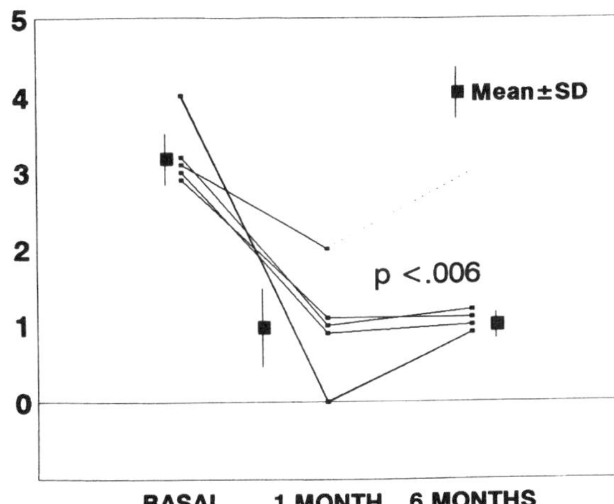

FIGURE 1.—Changes in symptom score after treatment with botulinum toxin. One of the patients has been lost at the follow-up after 4 months (*P* value obtained at 1 and 6 months in comparison with baseline). (Courtesy of Annese V, Basciani M, Lombardi G, et al: Perendoscopic injection of botulinum toxin is effective in achalasia after failure of myotomy or pneumatic dilation. *Gastrointest Endosc* 44:461–465, 1996.)

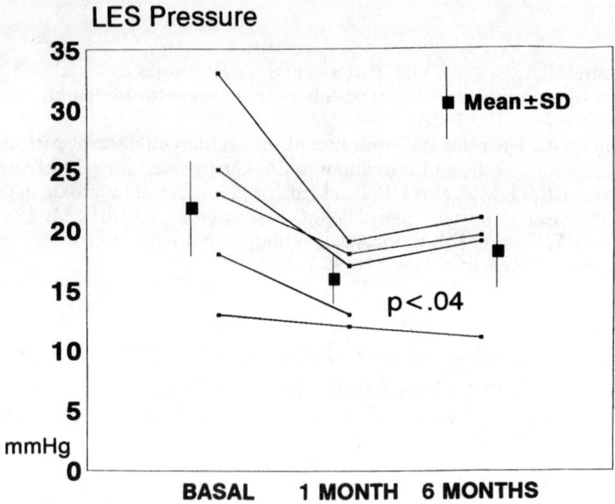

FIGURE 2.—Changes in basal values of LES pressure after treatment with botulinum toxin (*P* value obtained at 1 and 6 months in comparison with baseline). (Courtesy of Annese V, Basciani M, Lombardi G, et al: Perendoscopic injection of botulinum toxin is effective in achalasia after failure of myotomy or pneumatic dilation. *Gastrointest Endosc* 44:461–465, 1996.)

with achalasia. Thereafter, botulinum toxin was used in an open trial to treat patients who failed to benefit from myotomy or pneumatic dilation.

Methods.—The 5 patients, 2 men and 3 women with a mean age of 45, had experienced dysphagia and body weight loss over a mean period of 4.5 years. With the patient under conscious sedation, a flexible upper endoscopy was performed and botulinum toxin (total 100 U) was injected through a 4-mm sclerotherapy needle into the LES region. The procedure required 10 minutes and was performed on an outpatient basis. Patients were evaluated with esophageal manometry and esophageal retention studies.

Results.—One month after the botulinum injection, the mean symptom score decreased significantly from 3.2 to 1 (Fig 1). One patient's score improved from 3 to 2 and the patient decided to undergo surgical myotomy. Mean LES pressure decreased 30% from 22.4 mm Hg at baseline to 15.8 mm Hg after treatment (Fig 2). One month later, patients showed a mean decrease of 61% in esophageal retention 10 minutes after radionuclide bolus swallowing. Three patients required a second injection of botulinum toxin between 3 and 6 months after the initial procedure. The only side effect of treatment was mild postinjection chest pain in 1 patient.

Discussion.—Intrasphincteric injection of botulinum toxin is a simple and effective therapy for achalasia in patients who have failed to respond to standard treatment. Chemical denervation with botulinum toxin decreases LES pressure, with beneficial effects on symptoms of dysphagia and esophageal retention.

▶ Who would ever have thought that botulinum toxin would have found a useful place in the world? Pasricha and his colleagues[1] previously have shown that the direct injection of this toxin into the LES decreases its tone in patients with achalasia. Annese and his colleagues move a step further by demonstrating that it also can be used effectively in patients with achalasia who have failed to respond to myotomy or therapeutic bougienage. Apparently, botulinum toxin chemically denervates a variety of muscles, such as those that control the eyelids, larynx, and facial muscles. It now remains to develop a way to overcome the transience of the therapy.

F.G. Moody, M.D.

Reference

1. Pasricha PJ, Ravich WJ, Kalloo AN: Effects of intrasphincteric botulinum toxin on the lower esophageal sphincter in piglets. *Gastroenterology* 105:1045–1049, 1993.

5 Esophageal Carcinoma

Prognostic Factors of Resected Adenocarcinoma of the Esophagus
Hölscher AH, Bollschweiler E, Bumm R, et al (Technische Universität München, Germany)
Surgery 118:845–855, 1995   1–13

Introduction.—The incidence of adenocarcinoma of the esophagus seems to have increased in Europe and North America. Researchers examined the clinical and pathological characteristics, results of surgical treatment, and significance of prognostic factors in adenocarcinoma of the esophagus in a review of 165 patients treated during a 12.5-year period.

Methods.—In the study period, 186 of 538 patients who underwent resection with curative intention for esophageal cancer had adenocarcinomas. Not included in this review were the 21 patients who had chemotherapy before their operation for adenocarcinoma. The study group had a median age of 62.0 years and a male to female ratio of 8:1. Adenocarcinoma of the esophagus was defined as an adenocarcinoma centered more than 1 cm above the anatomical cardia. For tumors of the distal esophagus, treatment of choice was transhiatal radical subtotal esophagectomy. A right transthoracic en bloc esophagectomy with extended mediastinal lymphadenectomy was performed in cases with a quite oral extension of Barrett's esophagus and adenocarcinoma in the mid- or upper-esophageal part. Median follow-up was 4.6 years.

Results.—The most common symptoms reported were recent onset dysphagia (57.6%) and epigastric pain (21.8%). Preoperative endoscopy showed 82.4% of patients to have tumor development within Barrett's mucosa, which was histologically confirmed at resection. Transhiatal radical esophagectomy was performed in 78.8% of patients and transthoracic esophagectomy in 17.6%. Complete removal of tumor was achieved in 83% of patients. Interposition of a gastric tube was used for reconstruction in 93.9% of cases. Lymph node metastases were detected in submucosal cancer at rates that ranged from 18% in stage pT1b to 96% in stage pT4. Postoperative complications, the most common of which was cervical anastomotic leakage, occurred in 71 of 165 patients. The 30-day mortality rate was 6.1% and the overall 5-year survival rate was 34%. Survival among patients with no postoperative residual tumor (R0) was related to pT category. No patient with a pT1 tumor limited to the mucosa (pT1a)

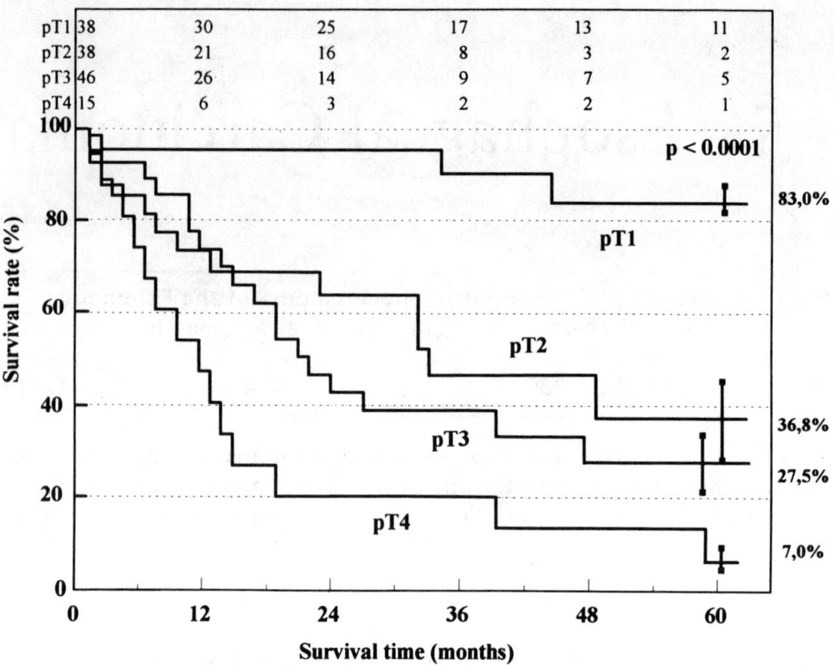

FIGURE 2.—Five-year survival curves of patients who underwent RO resection according to pT category (*n* = 137). *Abbreviation: RO*, no postoperative residual tumor. (Courtesy of Hölscher AH, Bollschweiler E, Bumm R, et al: Prognostic factors of resected adenocarcinoma of the esophagus. *Surgery* 118:845–855, 1995.)

died during follow-up (Fig 2), whereas none with ≥lymph node metastases achieved long-term survival.

Conclusion.—Lymph node ratio and pT were significant independent predictors of long-term survival in adenocarcinoma of the esophagus. Only patients with early stage cancer have a good prognosis after resection. Radical tumor removal with a margin of clearance in the lymphatic drainage may improve prognosis if the involved node ratio is less than 30%.

▶ Hölscher et al. at the Technische Universität in Munich have provided a thoughtful and informative report on their extensive surgical experience with adenocarcinoma of the esophagus. These cancers are usually located in the lower third of the esophagus and are amenable to a radical transhiatal esophagectomy. If the tumor is removed in its entirety, confined to the mucosa, and no nodes are involved, the 5-year survival rate exceeded 80%. The key is to identify these lesions in patients with Barrett's esophagitis early and have them removed by surgeons who perform transhiatal esophagectomies on a frequent basis.

F.G. Moody, M.D.

Impact of Clinicopathologic Parameters on Patient Survival in Carcinoma of the Cervical Esophagus
Kelley DJ, Wolf R, Shaha AR, et al (Mem Sloan-Kettering Cancer Ctr, New York)
Am J Surg 170:427–431, 1995   1–14

Introduction.—Even with adjuvant therapy and new reconstruction techniques, survival remains poor for patients with carcinoma of the cervical esophagus. In a previous study, the authors reported a 5-year cumulative survival of only 9%. The effects of new treatment approaches on survival and quality of life for patients with cervical esophageal carcinoma were retrospectively evaluated.

Patients.—A total of 82 patients treated for carcinoma of the cervical esophagus during a 13-year period were studied. There were 45 men and 22 women, and their mean age was 63 years. Dysphagia was present at the initial evaluation in 86% of patients, and only 19% had been treated previously. No physical abnormalities were detected in 56% of patients; 21% had a neck mass. Of patients in whom staging was possible, 9 had stage II disease, 38 had stage III disease, and 5 had stage IV disease.

Outcomes.—Twenty-two patients underwent curative surgery, and another 7 underwent palliative surgical procedures. Seven patients had unresectable disease and received palliative treatment only. Ten patients received radiation, with or without chemotherapy, as definitive treatment; another 4 received chemotherapy alone for cure, and 17 received palliative therapy. The mean survival was 17 months after diagnosis, and the cumulative 5-year survival was 12%. On multivariate analysis, factors significantly associated with decreased survival were persistent disease, having received chemotherapy before initial evaluation, and receiving chemotherapy for cure. Survival, disease-free interval, and swallowing function tended to be better in surgically treated patients.

Conclusions.—Survival continues to be poor for patients with carcinoma of the cervical esophagus. Survival and quality of life may be better for patients who undergo curative surgical resection. Curative surgery is still a possibility in patients with extraesophageal extension or nodal disease, although patients with persistent disease at the primary site after treatment are not likely to do well.

▶ Cancer of the cervical esophagus under the best of circumstances, which is surgical extirpation, is a bad disease. The authors use the power of multivariate analysis to show that chemotherapy is a detriment to a favorable outcome. Although radiation therapy appears to provide survival rates comparable to surgery, those who undergo surgery have a higher likelihood of being able to eat their food. Fortunately, this is a relatively uncommon malignancy.

F.G. Moody, M.D.

A Comparison of Multimodal Therapy and Surgery for Esophageal Adenocarcinoma

Walsh TN, Noonan N, Hollywood D, et al (St James's Hosp, Dublin; St Luke's Hosp, Dublin; Trinity College, Dublin)
N Engl J Med 335:462–467, 1996

1–15

Background.—In uncontrolled studies, combined chemotherapy and radiotherapy has been reported to improve survival in patients with esophageal adenocarcinoma. In a prospective, randomized study, surgery alone was compared with combined chemotherapy, radiotherapy, and surgery.

Methods.—Fifty-eight patients were initially assigned to multimodal therapy and 55 to surgery. Multimodal treatment consisted of 2 courses of fluorouracil (15 mg/kg of body weight every day for 5 days) and cisplatin (75 mg/m² of body surface area on day 7) in weeks 1 and 6 and a course of radiotherapy (40 Gy in 15 fractions during 3 weeks, beginning concurrently with the first chemotherapeutic course). Surgery was performed after chemotherapy and radiotherapy. Patients assigned to the surgery-only group received no treatment preoperatively.

Findings.—Seventeen percent of the patients receiving multimodal therapy had to be withdrawn for protocol violations. Forty-two percent of 55 evaluable patients in the multimodal treatment group had positive nodes or metastases at the time of surgery, compared with 82% of the 55 patients treated by surgery alone. Twenty-five percent of the patients undergoing surgery after multimodal treatment had complete pathologic responses. Patients treated by multimodal therapy had a median survival of 16 months, compared with 11 months for those treated with surgery alone.

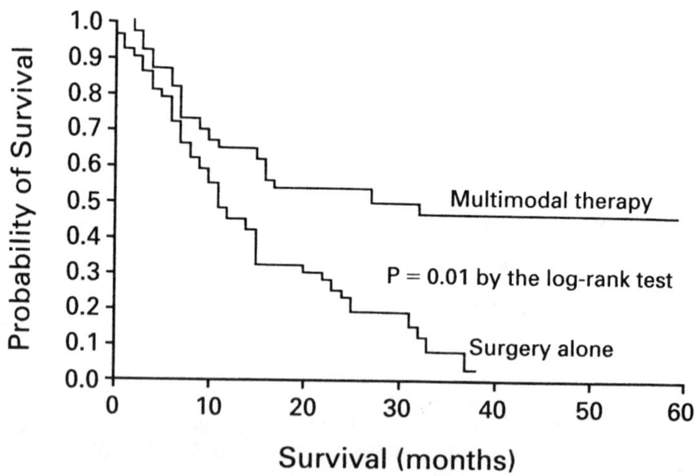

FIGURE 1.—Kaplan-Meier plot of survival of patients with esophageal adenocarcinoma, according to the intention-to-treat analysis. (Reprinted by permission of *The New England Journal of Medicine*, courtesy of Walsh TN, Noonan N, Hollywood D, et al: A comparison of multimodal therapy and surgery for esophageal adenocarcinoma. *N Engl J Med* 335:462–467. Copyright 1996, Massachusetts Medical Society. All rights reserved.)

Among patients receiving multimodal therapy, survival at 1 year was 52%; 2 years, 37%; and 3 years, 32%. Among those treated with surgery alone, the 1-, 2-, and 3-year survival rates were 44%, 26%, and 6%, respectively. The difference in survival was significant at 3 years (Fig 1).

Conclusion.—In patients with adenocarcinoma of the esophagus, multimodal treatment followed by surgery is associated with a significantly better survival than surgery alone at 3 years. Direct treatment-related toxic effects were minimal. Multimodal treatment should be considered in all patients with carcinoma confined to the esophagus and draining lymph nodes.

▶ This prospective, randomized, controlled trial presents data indicating that multimodal therapy consisting of 2 courses of chemotherapy and 1 course of radiotherapy followed by surgery provides a significant survival advantage over surgery alone at 3 years for patients with adenocarcinoma of the esophagus. Although the survival benefit of multimodal therapy in this study is impressive, several important questions arise: (1) Barrett's esophagus, which is frequently present in patients with esophageal adenocarcinoma, was found in less than 40% of the patients. (2) Staging of the tumor was not uniform in that not all patients had preoperative CT scans; endoscopic ultrasonography, which is accurate in assessing tumor stage, was not used. (3) The study included patients with early, as well as advanced, disease. The key question arises as to whether multimodal therapy is necessary in patients with early disease and no evidence of advanced local disease as primary resection appears to be the treatment of choice in patients with stage-1 and stage-2 adenocarcinoma of the esophagus. It would be helpful in this and similar studies if a subgroup analysis were provided. Such an analysis would clarify whether multimodal therapy can be widely recommended for patients with adenocarcinoma of the esophagus.

For a fine review of this subject, which amplifies many of the above points, see the editorial by Weke and Fink.[1]

N.J. Greenberger, M.D.

Reference

1. Weke HJ, Fink U: Multimodal therapy for adenocarcinoma of the esophagus and esophagogastric function. *New Engl J Med* 335:509–510, 1996.

Quality-of-life Assessment in Patients Undergoing Treatment for Oesophageal Carcinoma
O'Hanlon DM, Harkin M, Karat D, et al (Newcastle Gen Hosp, Newcastle upon Tyne, England)
Br J Surg 82:1682–1685, 1995   1–16

Introduction.—The traditional goal of treatment for esophageal cancer has been to prolong survival. However, given the distressing and debilitating symptoms of this tumor, it may be better to focus on the quality rather than the quantity of life. Specially selected instruments were used to prospectively assess quality of life in patients being treated for esophageal cancer.

Methods.—Sixty-nine consecutive patients undergoing treatment for carcinoma of the esophagus were studied. They were evaluated on the Rotterdam Symptom Checklist, a validated and cancer-specific tool; a dysphagia score; and an activities of daily living questionnaire, which was specially designed to address the unique problems of patients with esophageal cancer. Treatment consisted of surgery in 18 patients, radiotherapy or intubation in 43, and a combination of surgery and other treatments in 8.

Results.—The results of the 3 study instruments were significantly correlated with each other. Patients whose treatment included surgery were younger than those in the other groups and had significantly better scores for all preoperative parameters. These included scores for "knowledge and communication" and for "mobility and fatigue." Patients treated with surgery alone and those receiving palliative therapy had significant declines in their dysphagia scores after treatment. Among the activities of daily living assessed, two—self-care and eating and drinking—improved significantly in the surgically treated patients. In contrast, none of these parameters improved in the patients receiving palliative therapy.

Conclusions.—In patients with esophageal carcinoma, quality-of-life assessments such as the ones used in this study can help in evaluating quality of life and patient well-being. They can also help in identifying deficiencies in practice, such as the need for good communication and adequate analgesia in postoperative patients. Surgery or palliative therapy may bring an improvement in dysphagia scores.

▶ O'Hanlon and co-workers in the Oesophagogastric Cancer Unit of the Department of Surgical Gastroenterology at the Newcastle General Hospital discuss in a forthright way expected outcomes from the treatment of esophageal cancer. Their use of quality-of-life assessment parameters is refreshing. In fact, they go so far as to suggest that to put patients with incurable forms of the disease, which most are, through heroic efforts for a few more months of misery is unethical. I purposefully have chosen my words to be provocative to remind myself that aggressive palliative maneuvers by whatever modality may not be in the patient's best interest. Furthermore, it may be a misuse of expensive medical resources.

F.G. Moody, M.D.

p53 Protein Accumulation and Gene Mutations in Multifocal Esophageal Precancerous Lesions From Symptom Free Subjects in a High Incidence Area for Esophageal Carcinoma in Henan, China

Wang LD, Zhou Q, Hong J-Y, et al (Rutgers Univ, Piscataway, NJ; Henan Med Univ, Zhengzhou, Henan, China)
Cancer 77:1244–1249, 1996

1–17

Background.—Henan Province, China, has a high incidence of esophageal carcinoma. The multifocal occurrence of precancerous and cancerous lesions of the esophagus has been observed among the residents. p53 protein accumulation and mutation were analyzed in the middle and lower thirds of the esophagus in asymptomatic persons from this region.

Methods.—Fifty-five residents of Henan Province participated. Biopsy samples were obtained from the middle and lower thirds of the esophagus from each participant, and p53 protein accumulation and gene mutation were examined in multifocal esophageal precancerous lesions.

Findings.—Histopathologically, 20 of the 110 biopsy specimens had dysplasia, 72 had basal cell hyperplasia, and 18 had normal epithelia.

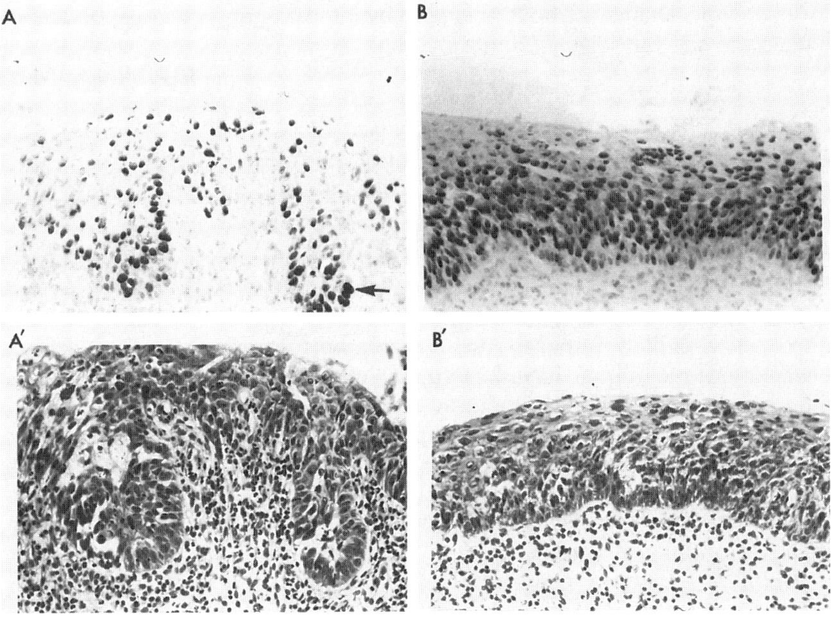

FIGURE 1.—Analysis of p53 protein immunostaining in a patient with concurrent dysplasia in the middle-third and the lower-third esophageal biopsy. Immunoreactivity is located in the nuclei of the dysplastic cells (*arrows*) from the middle-third biopsy (**A**) and the lower-third biopsy (**B**) (magnification ×600). The stroma cells are negative. H & E stain of serial sections corresponding to **A** and **B** are shown as **A'** and **B'**, respectively. (Courtesy of Wang LD, Zhou Q, Hong J-Y, et al: p53 protein accumulation and gene mutations in multifocal esophageal precancerous lesions from symptom free subjects in a high incidence area for esophageal carcinoma in Henan, China. *Cancer* 77:1244–1249, Copyright © 1996 American Cancer Society. Reprinted by permission of Wiley-Liss, Inc., a division of John Wiley & Sons, Inc.)

Concurrent lesions in the middle- and lower-third specimens were found in 4% of the patients with dysplasia and in 47% of those with basal cell hyperplasia (Fig 1). Immunohistochemical analysis revealed high concurrent rates of p53 protein accumulation. Missense mutations were found in 5 of 32 samples from 16 patients on p53 sequence analysis. Different mutations in the middle-third and lower-third specimens were observed in 1 patient. In the other 4 specimens, a single mutation was found in the middle- or lower-third sample.

Conclusions.—p53 protein accumulation and mutations occur in the early stages of esophageal carcinogenesis. Key molecular events in multifocal esophageal carcinogenesis may be independent somatic mutations of the p53 tumor suppressor gene and protein accumulation in different areas of the esophageal field.

▶ This article emphasizes the importance of global epidemiology to advance our knowledge of the pathogenesis of disease. The authors take advantage of patients at risk for esophageal cancer in Henan, China, and the technology for analysis at the laboratory of Cancer Research at Rutgers University. The techniques employed appear standard for p53 gene analysis, but the power of the study is in the availability of an asymptomatic population at high risk for esophageal cancer. Linear follow-up by interval biopsy of this population should provide further useful information.

F.G. Moody, M.D.

Oesophagectomy Without Thoracotomy: First 250 Patients
Gupta NM (Postgraduate Inst of Med, Education and Research, Chandigarh, India)
Eur J Surg 162:455–461, 1996   1–18

Introduction.—One-stage surgical resection is generally recognized as an effective palliative therapy for patients with esophageal cancer. However, several techniques have been used (left thoracoabdominal approach, left thoracotomy, right thoracotomy with laparotomy) and there is disagreement as to which approach is optimal. The high rate of complications and mortality associated with these procedures have focused interest on other approaches, such as transhiatal esophagectomy. Morbidity and mortality after transhiatal esophagectomy without thoracotomy in the treatment of esophageal carcinoma were described.

Methods.—Elective transhiatal esophagectomy without thoracotomy was performed on 250 patients with esophageal cancer during a 6.5-year period. Operative, postoperative, and late complications were identified, and mortality was determined.

Results.—Dysphagia was the primary complaint in all patients, with 45 patients experiencing complete dysphagia. Complications occurred in 58 patients (23%). During surgery, 8 patients sustained splenic injury, necessitating splenectomy. Recurrent laryngeal nerve palsy, anastomotic leak, and pleural effusion were the most common postoperative complications, occurring in 35, 38, and 13 patients, respectively. Laryngeal nerve damage was permanent in 2 patients. All patients with anastomotic leak were successfully treated with conservative therapy. Two patients required additional surgery because of postoperative internal hemorrhage. There were no deaths during surgery, but 14 patients died within 30 days of the procedure. None of the patients died as a result of anastomotic leak. Late complications included anastomotic stenosis in 44 patients and regurgitation in 12 patients. Ninety-two percent of patients survived for 6 months. The 1-year and 5-year survival rates were 45% and 5%, respectively.

Conclusion.—Transhiatal esophagectomy without thoracotomy is a safe procedure, with a low rate of complications and good functional results. However, mortality from esophageal cancer remains high.

▶ Gupta has provided a straightforward, concise, and well-documented description of the benefits and morbidity associated with transhiatal esophagectomy for esophageal cancer. The numbers support his almost across-the-board use of this approach as a means for establishing a way to eat as patients with the disease slowly succumb to its metastatic spread. Efforts should be made in Chandigarh to achieve earlier detection of what must be a common disease in the area. Preventive strategies would also greatly benefit people who must be exposed to a unique oncogenic stimulus, judging by the large number of cases treated over a relatively short period.

F.G. Moody, M.D.

Laparoscopic Mobilization of the Stomach for Oesophageal Replacement

Jagot P, Sauvanet A, Berthoux L, et al (Univ of Paris VII)
Br J Surg 83:540–542, 1996
1–19

Background.—The main cause of the morbidity and mortality associated with esophagectomy continues to be postoperative pulmonary complications. The laparoscopic approach for gastric mobilization in esophageal replacement was assessed in an attempt to improve the postoperative pulmonary course.

Patients and Methods.—Nine patients (mean age, 61 years) who had esophageal cancer were treated by esophagogastrectomy with laparoscopic gastric mobilization (Fig 1) and abdominal lymphadenectomy (Fig 2). All had moderate to severe airway obstruction. The mean forced expiratory flow rate at 1 second was 65% of the predicted value. In 6 patients, an abdominal laparoscopic approach was combined with a right open thoracotomy. In the other 3 patients, a laparoscopic abdominal and transhiatal approach was combined with a left cervictotomy. No one needed conversion to open laparotomy.

Outcomes.—All patients survived the procedure and had an uneventful postoperative course. One patient needed perioperative thoracic drainage

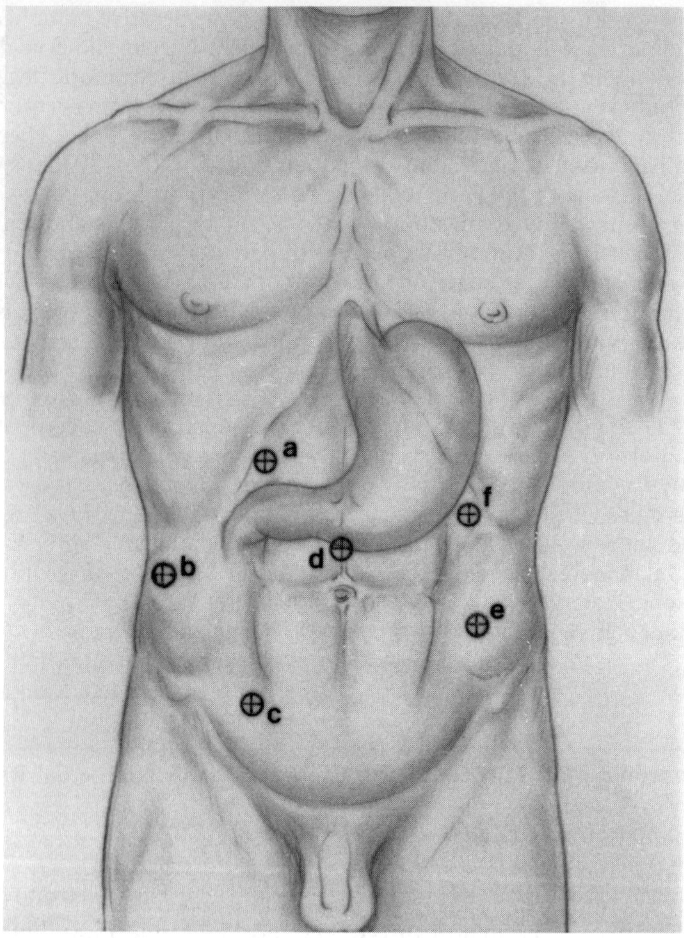

FIGURE 1.—Position of the cannulas for laparoscopic gastric mobilization. *a,* a retractor of the left liver lobe (5 mm); *b,* grasping forceps for retraction of the stomach (5 mm); *c,* grasping forceps for retraction of the greater omentum (5 mm); *d,* 0 degree laparoscope (10 mm); *e,* grasping forceps for traction of the encircled oesophagus and laparoscopic during division of the vasa brevia (10 mm); *f,* electrosurgical scissors, clip applicator (10 mm) or stapler in the transhiatal procedure (12 mm). (Courtesy of Jagot P, Sauvanet A, Berthoux L, et al: Laparoscopic mobilization of the stomach for oesophageal replacement. *Br J Surg* 83:540–542, 1996, Blackwell Science, Ltd.)

for pneumothorax. Postoperative extubation occurred at the end of surgery in 2 patients and on the day after surgery in 7. On the eighth postoperative day, the mean decrease in forced vital capacity was 15% of the preoperative value. The mean length of hospital stay was 10.3 days. None of the patients had delayed gastric emptying.

Conclusions.—Laparoscopy appears to be useful in the surgical treatment of esophageal cancer. Further studies are needed to better define the benefits of this technique on a patient's postoperative pulmonary course and long-term survival.

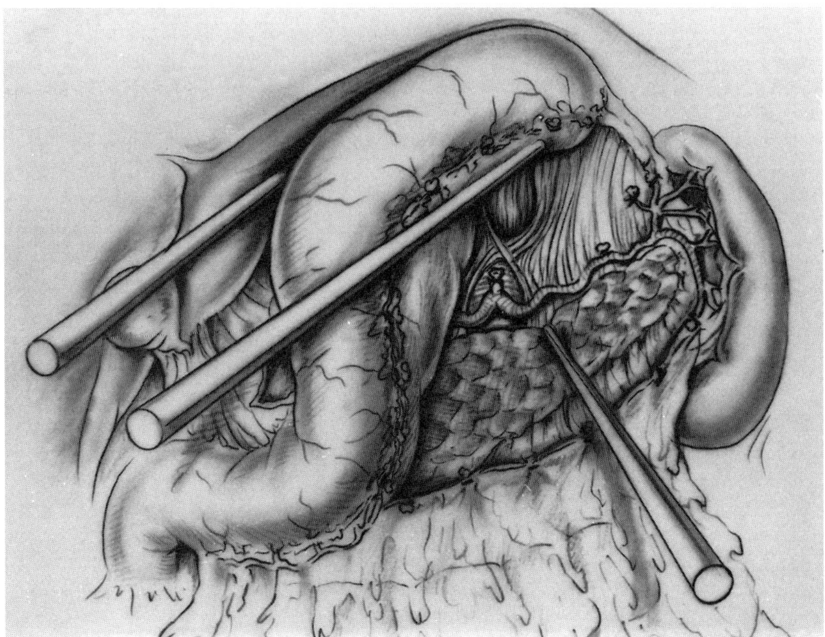

FIGURE 2.—Laparoscopic coeliac lymphadenectomy. (Courtesy of Jagot P, Sauvanet A, Berthoux L, et al: Laparoscopic mobilization of the stomach for oesophageal replacement. *Br J Surg* 83:540–542, 1996, Blackwell Science, Ltd.)

▶ This study of laparoscopic gastric mobilization for esophageal replacement is small, but it nonetheless clearly reveals the benefits of this approach. The lesser wounding incurred by this technique appeared to have a salutary effect on postoperative pulmonary function in that the patients were out of the hospital in 10 days. This likely would translate to 5 days in our current "boot and scoot" system in the United States.

F.G. Moody, M.D.

6 Miscellaneous

Esophageal Perforation

Delayed Primary Repair of Intrathoracic Esophageal Perforation: Is It Safe?

Wang N, Razzouk AJ, Safavi A, et al (Loma Linda Univ, Calif; Kaiser Permanente Med Ctr, Fontana, Calif)
J Thorac Cardiovasc Surg 111:114–122, 1996   1–20

Introduction.—Primary repair of the esophagus has not been recommended if an intrathoracic esophageal perforation is more than 24 hours old. Other approaches, however, require further reconstructive operations and have been associated with high mortality rates. The cases reported here demonstrate that the time interval between perforation and operative intervention need not in itself deter the surgeon from primary repair.

Methods.—A review of records from 2 institutions that use a similar approach to the management of esophageal perforation identified 22 patients treated between 1986 and 1994. Eighteen had a primary repair, 3 had esophageal exclusion, and 1 underwent esophageal resection. Among patients with primary repair, the cause of perforation was iatrogenic in 50%. Time between perforation and repair ranged from 4 hours to 13 days. Five patients (group A) were treated within 6 hours of esophageal perforation, 6 (group B) within 6 to 24 hours, and 7 (group C) after more than 24 hours. The perforation was approached via a left thoracotomy incision in 15 patients and a right thoracotomy incision in 3. Additional tissue was used to buttress the repair site in 13 patients; in 7, a fundic wrap reinforced the site of primary repair. Outcome variables analyzed in the 3 groups were esophageal leak, postoperative sepsis, overall morbidity, and mortality.

Results.—Postoperative leaks occurred in 0% of group A, 67% of group B, and 83% of group C. Although postoperative morbidity was high, group A had a lower rate (40%) than either group B (100%) or group C (86%). Four of the 5 patients in group A had iatrogenic perforation and were diagnosed immediately. Only 1 of the 7 patients treated by addition of a fundic wrap had a postoperative leak. Postoperative sepsis occurred in 11 patients and was associated with the presence of preoperative sepsis, but unrelated to the interval between perforation and repair. Esophageal leak and postoperative morbidity were not associated with increased mortality; there was 1 death in each group. Thirteen of the 15 survivors were followed for a mean period of 65 months. The single late death, 4 years after perforation repair, was the result of myocardial infarction.

Conclusion.—With advances in intensive care, most patients with intrathoracic esophageal perforation can be safely managed with primary repair. Despite postoperative morbidity and leakage at the suture site, which is most common when repair is delayed, outcome can be favorable. Potential contraindications to primary repair include malignant disease, a severely damaged esophagus, and preoperative sepsis accompanied by hemodynamic and respiratory instability.

▶ The numbers are small, but the message is clear. The repair of intrathoracic esophageal perforations can be accomplished successfully at the time they are identified, even if a delay in diagnosis has occurred. The results suggest, however, that repairs performed early (less than 6 hours after the event) will have fewer leaks from the site of repair in the postoperative period.

F.G. Moody, M.D.

PART TWO

THE STOMACH AND DUODENUM

Introduction

Five articles in this section deal with *Helicobacter pylori*. It appears that *H. pylori* interferes with duodenal bicarbonate production as well facilitating the delivery of an increased acid load into the duodenum and that both abnormalities are reversed by eradication of *H. pylori*. A provocative article documents that *H. pylori* can be transmitted between spouses. Three articles attest to the efficacy of 1 week of triple therapy in eradicating *H. pylori* in approximately 90% of patients. The triple therapy drug regimens consist of 2 antibiotics and 1 antisecretory drug. The role of *H. pylori* in gastric carcinogenesis is also reviewed.

Five articles deal with pharmacologic considerations. Over the counter (OTC) famotidine was compared with OTC calcium carbonate in reducing gastric acid secretion. Both preparations were found to be equivalent with regard to the amount of acid neutralized, but there were important differences. The OTC calcium carbonate has a short duration of action compared with OTC famotidine, which had a slower onset of action but a much more prolonged duration of effect.

Accumulating evidence indicates that long-term use of proton pump inhibitors in patients with *H. pylori* infection increases the likelihood of atrophic gastritis developing along with micronodular hyperplasia. The practical implication is that patients being considered for long-term treatment with proton pump inhibitors should be checked for *H. pylori*. If infection is present, it should be eradicated.

Two recent studies indicate that between one fifth and one fourth of patients seen originally for dyspepsia will be found to have peptic ulcer disease. Equally important, one fourth to one third of the patients will be found to have endoscopically verified non-ulcer dyspepsia. Such patients are likely to be female and to complain of nausea and emesis, but not to experience severe abdominal pain. A review article describing over 300 such patients provides new insights into this incompletely understood disorder.

Somatostatin receptor scintigraphy (SRS) has emerged as the diagnostic procedure of choice in patients with suspected gastrinomas. This test identified both gastrinomas and metastatic lesions more accurately than a combination of tests including endoscopy, ultrasound, CT scan, MRI, and angiography.

Two articles deal with acute upper gastrointestinal hemorrhage, 1 providing guidelines for identifying patients at low risk of continued bleeding and another comparing the cost incurred in teaching vs. non-teaching hospitals. An interesting study on vitamin B_{12} deficiency after gastric surgery indicates that as many as 2% of the population more than 65 years old have occult B_{12} deficiency and that this diagnosis can be facilitated by determining methylmalonic acid in the urine and blood homocysteine levels.

Norton J. Greenberger, M.D.

7 Helicobacter Pylori

Pathophysiology of Peptic Ulcers

The Influence of *Helicobacter pylori* Infection on Postprandial Duodenal Acid Load and Duodenal Bulb pH in Humans

Hamlet A, Olbe L (Univ of Göteborg, Sweden)
Gastroenterology 111:391–400, 1996   2–1

Background.—The authors of this study recently postulated a new concept of duodenal ulcer (DU) pathogenesis, in which it is suggested that *Helicobacter pylori* infection, located mainly in the gastric antrum, contributes to the hypergastrinemia and increased, prolonged gastric acid response to meals through selective blockade of inhibitory reflex pathways from the antrum to the gastrin and parietal cells. The blockade of the inhibitory pathways induced by antral *H. pylori* infection would, thus, increase duodenal acid load and reduce pH in the duodenal bulb as a general prerequisite for DU development. Duodenal acid load and duodenal bulb pH after a meal were investigated before and after *H. pylori* eradication.

Methods.—A marker-dilution method and a pH electrode in the duodenal bulb were used to determine gastric emptying, acid secretion, gastrin release, duodenal acid load, and duodenal bulb pH in 8 *H. pylori*–negative controls and 8 *H. pylori*–infected patients. Assessments were made during the first 2 hours after peptone meals of pH 7.0 and 2.0 before and 6 months after infection eradication.

Findings.—Patients with *H. pylori* infection had increased gastric emptying, gastrin release, and acid secretion; a greater duodenal acid load; and lower duodenal bulb pH after meals. Eradicating the infection normalized these responses (Figs 2–4).

Conclusion.—An increased, prolonged postprandial acid secretion is a general prerequisite for DU development in patients with *H. pylori* infection. Such postprandial acid secretion is caused, in part, by an impaired low pH inhibition of acid secretion, gastrin release, and gastric emptying, resulting in an increased duodenal acid load and prolongation of low pH in the duodenal bulb.

▶ Although it is now clearly established that *H. pylori* is the primary causal factor in duodenal ulcer disease, the pathogenetic mechanisms remain

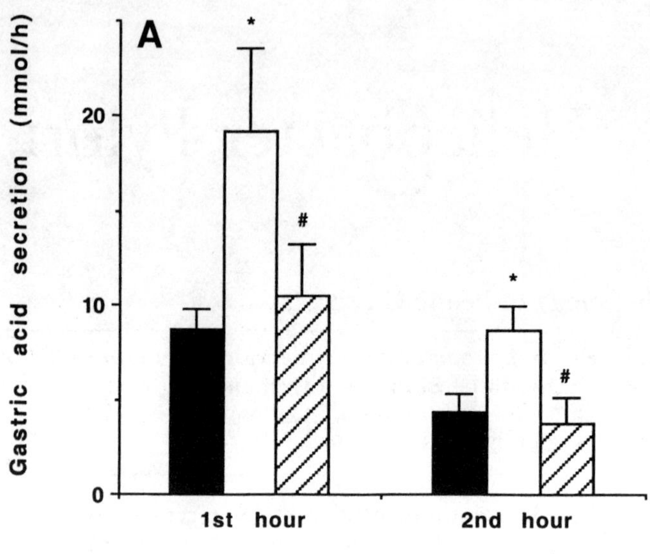

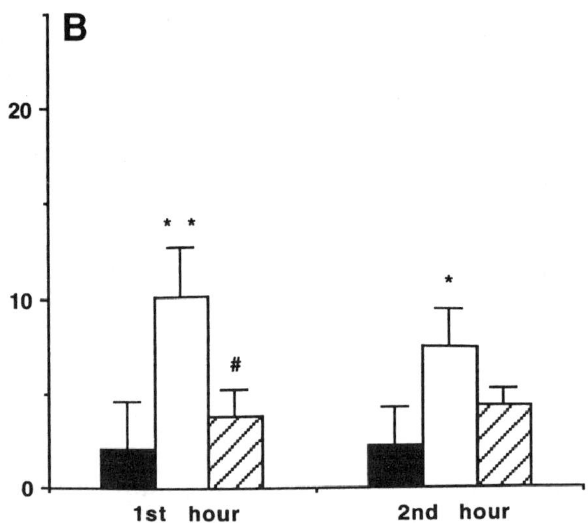

FIGURE 2.—Mean ± standard error of the mean cumulative gastric acid secretion (in millimoles per hour) after a liquid peptone meal of (**A**) pH 7.0 and (**B**) pH 2.0 in 8 *H. pylori*–negative (*black bar*) and 8 *H. pylori*–infected (*white bar*) patients before and 6 months after successful eradication therapy (*striped bar*). *Asterisk* indicates $P < 0.05$ and *double asterisk* indicates $P < 0.01$ compared with the *H. pylori* –negative control group; *Sharp* indicates $P < 0.05$ compared with the corresponding values before treatment. (Courtesy of Hamlet A, Olbe L: The influence of *Helicobacter pylori* infection on postprandial duodenal acid load and duodenal bulb pH in humans. *Gastroenterology* 111:391–400, 1996.

incompletely defined. Previous studies have demonstrated that *H. pylori* infection is associated with increased basal and meal-stimulated serum gastrin levels and increased basal gastric acid secretion and that successful eradication of *H. pylori* results in reversal of these 3 abnormalities. Previous

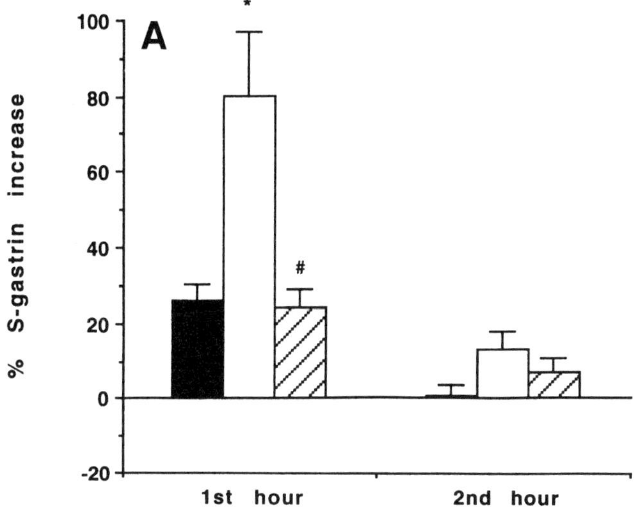

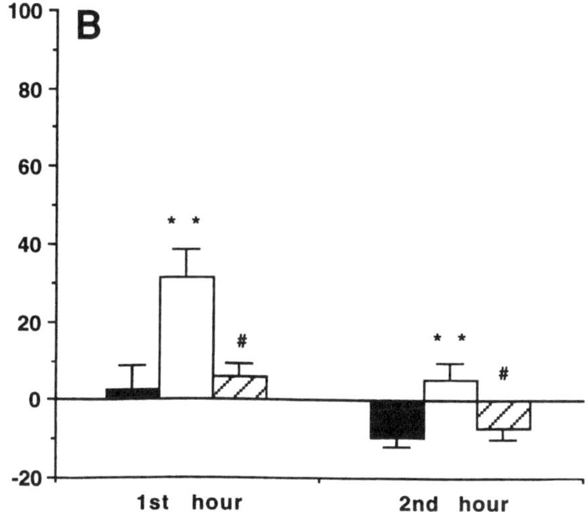

FIGURE 3.—Mean ± standard error of the mean baseline-adjusted percentage increase of cumulated serum gastrin levels as a response to a liquid peptone meal of (**A**) pH 7.0 and (**B**) pH 2.0 in 8 *H. pylori*–negative (*black bar*) and 8 *H. pylori*–infected (*white bar*) patients before and 6 months after successful eradication therapy (*striped bar*). *Asterisk* indicates $P < 0.05$ and *double asterisk* indicates $P < 0.01$ compared with the *H. pylori*–negative control group; *Sharp* indicates $P < 0.05$ compared with the corresponding values before treatment. (Courtesy of Hamlet A, Olbe L: The influence of *Helicobacter pylori* infection on postprandial duodenal acid load and duodenal bulb pH in humans. *Gastroenterology* 111:391–400, 1996.)

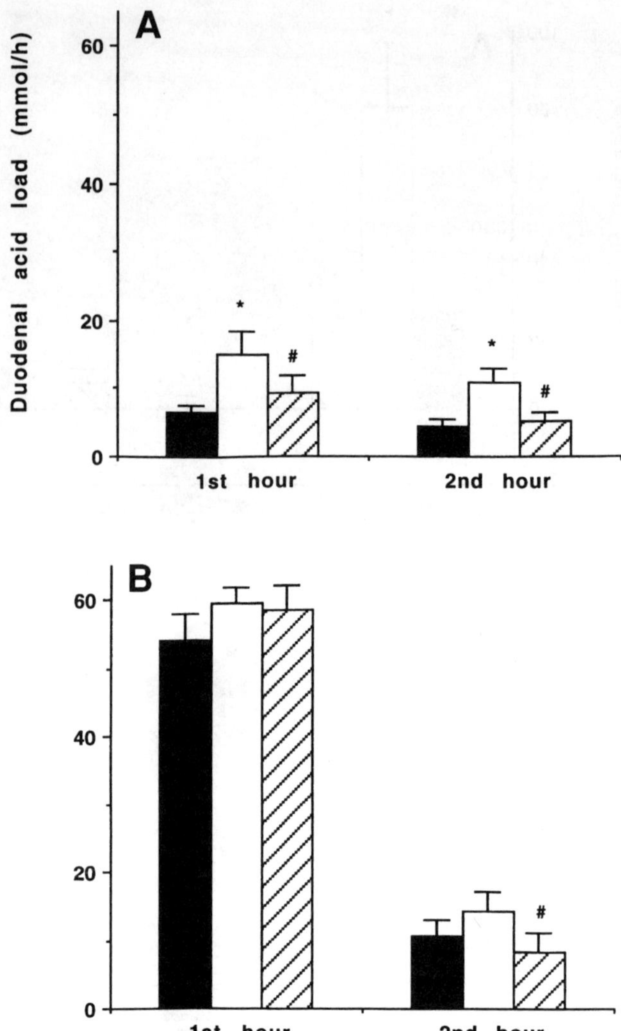

FIGURE 4.—Mean ± standard error of the mean duodenal acid load (in millimoles per hour) after a liquid peptone meal of (**A**) pH 7.0 and (**B**) pH 2.0 in 8 *H. pylori*–negative (*black bar*) and 8 *H. pylori* –infected (*white bar*) patients before and 6 months after successful eradication therapy (*striped bar*). *Asterisk* indicates $P < 0.05$ compared with the *H. pylori*–negative control group; *Sharp* indicates $P < 0.05$ compared with the corresponding value pre treatment. (Courtesy of Hamlet A, Olbe L: The influence of *Helicobacter pylori* infection on postprandial duodenal acid load and duodenal bulb pH in humans. *Gastroenterology* 111:391–400, 1996.)

studies by Olbe et al.[1] showed that inhibition of gastrin release and acid secretion in response to antral distention were inhibited by *H. pylori* infection; eradication of *H. pylori* corrected both of these abnormalities.

The authors have put forth a new concept of duodenal ulcer pathogenesis. They postulate that *H. pylori* infection, which is usually localized in the gastric antrum, blocks inhibitory reflex pathways from the antrum to gastrin and parietal cells, which, in turn, results in an increased duodenal acid load and a reduced pH in the duodenal bulb. In this connection, earlier studies have demonstrated that patients with duodenal ulcer disease have an increased and prolonged acid response to a meal. The aim of this study was to clarify whether this is related to *H. pylori* infection by determining duodenal acid load and duodenal bulb pH after a meal *before* and *after* eradication of *H. pylori.*

The key findings can be summarized as follows: (1) *H. pylori*–infected patients had increased gastrin release, increased gastric acid secretion, high duodenal acid load, and lower duodenal bulb pH (see figures); and (2) these abnormalities were normalized after eradication of *H. pylori.* These observations provide further insights into the mechanisms whereby *H. pylori* infection results in duodenal ulcer disease.

N.J. Greenberger, M.D.

Reference

1. Olbe L, Hamlet A, Dalenbreck J, et al: A mechanism by which *Helicobacter pylori* infection of the antrum contributes to the development of duodenal ulcer. *Gastroenterology* 110:1386–1394, 1996.

Epidemiology

Prevalence of *Helicobacter pylori* Infection and Related Gastroduodenal Lesions in Spouses of *Helicobacter pylori* Positive Patients With Duodenal Ulcer
Parente F, Maconi G, Sangaletti O, et al (I Sacco Univ, Milan, Italy)
Gut 39:629–633, 1996
2–2

Background.—Few studies have assessed the risk of infection among spouses of patients infected with *Helicobacter pylori.* The studies that do exist have yielded conflicting findings. The seroprevalence of *H. pylori* infection and the frequency of gastroduodenal lesions was assessed in the spouses of patients with *H. pylori* infection.

Methods.—One hundred twenty-four spouses (52% female) of patients with duodenal ulcers seen consecutively during 10 months were studied. The spouses were screened for serum IgG anti–*H. pylori* antibodies and completed a questionnaire eliciting information on the presence of chronic or recurrent dyspepsia. The control group consisted of 249 volunteer blood donors matched for age, sex, origin, and socioeconomic status.

Findings.—The seroprevalence of *H. pylori* infection was significantly higher in spouses (71%) than in control subjects (58%). Thirty-four percent of the 88 seropositive spouses reported dyspeptic symptoms, compared with only 12% of the 34 seronegative spouses. Ninety-eight percent of the 49 seropositive spouses undergoing endoscopy had confirmation of *H. pylori* infection. Among those spouses, endoscopic findings demonstrated active duodenal ulcer in 17%, duodenal scar and cap deformity in 4%, active gastric ulcer in 4%, erosive duodenitis in 6%, antral erosions

TABLE 2.—Endoscopic Findings in *Helicobacter pylori*–Positive Spouses According to the Presence or Absence of Upper Gastrointestinal Symptoms

Symptomatic spouses	No	Never symptomatic spouses	No
Active duodenal ulcer	8 (31)	Active gastric ulcer	1 (5)
Scar+cap deformity	2 (8)	Antral erosions	1 (5)
Erosive duodenitis	2 (8)	Erosive duodenitis	1 (5)
Active gastric ulcer	1 (4)		
Antral erosions	1 (4)		
Antral erosions+erosive duodenitis	1 (4)		
Peptic oesophagitis	1 (4)		
Normal findings	10 (38)	Normal findings	19 (86)
Total	26	Total	22

Note: Values in parentheses are percentages. For the percentage of endoscopic lesions in symptomatic vs. never symptomatic spouses, $P = 0.002$ (χ^2 test with Yates correction).

(Courtesy of Parente F, Maconi G, Sangaletti O, et al: Prevalence of *Helicobacter pylori* infection and related gastroduodenal lesions in spouses of *Helicobacter pylori* positive patients with duodenal ulcer. *Gut* 39:629–633, 1996.)

in 4%, and antral erosions plus duodenitis and peptic esophagitis in 1 patient each. Compared with spouses who had never had symptoms, spouses with symptoms had a significantly greater prevalence of major endoscopic lesions (Table 2).

Conclusions.—Spouses of *H. pylori*–positive patients with duodenal ulcer may be at increased risk for *H. pylori* colonization and possibly for peptic ulcer disease. There may be a need for serologic screening of the co-habitating partners of such patients.

▶ Two recent studies examined the possibility of spouse-to-spouse transmission of *H. pylori*. In the above study, Parente and colleagues reported (1) that there was a higher prevalence of infection in spouses of patients with duodenal ulcers than in a matched control population; (2) that infected spouses were more likely to have dyspeptic symptoms than those without infection; and (3) that infected spouses with dyspeptic symptoms had an appreciable prevalence of active peptic ulceration (9 of 26 patients, or 35%).

The second study, by Georgopoulos and associates,[1] also demonstrated that spouses of *H. pylori*–infected patients with duodenal ulcer disease are more likely to harbor *H. pylori* infection than are spouses of *H. pylori*–negative patients with duodenal ulcer (42 of 58 or 78% vs. 2 of 10, or 20%, respectively). They extended this observation by examining the ribosomal patterns of *H. pylori* strains derived from 18 patients with duodenal ulcer disease and their spouses. In each of 8 couples, a single strain had colonized both partners, whereas in the remaining 10 couples, each partner was colonized by a distinct *H. pylori* strain. This study provides more direct evidence for some *H. pylori* infection being transmitted from spouse to spouse.

Together, these 2 studies suggest that dyspeptic spouses of *H. pylori*–infected patients with peptic ulcer disease should be investigated further for active peptic ulcer disease. For an authoritative editorial on spousal transmission of H. pylori, see the article by Collins.[2]

N.J. Greenberger, M.D.

References

1. Georgopoulos SD, Metis AF, Spiliadis CA: *Helicobacter pylori* infection in spouses of patients with duodenal ulcer and comparison of ribosomal RNA gene patterns. *Gut* 39:634–638,1996.
2. Collins BJ: *Helicobacter pylori*? Is it all in the family? *Gut* 39: 768, 1996.

Treatment Regimens

One-week Low-dose Triple Therapy for *Helicobacter pylori* Is Sufficient for Relief From Symptoms and Healing of Duodenal Ulcers

Labenz J, Idström J-P, Tillenburg B, et al (Elisabeth Hosp, Essen, Germany; Ruhr Univ of Bochum, Germany)
Aliment Pharmacol Ther 11:89–93, 1997   2–3

Background.—Few studies of short-term treatment for *Helicobacter pylori* have appeared in the literature. The efficacy of 1-week low-dose triple therapy for *H. pylori* infection in relieving dyspeptic symptoms and healing duodenal ulcers was investigated.

Methods.—Fifty-nine patients were enrolled in the randomized, double-blind, 2-center trial. All had duodenal ulcers and positive rapid urease test results. For 1 week, treatment consisted of omeprazole, 20 mg twice a day; clarithromycin, 250 mg twice a day; and metronidazole, 400 mg twice a day. Patients were then treated for another 3 weeks with omeprazole, 20 mg once a day, or placebo. Endoscopy was performed before treatment and after 2 and 4 weeks of treatment.

Findings.—The overall cure rate was 96%. Cure rates were comparable in the 2 groups. After 2 weeks, duodenal healing was confirmed in 91% of those given omeprazole and in 76% given placebo. All ulcers had healed after 4 weeks. The 2 groups had comparable relief from dyspeptic symptoms and adverse events.

Conclusions.—One week of treatment with omeprazole, clarithromycin, and metronidazole is effective and well tolerated in patients with *H. pylori* infection and duodenal ulcer. Continuing antisecretory therapy past anti-*H. pylori* treatment appears to be unnecessary.

▶ This study indicates that a 1-week triple therapy regimen consisting of omeprazole, 20 mg twice a day; clarithromycin, 250 mg twice a day; and metronidazole, 400 mg twice a day, is a simple, convenient, and highly effective treatment for *Helicobacter pylori*–associated duodenal ulcers.

Additional support for a 3-drug regimen consisting of 1 antisecretory drug and 2 antimicrobial agents is provided by a study by Labenz et al.[1] In an open-label study, 60 patients with duodenal ulcer were treated for 1 week with pantoprazole, 40 mg twice a day; clarithromycin, 500 mg twice a day; and amoxycillin, 1.0 g twice a day. During the second week, patients received pantoprazole, 40 mg every morning. *Helicobacter pylori* infection was cured in 47 (89%) of 53 patients who completed the trial according to protocol. Four weeks after drug treatment 55 (92%) of 60 patients had healed ulcers.

N.J. Greenberger, M.D.

Reference

1. Labenz J, Tillenburg B, Worsmulle J, et al: Efficacy and tolerability after one week triple therapy consisting of pantoprazole, clarithromycin, and amoxycillin for cure of *Helicobacter pylori* infection in patients with duodenal ulcer. *Aliment Pharmacol Ther* 11:95–100, 1997.

Long-term Follow-up After Cure of *Helicobacter pylori* Infection With 4 Days of Quadruple Therapy

Lai JYL, de Boer WA, Driessen WMM, et al (Sint Anna Hosp, Oss, The Netherlands; Sint Joseph Hosp, Veldhoven, The Netherlands)
Aliment Pharmacol Ther 10:645–650, 1996

2–4

Background.—Four days of quadruple treatment after omeprazole pretreatment is effective in patients with *Helicobacter pylori* infection. The long-term benefits of this treatment were studied.

Methods.—All 49 patients participating in a previous study were invited to return for ^{14}C-urea breath and serologic testing. Between January and December, 1994, these patients had been treated with omeprazole, 20 mg before breakfast and before dinner on days 1–7; tripotassium dicitrato

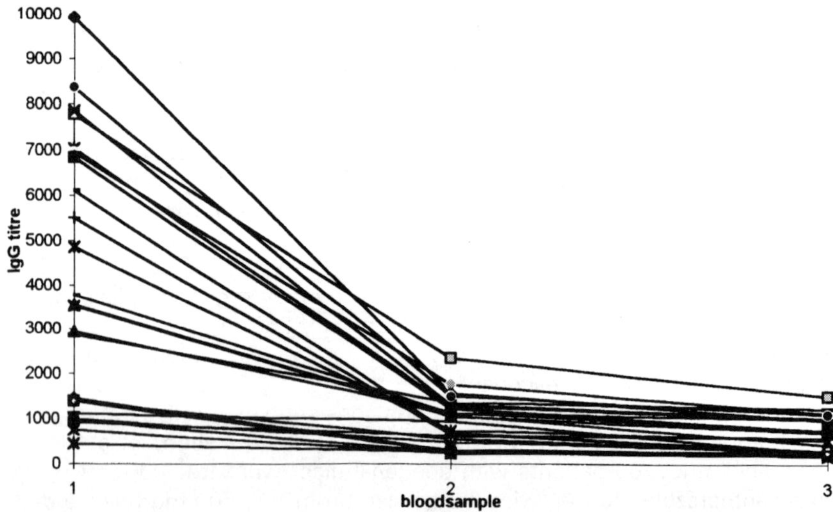

FIGURE 1.—Decline in IgG titer in 24 patients after successful cure of *H. pylori* infection. Blood sample 1 was taken before treatment; blood sample 2 was taken 6 months after treatment; and blood sample 3 was taken at the end of the follow-up (range, 11.4–23.6 months). The cut-off level is 300. (Courtesy of Lai JYL, de Boer WA, Driessen WMM, et al: Long-term follow-up after cure of *Helicobacter pylori* infection with 4 days of quadruple therapy. *Aliment Pharmacol Ther* 10:645–650, 1996.)

bismuthate, 120 mg 4 times a day before each meal and before bed on days 4–7; tetracycline hydrochloride, 500 mg 4 times a day during each of 3 meals on days 4–7; and metronidazole, 500 mg 3 times a day during each of 3 meals on days 4–7. Thirty-seven patients, or 76%, were willing to return. The mean follow-up was 14.7 months.

Findings.—All patients had a negative urea breath test result. In addition, all had steadily declining IgG antibody titres. At the end of follow-up, the mean decrease was 83%. Titres were not increased in any of the patients. Thus, the rate of reinfection was 0% (Fig 1).

Conclusion.—Four-day quadruple treatment effectively eradicates *H. pylori* infection in the long term. The biopsy method used was found to be reliable for identifying treatment failures 5–6 weeks after therapy.

▶ The authors previously reported that 4 days of quadruple therapy after a 3-day pretreatment with omprazole is an effective therapy for *H. pylori* infection.[1] They now report that after a mean follow up of 14.7 months, none of 37 patients had evidence of reinfection. This was demonstrated by negative urea breath tests as well as by a sharp decrease in serum IgG antibody titers.

Many useful treatment regimens for *H. pylori* infections are now available, with cure rates above 90%. Treatments with less than a 90% overall cure rate should probably no longer be used. A popular regimen, abbreviated MOC, includes metronidazole, omeprazole, and clarithromycin given for 7 days. This regimen is clearly superior to the dual regimen of omeprazole and clarithromycin, which yields *H. pylori* eradication rates in the 35% to 75% range.

The importance of metronidazole in treatment regimens is underscored by 2 recent studies. Yousfi et al. reported that 1 week of triple therapy with omeprazole, amoxicillin, and clarithromycin for treatment of *H. pylori* infection resulted in a cure rate (intention to treat analysis) of only 77%.[2] Bell et al. determined the effect of *H. pylori* eradication with omeprazole and amoxicillin, with or without metronidazole, in the 12-month course of duodenal ulcer disease in 105 patients.[3] During the 12-month untreated follow-up, the life table endoscopic relapse rates were 12% for omeprazole-amoxicillin and 2% for omeprazole-amoxicillin-metronidazole. Thus, a triple regimen including metronidazole eradicates *H. pylori* in significantly more patients than the dual regimen of omeprazole-amoxicillin.

Finally, a recent article provides further understanding of the role of omeprazole in treatment regimens.[4] In addition to its acid suppression effect, omeprazole increases intragastric concentrations of amoxicillin, in part by reducing gastric juice volume. Interestingly, concentrations of clarithromycin were not changed significantly by omeprazole treatment.

N.J. Greenberger, M.D.

References

1. de Boer WA, Diressen WMM, Tytgat GNJ: Only findings of quadruple therapy can effectively cure *Helicobacter pylori* infection. *Aliment Pharmacol Ther* 9:633–638, 1995.
2. Yosfi MD, El-Zimaity HMT, Genta RM, et al: One week triple therapy with omeprazole amoxicillin and clarithromycin for treatment of *Helicobacter pylori* infection. *Aliment Pharmacol Ther* 10:617–621, 1996.
3. Bell GD, Bate CM, Axon ATR, et al: Symptomatic and endoscopic duodenal ulcer relapse rates 12 months following *Helicobacter pylori* eradication treatment with omeprazole and amoxicillin with or without metronidazole. *Aliment Pharmacol Ther* 10:637–644, 1996.
4. Goddard AF, Jessa MJ, Barret DA, et al: Effect of omeprazole on the distribution of metronidazole, amoxicillin and clarithromycin in gastric juice. *Gastroenterology*, 111:358–367, 1996.

Lansoprazole, Clarithromycin and Metronidazole for Seven Days in *Helicobacter pylori* Infection

Harris AW, Pryce DI, Gabe SM, et al (St Mary's Hosps, London; Lederle Labs, Gosport, England)
Aliment Pharmacol Ther 10:1005–1008, 1996

2–5

Background.—A 1-week low-dose regimen of omeprazole, clarithromycin, and either a nitroimidazole or amoxicillin has been proved effective in eradicating *Helicobacter pylori*. However, the efficacy of a nitroimidazole-containing regimen against *H. pylori* resistant to this antimicrobial agent must be established before it can be recommended for use in regions with a high prevalence of pretreatment nitroimidazole resistance. The efficacy and safety of a triple therapy antimicrobial regimen in such a region was evaluated in an open study.

Methods.—Seventy-five patients positive for *H. pylori* and with gastritis or duodenal ulcer were enrolled in a study of lansoprazole, 30 mg every morning; clarithromycin, 250 mg twice a day; and metronidazole, 400 mg twice a day. CLOtest, histology, culture, and ^{13}C-urea breath test were used to determine *H. pylori* status. Seventy-one patients completed treatment and were available for follow-up.

Findings.—*H. pylori* was eradicated in 86% of the patients in a per-protocol analysis and in 81% in an intention-to-treat analysis. *H. pylori* was eradicated in 75% of the patients with metronidazole-resistant strains and in 92% of those with metronidazole-sensitive strains. At least 1 adverse effect occurred in 45 patients, including 3 who quit treatment because of such effects.

Conclusions.—The regimen described eradicates *H. pylori* in up to 86% of patients with gastritis or duodenal ulcer. Patients with pretreatment metronidazole-resistant strains of *H. pylori* also benefit from this treatment.

▶ This study demonstrated that a 1-week course of lansoprazole 30 mg daily, clarithromycin 250 mg twice daily, and metronidazole 400 mg twice daily eradicated *H. pylori* in 86% of patients. Further, it proved effective in patients known to harbor metronidazole-resistant strains of *H. pylori*. Almost identical results using a similar triple therapy regimen for 1 week have been reported by Goddard and Speller.[1] Successful eradication of *H. pylori* was achieved in 96 of 111 patients (87%) receiving omeprazole 20 mg twice daily, clarithromycin 250 mg twice daily, and either metronidazole 400 mg or tinidazole 500 mg twice daily for 7 days. An additional observation was the demonstration that treatment failure in patients receiving omeprazole-based treatments was associated with smoking.

N.J. Greenberger, M.D.

Reference

1. Goddard AP, Speller RC: *H. pylori* eradication in clinical practice: One week low dose triple therapy is preferable to classical bismuth based triple therapy. *Aliment Pharmacol Ther* 10:1005–1008, 1996.

Gastric Carcinogenesis

Helicobacter pylori in Promotion of Gastric Carcinogenesis
Rugge M, Cassaro M, Leandro G, et al (Univ of Padova, Italy; Gastroenterology Hosp DeBellis, Castellana Grotte, Italy; Univ of Udine, Italy; et al)
Dig Dis Sci 41:950–955, 1996   2–6

Background.—In the multistep hypothesis of intestinal-type gastric carcinogenesis, the identification of the microenvironmental agents that induce gastric atrophy and intestinal metaplasia (IM) is crucial, as both are thought to be early precursors of gastric cancers. Epidemiologic evidence suggests that *Helicobacter pylori* is associated with gastric epithelial malignancies. Gastric abnormalities were assessed in consecutive nonulcerous dyspeptic patients, with a focus on the relationship between *H. pylori* infection and atrophic metaplastic lesions.

Methods.—Two hundred sixty-seven consecutive nonulcerous, untreated subjects were included in the study. Histological and histochemical analyses were performed, and the phenotypes of intestinal metaplasia documented.

Findings.—Helicobacter pylori infection was found in 61% of the subjects. Intestinal metaplasia, especially types II and III, was significantly correlated with both *H. pylori* detection and advanced age. In a logistic regression analysis, IM development was more significantly associated with *H. pylori* infection than with age, with no interactions.

Conclusions.—Helicobacter pylori is 1 of the major causes of mucosal lesions involved in the multistep process of gastric carcinogenesis. Any attempt to eradicate this infection is justified. In the nonulcerous dyspeptic patients assessed in the current study, the prevalence of *H. pylori* infection was significantly lower than in patients with gastric dysplasia and a high risk of cancer development.

▶ It is logical to think (but not conclude) that *H. pylori* may be an etiologic vector in the pathogenesis of gastric cancer. This study attempts to move along this path as it relates by regression analysis the presence of *H. pylori* to IM in non-ulcer bearing patients. It was unexpected that age was less significant than *H. pylori* in odds ratio analysis.

F.G. Moody, M.D.

8 Pharmacologic Considerations

Omeprazole and Duodenal Bicarbonate Secretion

Atrophic Gastritis and *Helicobacter pylori* Infection in Patients With Reflux Esophagitis Treated With Omeprazole or Fundoplication
Kuipers EJ, Lundell L, Klinkenberg-Knol EC, et al (Free Univ Hosp, Amsterdam: Univ Hosp, Leiden, The Netherlands; Univ Hosp, Nijmegen, The Netherlands; et al)
N Engl J Med 334:1018–1022, 1996   2–7

Background.—Drug therapy administered for the eradication of *Helicobacter pylori* infection is often ineffective and can promote an increase in the activity of corpus gastritis, an effect that may speed atrophic changes of the gastric mucosa and lead to gastric cancer. Patients with reflux esophagitis, some treated with omeprazole and others with fundoplication, were compared for the development of atrophic gastritis.

Patients and Methods.—Study participants were patients from 2 separate cohorts: 72 treated with fundoplication and 105 with omeprazole (40 mg once daily until healing was verified, followed by a maintenance dose of 20–40 mg daily). All had endoscopically confirmed reflux esophagitis ranging from grade I to grade IV. Patients were followed for an average of 5 years and monitored for the presence of *H. pylori* and the development of atrophic gastritis. Biopsy samples for histologic evaluation were obtained at follow-up gastroscopy.

Results.—At baseline, 31 patients in the fundoplication group were infected with *H. pylori* and 41 were not infected. A single patient who was infected with *H. pylori* had atrophic gastritis before fundoplication, and this condition persisted after surgery. None of the *H. pylori*–negative patients had histologic signs of active gastritis preoperatively, and none were subsequently found to have the infection or to have inflammation or atrophy of the gastric mucosa. In the omeprazole group, however, atrophic gastritis was diagnosed in 18 of 59 patients who had *H. pylori* infection at baseline and in 2 of 46 who were not infected; no patient in this group had atrophic gastritis before the start of treatment.

Conclusion.—Among patients with reflux esophagitis and *H. pylori* infection at baseline, there was a significant association between omeprazole treatment and the development of atrophic gastritis. Long-term acid-suppressive therapy with omeprazole fails to eradicate *H. pylori* in infected patients and leads to the development of atrophic gastritis and argyrophil-cell hyperplasia in patients with the infection. Fundoplication did not promote the development of atrophic gastritis.

▶ This study confirmed earlier reports indicating that long-term use of proton pump inhibitors in patients with concurrent infection with *H. pylori* is associated with a considerable risk of atrophic gastritis developing. Further, this study clearly demonstrates that fundoplication carried out in patients who are *H. pylori*–positive does not result in atrophic gastritis. The therapeutic implications seem clear. Patients who are to be placed on long-term maintenance therapy with proton pump inhibitors should be checked for the presence of *H. pylori*, and if tests are positive, should undergo appropriate treatment to eradicate *H. pylori*. Importantly, eradication of *H. pylori* should be documented by either a urea breath test or by a significant decrease in either IgA or IgG *H. pylori* antibody titers at 3 and 6 months after completion of treatment.[1] Treatment regimens that have been shown to result in a greater than 90% eradication rate of *H. pylori* include omeprazole, bismuth, metronidazole, and tetracycline given for 1 week or metronidazole, omeprazole, and clarithromycin also given for 1 week. Alternatives include omeprazole, amoxicillin, and clarithromycin given for 1 week. Recent studies indicate that 1 week of treatment with lansoprazole, clarithromycin, and metronidazole also effectively eradicates *H. pylori*. Patients on long-term maintenance therapy with proton pump inhibitors should also have their serum vitamin B_{12} levels checked because B_{12} stores can be depleted during a 3- to 5-year periods of continuous therapy with proton pump inhibitors. Another complication, albeit infrequent, of long-term use of proton pump inhibitors is the development of bacterial overgrowth in the proximal small bowel.

N.J. Greenberger, M.D.

Reference

1. Fallone CA, Barkun AN, Loo V, et al: Usefulness of serology and determination of *Helicobacter pylori* eradication after therapy. *Gastroenterology* 110:106A, 1996.

Omeprazole and Atrophic Gastritis

Omeprazole Promotes Proximal Duodenal Mucosal Bicarbonate Secretion in Humans

Mertz-Nielsen A, Hillingsø J, Bukhave K, et al (Univ of Copenhagen; Technical Univ of Denmark)
Gut 38:6–10, 1996   2–8

Introduction.—Research has focused on mucosal bicarbonate transport mechanisms because bicarbonate is the first line of defense against luminal acid and pepsin. Several studies have concentrated on the effect of various antiulcer drugs on gastroduodenal bicarbonate secretion, including the proton pump inhibitor and omeprazole in animals; however, no studies on humans have been done with omeprazole. These studies showed that there were higher rates of proximal duodenal mucosal bicarbonate secretion than with an H_2 receptor antagonist for gastric acid inhibition. Heathy volunteers participated in experiments without acid inhibition and after the administration of omeprazole and ranitidine in supramaximal equipotent doses large enough to obtain total inhibition of gastric acid secretion. The combination of omeprazole and ranitidine on basal duodenal mucosal bicarbonate secretion was also examined.

Methods.—Gastroduodenal perfusions were performed in healthy volunteers who were divided into 4 groups: 17 were in the control experiments, 17 were pretreated with high-dose omeprazole, 9 were pretreated with ranitidine, and 4 received a combination of omeprazole and ranitidine. Measurements were taken of basal and stimulated gastric and duodenal bicarbonate secretion rates.

Results.—Gastric acid secretion was completely inhibited by omeprazole and ranitidine (pH 6.9 vs. 6.8). Higher rates of basal stimulated duodenal bicarbonate secretion were found with omeprazole than with controls (597 vs. 351 µmol/hr). Higher rates of vagally stimulated duodenal bicarbonate secretion were also found with omeprazole than with controls (834 vs. 474 µmol/hr) (Table 2). This was not the case with acid-stimulated duodenal bicarbonate secretion (3,351 vs. 2,550 µmol/hr). An increase in duodenal bicarbonate secretion was found with the combination of omeprazole and ranitidine, whereas no change in either basal or stimulated secretion was found with ranitidine alone (Fig). Basal and vagally stimulated bicarbonate secretion was independent of the means of acid inhibition in the stomach.

Conclusion.—Proximal duodenal mucosal bicarbonate secretion, promoted by the proton pump inhibitor omeprazole, is apparently independent of its gastric acid–inhibitory effect. In duodenal ulcer healing, the observed increase in duodenal neutralizing capacity caused by omeprazole

TABLE 2.—Effect of Ranitidine, Omeprazole, and the Combination of Omeprazole and Ranitidine (*Ome + Ran*) on Gastric and Proximal Duodenal Mucosal Bicarbonate Secretion Rates in Healthy Volunteers During Basal Conditions and After Stimulation With Modified Sham Feeding and Luminal Acid (0.1 mol/L, 20 mL, 5 min)

	Gastric HCO_3^- (*μmol/hr*)			Duodenal HCO_3^- (*μmol/h × 3 cm*)				
	Number	*Basal*	*Sham Feeding*	*Number*	*Basal*	*Sham Feeding*	*Number*	*Luminal Acid*
Control	17	—	—	17	351 (39)	474 (66)*	9	2,550 (456)*
Ranitidine	9	401 (56)	1,316 (412)*	9	363 (63)	582 (204)*	9	1,752 (573)*
Omeprazole	17	500 (104)	916 (196)*	17	597 (48)†	834 (72)*†	9	3,351 (678)*
Ome+Ran	4	—	—	4	528 (78)‡	—		—

Note: Values are means (SEM).
*$P < 0.05$ vs. basal values.
†$P < 0.02$ vs. control and ranitidine treatment (Student-Newman-Keul test)
‡$P = 0.05$ vs. control (Student's *t* test).
(Courtesy of Mertz-Nielsen A, Hillingsø J, Bukhave K, et al: Omeprazole promotes proximal duodenal mucosal bicarbonate secretion in humans. *Gut* 38:6–10, 1996.)

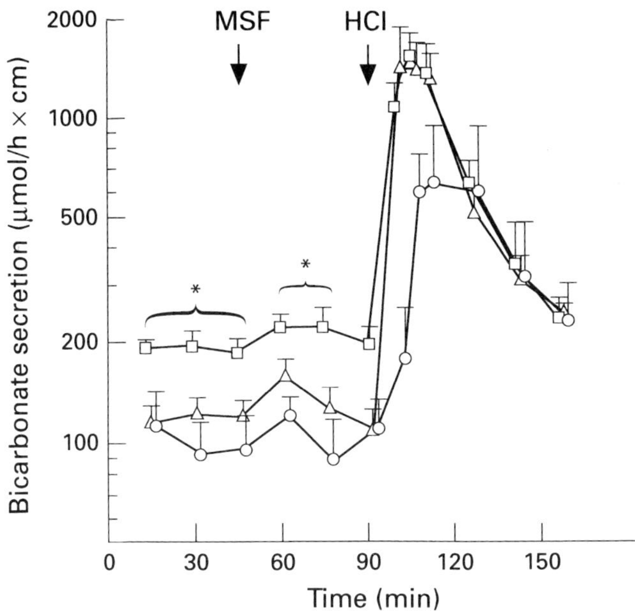

FIGURE.—Effects of omeprazole (*squares*) and ranitidine (*circles*) on basal and stimulated proximal duodenal mucosal bicarbonate secretion in healthy volunteers compared with no treatment (*triangles*), mean (SEM). *$P < 0.02$ vs. control and ranitidine treatment (Student-Newman-Keul multiple comparison test). *Abbreviations: MSF,* modified sham feeding; *HCl,* acid load. (Courtesy of Mertz-Nielsen A, Hillingsø J, Bukhave K, et al: Omeprazole promotes proximal duodenal mucosal bicarbonate secretion in humans. *Gut* 38:6–10, 1996.)

is likely to add to the documented superiority of omeprazole compared with histamine H_2 receptor antagonists.

▶ These results demonstrate that omeprazole promotes proximal duodenal mucosal bicarbonate secretion but not gastric bicarbonate secretion in healthy volunteers, apparently independent of its inhibitory effect on gastric acid secretion. In their discussion the authors put this in a practical perspective by calculating the acid-neutralizing potential for such duodenal bicarbonate secretion. They calculate that the normal basal output of bicarbonate from the duodenum approximates 1,000 µmol/hr, or 25% of the basal acid secretion. However, omeprazole-induced duodenal bicarbonate output amounts to approximately 1,800 µmol/hr, or 40% of the basal gastric acid secretion that can be neutralized by this alkali. The increase in duodenal acid-neutralizing capacity induced by omeprazole, coupled with a more potent inhibitory effect on acid secretion, helps account for its superiority over histamine H_2 antagonists in duodenal ulcer healing.

N.J. Greenberger, M.D.

Omeprazole and Acid Secretory Capacity

Marked Increase in Gastric Acid Secretory Capacity After Omeprazole Treatment

Waldum HL, Arnestad JS, Brenna E, et al (Norwegian Univ, Trondheim)
Gut 39:649–653, 1996   2–9

Background.—Unlike histamine$_2$ blockers, proton pump inhibitors have not been found to give rebound hypersecretion of acid. Because of the hyperplasia of the enterochromaffin-like (ECL) cell provoked by hypergastrinemia caused by profound acid inhibition and the central role of histamine from ECL cells in the regulation of acid secretion, the lack of any rebound acid hypersecretion after treatment with proton pump inhibitors has been questioned. The effect of omeprazole therapy on post-treatment acid secretion was investigated.

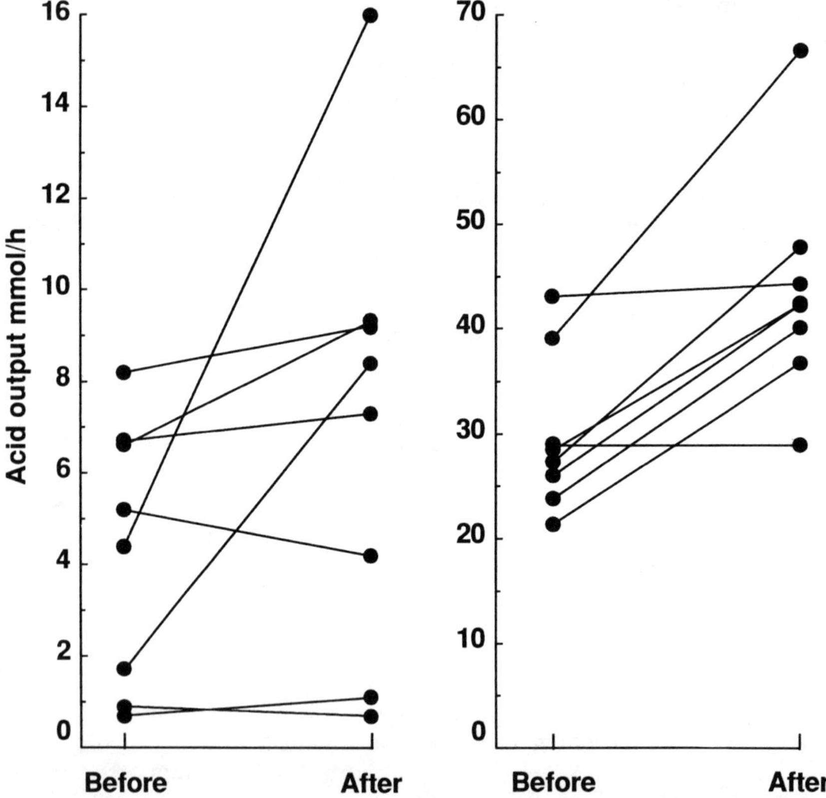

FIGURE.—Basal (left) and pentagastrin-stimulated (right) acid secretion before and 14 days after a 90-day treatment period with omeprazole 40 mg daily. (Courtesy of Waldum HL, Arnestad JS, Brenna E, et al: Marked increase in gastric acid secretory capacity after omeprazole treatment. *Gut* 39:649–653, 1996.)

Methods.—Nine patients with reflux esophagitis participated in the study. Basal and pentagastrin-stimulated acid secretion were determined before and 14 days after a 90-day treatment with the proton pump inhibitor omeprazole. Basal gastrin values and meal-stimulated gastrin release were assessed before and during omeprazole therapy. Biopsy samples were obtained from the oxyntic mucosa before and at the end of the treatment period for chemical assessment of the ECL cell mass.

Findings.—A marked increase in meal-stimulated gastrin release during omeprazole therapy resulted in a greater ECL cell mass. Chromogranin A (CgA) was increased in serum during omeprazole therapy, suggesting that serum CgA may be used to test ECL cell hyperplasia. There were significant increases in basal and pentagastrin-stimulated acid secretion after omeprazole therapy (Fig).

Conclusions.—Acid secretion is increased after a conventional treatment period with a proton pump inhibitor. This probably is the result of ECL cell hyperplasia. It may have adverse consequences for acid-related diseases.

▶ This study shows for the first time that treatment with a proton pump inhibitor (omeprazole) in conventional dosage (40 mg/day) for 3 months induces posttreatment gastric acid hypersecretion. Basal acid secretion increased significantly after omeprazole therapy, as did pentagastrin-stimulated acid secretion. Meal-stimulated gastric gastrin and peak meal-stimulated gastrin secretion both increased fourfold during treatment with omeprazole. The finding that hypergastrinemia resulted in hyperplasia of the ECL cell is supported by 2 lines of evidence. First, the histamine concentration increased significantly in the oxyntic mucosa after 3 months of omeprazole therapy. Second, there also was a fourfold increase in the CgA concentration in the oxyntic mucosa after 3 months of omeprazole treatment. Taken together, these changes most likely reflect an increase in the ECL cell mass.

Whether the increase in gastric and secretory capacity *persists* is still an open question. Because this study was done 14 days after the completion of a 3-month course of omeprazole therapy, it will be important for these patients to be studied again after a more extended period.

N.J. Greenberger, M.D.

Effects of OTC CaCO$_3$ and Famotidine

Comparison of the Effects of Over-the-counter Famotidine and Calcium Carbonate Antacid on Postprandial Gastric Acid: A Randomized Controlled Trial
Feldman M (Univ of Texas Southwestern Med Ctr, Dallas)
JAMA 275:1428–1431, 1996   2–10

Introduction.—Because the amount of acid titrated by antacids in vivo has not been determined, it is uncertain how effectively and rapidly various antacids neutralize acid within the human stomach. The acid-reducing properties of an antacid (Tums, 1,000 mg) were compared with those of an over-the-counter histamine$_2$-receptor antagonist (Pepcid AC, 10 mg).

Methods.—In a randomized, double-blinded, placebo-controlled cross-over trial, 18 healthy adults with a mean age of 39 years received each of 3 treatments: placebo, calcium carbonate, and famotidine. All participants had normal gastric acid secretion rates. Medications were taken 1 hour after a test meal that was infused into the stomach through a nasogastric tube. Two identical meals were infused 2.5 and 6.0 hours after the treatments. Intragastric pH was maintained at 4.0 for 1 hour before and 9 hours after the medication by means of in vivo intragastric titration with 0.3N sodium bicarbonate. Treatment groups were evaluated for the number of milliequivalents of titrant required to maintain gastric pH at 4.0.

Results.—Calcium carbonate had a rapid onset of action, neutralizing 6.7 mmol of acid in the first 30 minutes, but ceased to be effective after 60 minutes. Famotidine had a delayed onset of action (>90 minutes) compared with calcium carbonate but was effective for at least 540 minutes. The peak of famotidine's effect was observed at 210 minutes, when acid secretion was reduced by 7.3 mmol per 30 minutes. Famotidine reduced the total titrant requirement, relative to placebo and antacid, in all 18 participants. The mean pH during continuous titration was 4.04 after placebo, 4.08 after calcium carbonate, and 4.26 after famotidine. This difference between famotidine and placebo and antacid was significant, especially after the first 2 meals.

Conclusion.—The antacid and histamine$_2$-receptor antagonist both reduced gastric acid after a meal, but their pharmacokinetic profiles differed. Whereas gastric acid was reduced rapidly with the antacid, this agent had a short duration of action. Famotidine was not effective until approximately 90 minutes, but its action continued at least 540 minutes.

▶ It is estimated that 60 million Americans have heartburn and that as many as 7% of the population have heartburn daily. Not surprisingly the public has been deluged with television advertisements touting the benefits of over-the-counter histamine$_2$-receptor antagonists (H$_2$RAs) as well as antacids. This carefully done study by Feldman comparing the effects of over-the-counter famotidine and calcium carbonate antacid provides some much needed objective information to the claims being made.

Both antacids and H$_2$RAs, taken in recommended over-the-counter doses, reduce gastric acid and relieve heartburn more effectively than placebo. However, the pharmacokinetic profile of an over-the-counter H$_2$RA such as famotidine is different from that of a calcium carbonate antacid such as Tums. If either are taken postprandially, peak potencies of the 2 medications are similar in terms of their reduction in gastric acid secretion. Calcium carbonate tablets have a more rapid onset of action, but the duration of action is short compared with famotidine, which has a delayed onset of action but a more prolonged duration of effect. The author speculates that a preparation containing both an antacid and an H$_2$RA might prove to be more efficacious than either agent used alone. It bears emphasizing that heartburn in most cases invariably subsides within a 3- to 6-hour period. This helps to explain why both antacids and over-the-counter H_2RAs fare better than placebo in accelerating relief of symptoms, if the time frame chosen for study is 1–3 hours postprandially.

N.J. Greenberger, M.D.

Famotidine for Prevention of NSAID Induced Ulcers

Famotidine for the Prevention of Gastric and Duodenal Ulcers Caused by Nonsteroidal Antiinflammatory Drugs
Taha AS, Hudson N, Hawkey CJ, et al (Glasgow Royal Infirmary, Scotland; Univ Hosp, Nottingham, England; Merck Sharp & Dohme, Hoddesdon, England; et al)
N Engl J Med 334:1435–1439, 1996   2–11

Introduction.—The H_2-receptor antagonist famotidine can protect against gastric mucosal injury in normal patients receiving short-course therapy with aspirin or naproxen. However, the safety and effectiveness of famotidine in patients receiving long-term nonsteroidal anti-inflammatory drugs (NSAIDs) are unknown. Famotidine was evaluated for its ability to prevent NSAID-related gastric and duodenal ulcers in patients with arthritis.

Methods.—The randomized, placebo-controlled study included 285 patients who were receiving long-term NSAID therapy for rheumatoid arthritis or osteoarthritis. All were free of peptic ulcers at the start of the study. The patients were assigned to receive oral famotidine in a 20-mg or 40-mg twice-daily dose or placebo. Clinical and endoscopic evaluations were performed in blinded fashion using standardized criteria at baseline and after 4, 12, and 24 weeks of treatment. The 24-week cumulative incidence of gastric and duodenal ulcers was compared between groups.

Results.—Gastric ulcers developed in 20% of the placebo group, 13% of the patients receiving 20 mg of famotidine twice daily, and 8% of the patients receiving 40 mg of famotidine twice daily. Duodenal ulcers developed in 13%, 4%, and 2% of these groups, respectively. The higher dose of famotidine significantly reduced the incidence of ulcers at both sites, although the lower dose only reduced the rate of duodenal ulcers (Fig 1). Factors associated with an increased risk of ulcers were an increased peripheral white blood cell count and duodenal erosions with submucosal hemorrhage. Both famotidine doses were well tolerated.

Conclusions.—Famotidine, in a dosage of 40 mg twice daily, can safely reduce the incidence of gastric and duodenal ulcers in patients with arthritis who are receiving long-term NSAID therapy. A lower dose of famotidine may not reduce the incidence of gastric ulcers. Famotidine may also reduce problems with dyspepsia, which is not always present in patients with NSAID-induced ulcers.

▶ The results of this study demonstrate that treatment with a high dose of famotidine significantly reduced the cumulative incidence of both gastric and duodenal ulcers in patients with arthritis receiving long-term NSAID therapy.

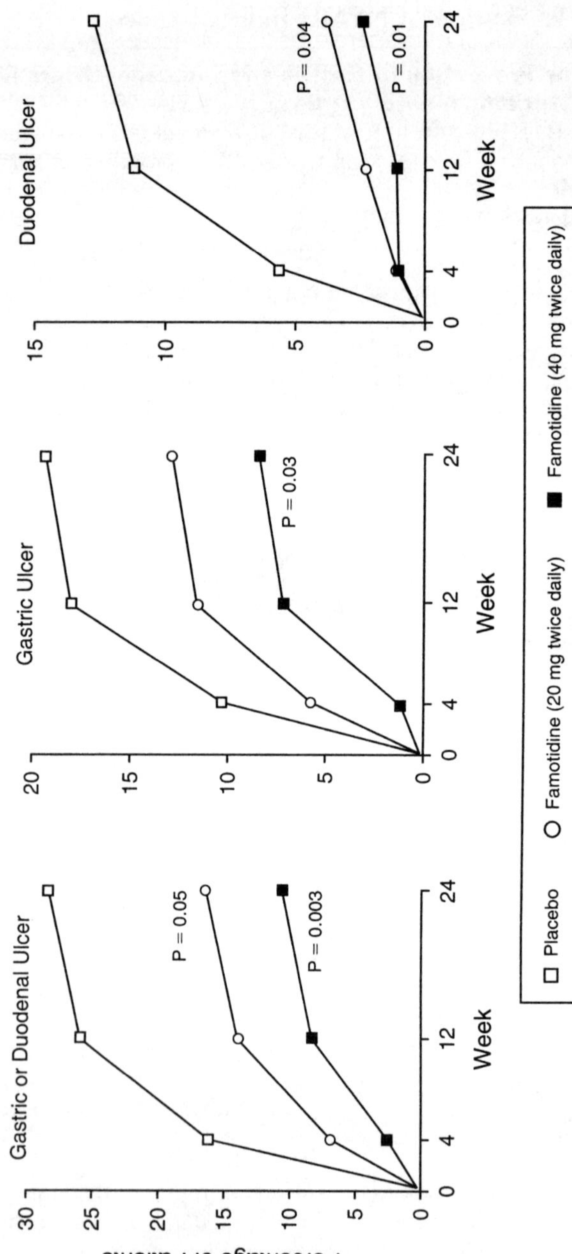

FIGURE 1.—Cumulative incidence of gastric and duodenal ulcers at 4, 12, and 24 weeks in patients with arthritis receiving long-term NSAID therapy, according to the group assignment. Data are from the intention-to-treat analysis. P values are for comparisons with the placebo group. (Courtesy of Taha AS, Hudson N, Hawkey CJ, et al: Famotidine for the prevention of gastric and duodenal ulcers caused by nonsteroidal antiinflammatory drugs. *N Engl J Med* 334:1435–1439. Copyright 1996, Massachusetts Medical Society. Reprinted by permission of *The New England Journal of Medicine*.)

This is particularly important because gastroduodenal damage has been demonstrated on endoscopic examination in 20% to 40% of patients taking NSAIDs. Further, gastrointestinal bleeding occurs in 1% of individuals who use NSAIDs regularly. Age older than 60 years, female gender, and prior ulcer disease or gastrointestinal bleeding increase this risk to approximately 3% and, in addition, if a patient has cardiovascular disease, the risk increases to approximately 9%. Although misoprostol has been shown to prevent NSAID-associated gastric and duodenal ulcer, it also may cause diarrhea and abdominal pain, and is unsuitable for women of childbearing potential. Thus, the report of Taha et al. is welcome because it provides a rationale for resumption or continuation of NSAID treatment in patients who require these medications and who may have had prior acid peptic disease or dyspepsia. In this connection, Taha et al. reported that about 30% of their patients had abdominal pain at baseline; at the end of the study, 29% of the patients in the placebo group had abdominal pain, as compared with 19% of the patients in the low-dose famotidine group and 17% of those in the high-dose group.

N.J. Greenberger, M.D.

9 Non-Ulcer Dyspepsia

Risk Indicators of Delayed Gastric Emptying of Solids in Patients With Functional Dyspepsia
Stanghellini V, Tosetti C, Paternicò A, et al (Univ of Bologna, Italy; Azienda Ospedaliera Policlinico Sant'Orsola-Malpighi, Bologna, Italy)
Gastroenterology 110:1036–1042, 1996   2–12

Background.—Functional or idiopathic dyspepsia is characterized by long-term or recurrent symptoms arising from the stomach or proximal small bowel that are not associated with organic, metabolic, or systemic disease. The relationship between gastric dysmotility and functional dyspepsia was examined to determine whether patients with functional dyspepsia have delayed gastric emptying of solids, whether gastric emptying abnormalities and symptoms of dyspepsia are related, and what clinical features might influence this relationship.

Methods.—Of 1,057 patients referred for investigation of chronic dyspepsia, 343 received a final diagnosis of functional dyspepsia (Table 1). In these 343 patients, gastric emptying was measured via a radioisotopic technique and the recording of 4 dyspeptic symptoms (nausea, vomiting, epigastric pain and burning, and postprandial fullness) as either absent, mild, relevant, or severe (depending on their effect on the patient's typical activities).

Results.—Delayed gastric emptying was diagnosed in 33.5% of the patients. Female sex, low body weight, presence of relevant and severe postprandial fullness, nausea, vomiting, and absence of relevant and severe epigastric pain were associated with greater frequency of delayed gastric emptying. With logistic regression, the factors independently associated with delayed gastric emptying were female sex, relevant and severe postprandial fullness, and severe vomiting.

Discussion.—In patients with chronic functional dyspepsia evaluated in a referral center, gastric emptying of solid components of caloric mixed meals was delayed. Dyspeptic symptoms were not directly correlated with delayed gastric emptying, however; many dyspeptic patients did not show an abnormality of gastric emptying. Other studies have also found a higher risk of gastric dysmotility in females as opposed to males, but the mechanism for this difference remains unclear. Studies of digestive symptoms

TABLE 1.—Final Diagnosis Formulated After Thorough Investigation of 1,057 Patients Referred for Chronic Dyspepsia

Diseases	No.	%
Peptic ulcer	226	21.4
Esophagitis	99	9.4
Biliary tree surgeries	58	5.5
Biliary lithiasis	48	4.5
Atrophic gastritis	46	4.4
Major abdominal surgeries	34	3.2
Gastric malignancies	6	0.6
Other gastrointestinal diseases (chronic liver diseases, pancreatitis, malabsorption, food allergy, etc.)	56	5.3
Diabetes	22	2.1
Metabolic/endocrine diseases (Zollinger-Ellison syndrome, Addison's disease, thyroid diseases, obesity)	33	3.1
Organic/systemic diseases (neoplasms, connective diseases, severe heart or respiratory failure)	28	2.6
Gynecologic diseases	22	2.1
Psychiatric diseases (anorexia nervosa, psychosis, severe anxiety)	36	3.4
Functional (idiopathic) dyspepsia	343	32.5
Total	1057	100

(Courtesy of Stanghellini V, Tosetti C, Paternicò A, et al: Risk indicators of delayed gastric emptying of solids in patients with functional dyspepsia. *Gastroenterology* 110:1036–1042, 1996.)

should take into account the intensity of such symptoms, not just their presence or absence.

▶ Dyspepsia can be broadly defined as episodic recurrent or persistent abdominal pain or discomfort referred to the upper abdomen. There are 3 subsets of dyspepsia: dyspepsia with gastroesophogeal reflux symptoms (GERD); dyspepsia with ulcer-like symptoms; and dysmotility-type dyspepsia manifested by symptoms of postprandial bloating, fullness, and distention. Up to one third of patients with dyspepsia may have all 3 types of symptoms. The term nonulcer dyspepsia refers to a complex and confusing disorder defined by a nondiagnostic esophagogastroduodenoscopy (EGD).

That functional dyspepsia (again defined by a normal EGD) is common is evident from the data in Table 1. Note that 32.5% of 1,057 patients were given a diagnosis of functional dyspepsia. No doubt this included patients with nonulcer dyspepsia and dysmotility-type symptoms. Stanghellini, et al. provide important information that will permit clinicians to identify the subset of patients with functional dyspepsia and delayed gastric emptying. Thus, female patients with low body weight, postprandial fullness, distention, bloating, nausea, and absence of *severe* epigastric pain are very likely to have delayed gastric emptying, especially for solids. Such patients are more likely to respond to treatment with promotility drugs such as cisapride rather than histamine H_2 receptor antagonists (H_2RAs) or proton pump inhibitors (PPIs). This is in contrast to patients with GERD-like dyspepsia and nonulcer dyspepsia with severe epigastric pain who are more likely to respond to H₂ RAs or PPIs.

N.J. Greenberger, M.D.

Long-term Follow-up of *Helicobacter pylori* Treatment in Non-ulcer Dyspepsia Patients
Elta GH, Scheiman JM, Barnett JL, et al (Univ of Michigan, Ann Arbor)
Am J Gastroenterol 90:1089–1093, 1995   2–13

Introduction.—About 15% of adults are affected by chronic dyspepsia. Although previous research has shown a strong link between *Helicobacter pylori* and non–ulcer-associated dyspepsia, conflicting results have occurred in some studies. In the absence of ulcer disease, routine testing for *H. pylori* may not be warranted, and more research is necessary to study the relationship between nonulcerative dyspepsia and *H. pylori*. Patients who had nonulcerative dyspepsia and were treated as though they had *H. pylori* infection with metronidazole and bismuth subsalicylate were described.

Methods.—Unexplained epigastric discomfort lasting for at least 4 weeks was the definition for non–ulcer-associated dyspepsia. Patients, regardless of their *H. pylori* status, were treated with metronidazole (250 mg 4 times daily) for 2 weeks and with bismuth subsalicylate tablets (524 mg 4 times daily) for 4 weeks. Another group of patients who were definitely infected with *H. pylori* according to an endoscopic examination were treated.

Results.—In this group, 67 were not infected and 33 were infected with *H. pylori*. During the latter part of the trial, 36 patients who were not infected were not treated. Treatment was completed by 21 uninfected patients and 19 infected patients. *Helicobacter pylori* was eradicated in 13 of 19 infected patients (68%). Symptoms improved in 8 of 13 (61%) *H. pylori*–eradicated patients and in 4 of 6 (66%) *H. pylori*–persistent patients; symptoms also improved in 14 of 21 (66%) uninfected patients. The 2 treatment groups had a similar long-term outcome after a mean of 34 months.

Conclusion.—The symptoms of non–ulcer-associated dyspepsia are not related to *H. pylori* infection. In up to 66% of the patients with nonulcerative dyspepsia, treatment with bismuth subsalicylate and metronidazole resulted in symptomatic improvement, regardless of whether *H. pylori* infection was diagnosed. Similar results were found after long-term follow-up of the uninfected and the infected groups. It is still necessary to conduct larger controlled studies to rule out a small, but potentially clinically significant benefit from *H. pylori* treatment in nonulcerative dyspepsia.

▶ This controlled study with a long-term follow-up (mean, 34 months) showed that treatment with bismuth subsalicylate and metronidazole resulted in symptomatic improvement in 61% to 66% of non–ulcer-associated dyspepsia patients regardless of initial or past treatment *and Helicobacter pylori* status. In 13 of 19 patients (68%) *H. pylori* was eradicated, yet symptom improvement was comparable in patients with (61%) and without (60%) successful *H. pylori* eradication and in uninfected patients (66%). Although the total number of patients studied was small and a beta or type II error cannot be excluded, the results are in accord with previous studies that have failed to demonstrate that eradication of *H. pylori* influences the natural history of nonulcerative dyspepsia.

N.J. Greenberger, M.D.

10 Peptic Ulcer Disease— Surgical Aspects

Type I Gastric Ulcer Treated by Parietal Cell Vagotomy and Mucosal Ulcerectomy

Jordan PH Jr (Baylor College of Medicine, Houston; VA Hosp, Houston)

J Am Coll Surg 182:388–393, 1996   2–14

Background.—Type I gastric ulcers, which occur at the gastric incisura, do not coexist with duodenal or pyloric ulcers. The most common surgical treatments for type I gastric ulcers are antrectomy and Billroth I anastomosis. The current study determined whether a less destructive acid-reduction operation, such as parietal cell vagotomy (PCV) and mucosal ulcerectomy, would yield outcomes equal to or better than those of antrectomy in patients with type I gastric ulcers.

Methods.—Forty-eight patients underwent parietal cell vagotomy and mucosal excision of the ulcer. The mean follow-up was 8 years.

Findings.—No operative mortality or major complications occurred in these patients. At the last follow-up, all but 4 patients were in Visick I and II classes. The 4 patients categorized as Visick IV needed a second gastric operation. The cumulative probability of recurrent ulcer rate determined by life-table analysis was 6.5% at 9 years.

Conclusions.—The PCV and ulcerectomy procedure is excellent for patients with Type I gastric ulcers. Clinicians can consider the operation as an alternative to antrectomy in this patient population.

▶ Paul Jordan, my colleague and dear friend here in Houston, continues to make important contributions to our surgical armamentarium for the treatment of acid peptic disease of the upper gastrointestinal tract. In this article, he establishes the safety and efficacy of treatment for garden variety gastric ulcers (Type 1) with PCV and mucosal excision of the ulcer. As is customary of Jordan's work, the follow-up is long and complete.

F.G. Moody, M.D.

Acute Surgical Treatment of Complicated Peptic Ulcers With Special Reference to the Elderly

Bulut O, Rasmussen C, Fischer A (Univ of Copenhagen)
World J Surg 20:574–577, 1996

Background.—Surgery for uncomplicated peptic ulcer disease has declined markedly since the introduction of H_2-receptor antagonists and proton pump inhibitors. However, the number of acute operative procedures in patients with complicated peptic ulcer has apparently not changed. The increased use of nonsteroidal anti-inflammatory drugs (NSAIDs) and other anti-inflammatory agents among elderly people has contributed to a significant increase in the number of hospital admissions for complicated peptic ulcer. The results of acute operative treatment in elderly patients with complicated peptic ulcer were reported.

Methods and Findings.—One hundred thirty-six consecutive patients undergoing surgery for acute complications of peptic ulcers between 1990 and 1993 were included in the review. Urgent surgery was needed in all patients. Ninety-one had perforations, 42 had hemorrhage, and 3 had a penetrated peptic ulcer. The median patient age was 77 years. Ninety-two patients had concurrent disease necessitating medical treatment. Fifty-eight percent of the patients were currently taking or recently had been taking anti-inflammatory agents at the time of admission. Sixty-six percent had duodenal ulcers. Only 34% were free of postoperative complications. The most common complications were pneumonia, arrhythmia, bleeding, and sepsis. Overall, 30% of the patients died, most from sepsis and multiorgan failure (Fig 1).

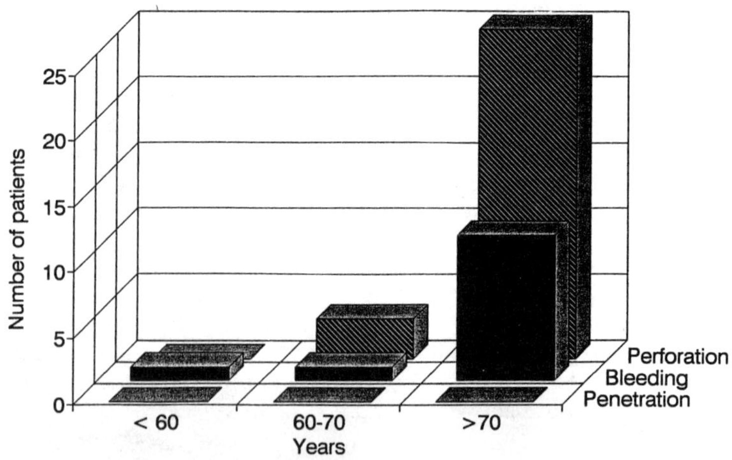

FIGURE 1.—Postoperative mortality in relation to age. (Courtesy of Bulut O, Rasmussen C, Fischer A: Acute surgical treatment of complicated peptic ulcers with special reference to the elderly. *World J Surg* 20:574–577, Copyright 1996, Springer-Verlag.)

Conclusion.—Peptic ulcer may develop in elderly persons taking 2 or more anti-inflammatory agents. Such patients should be treated prophylactically with ulcer-healing drugs.

▶ Fortunately, severe complications of peptic ulcer disease are decreasing in frequency in the general population but remain devastating in elderly patients who require anti-inflammatory agents for their comfort. Bulut's report displays the complexity of failing to identify such patients at risk and giving them peptic ulcer prophylaxis. Could it be that even in an advanced, socialized medical system, such as exists in Denmark, cost factors preclude the use of expensive antacid secretory drugs? H_2-blockers, omeprazole, sucralfate, and even *Helicobacter pylori* prophylaxis were available during this period of study. Or is the problem related to the fact that old people don't take their pills?

F.G. Moody, M.D.

Laparoscopic Truncal Vagotomy and Gastroenterostomy for Pyloric Stenosis
Wyman A, Stuart RC, Ng EKW, et al (Prince of Wales Hosp, Shatin, Hong Kong)
Am J Surg 171:600–603, 1996

2–16

Introduction.—The development of pyloric stenosis secondary to chronic ulceration in patients with peptic ulcer disease is an indication for surgery. The use of laparoscopic truncal vagotomy and gastroenterostomy, a new alternative to the standard operation of truncal vagotomy and a drainage procedure, was reported.

Methods.—The 12 patients, all men, were aged 22 to 56. All had a history of duodenal ulceration, ranging in duration from 2 to 10 years. Median duration of vomiting before admission was 4 weeks. With the patient under general anesthesia, the laparoscope is introduced and cannulae are inserted for retraction of the liver and dissection of the vagus nerves. The anterior vagus is identified and titanium clips are applied to each vagal trunk. A section is excised and sent for histologic examination. Although the principles of laparoscopic truncal vagotomy are the same as those of open surgery, with the magnified exposure of the esophagus, it is important not to mistake the longitudinal muscle bundles of the esophagus for vagal fibers. By retracting the transverse colon and omentum cephalad, the duodenojejunal flexure is exposed and a suitable segment of jejunum identified. This segment then is lifted over the transverse colon and apposed to the gastric antrum. Median operating time for the truncal vagotomy and gastroenterostomy was 210 minutes.

Results.—All patients were mobilized and required only oral analgesics after the first 24 hours. One patient remained hospitalized for 41 days because of delayed gastric emptying, but all others were discharged within 7 days. Conversion to laparotomy was required in 1 case near the end of the laparoscopic procedure. Two patients were readmitted, one with recurrent vomiting because of gastric stasis and another with peritonitis; both problems resolved with treatment. At a median follow-up of 6 months, symptomatic outcome was good in all 10 patients who had a totally laparoscopic procedure.

Discussion.—Laparoscopic techniques for the management of pyloric stenosis provide several advantages over open surgery: decreased pain, early mobilization, and avoidance of an upper abdominal incision with wound healing problems. The hospital stay is not significantly shortened, however, and longer follow-up is required before the procedure can be recommended routinely.

▶ Surgeons at the Prince of Wales Hospital in Hong Kong report on a small, but important, experience with the treatment of pyloric stenosis from acid-peptic disease by a truncal vagotomy and gastroenterostomy performed laparoscopically. They provide a detailed description of how to perform this operation. Important features of their approach are insertion of the laparoscope through the enterostomy to inspect the staple line of the gastroenterostomy for bleeding, and peroneal endoscopic examination of the gastroenterostomy at the completion of the procedure to ensure its patency.

F.G. Moody, M.D.

11 Gastrinomas

Somatostatin Receptor Scintigraphy

Somatostatin Receptor Scintigraphy: Its Sensitivity Compared With That of Other Imaging Methods in Detecting Primary and Metastatic Gastrinomas: A Prospective Study

Gibril F, Reynolds JC, Doppman JL, et al (NIH, Bethesda, Md)
Ann Intern Med 125:26–34, 1996
2–17

Background.—Accurate localization of primary neuroendocrine tumors, which are often small and difficult to find, is important. Because gastrinomas are an excellent model for obtaining information pertinent to less common pancreatic endocrine tumors, the localization of primary and metastatic gastrinoma in patients with Zollinger-Ellison syndrome was undertaken in a prospective comparison of the localizing abilities of ultrasonography, CT, MRI, bone scanning, selective angiography, and somatostatin receptor scintigraphy (SRS).

Methods.—Participating in the study were 80 consecutive patients with Zollinger-Ellison syndrome who were undergoing conventional tumor localization studies in addition to SRS using [^{111}In-DTPA-DPhe^1]octreotide with single-photon emission CT imaging at 4 and 24 hours. Fifteen patients also underwent exploratory laparotomy. Biopsies were performed for confirmation in patients with suspected liver metastases.

Results.—Somatostatin receptor scintigraphy identified extrahepatic gastrinomas or liver metastases in 70% of patients; angiography, in 40%; MRI, in 45%; CT, in 38%; and ultrasonography, in 19% . The sensitivity of SRS equalled that of all other tests combined. Somatostatin receptor scintigraphy yielded positive results in 58% of patients with suspected primary tumor, again proving as sensitive as all other tests combined (Fig 2). Sensitivity at detection of metastatic liver disease (histologically proven in 24 patients) was again highest for SRS (92%) and lower for MRI (71%), angiography (62%), ultrasonography (46%), and CT (42%). The SRS diagnosed 24 of 29 gastrinomas identified at later surgery, more than were evident with CT, MRI, ultrasonography, and angiography combined.

Conclusion.—These data show that for patients with Zollinger-Ellison syndrome, SRS is the single most sensitive method for detection of either primary or metastatic liver lesions. Somatostatin receptor scintigraphy should be the initial tumor localization study performed for patients with

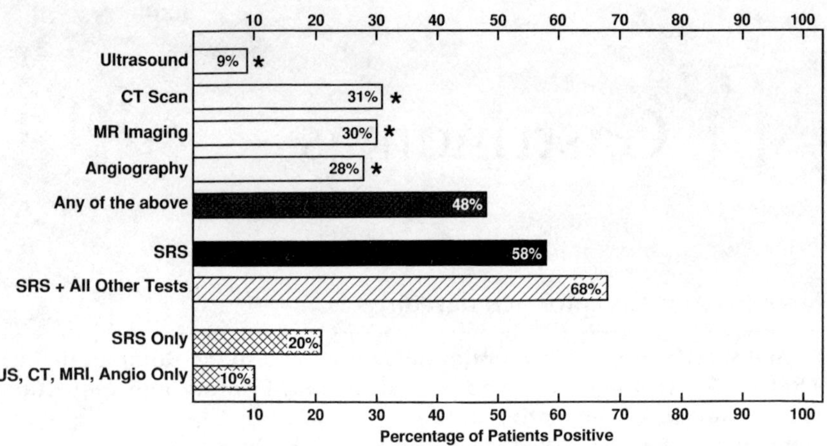

FIGURE 2.—Results of tumor localization studies for identification of an extrahepatic tumor in patients with Zollinger-Ellison syndrome. Results are expressed as the percentage of the 80 patients in whom any extrahepatic tumor was localized. Each patient was counted only once. *Triple asterisk* indicates $P < 0.001$ for the method compared with somatostatin receptor scintigraphy alone. *Abbreviations: Angio*, angiography; *SRS*, somatostatin receptor scintigraphy; *US*, ultrasonography. (Courtesy of Gibril F, Reynolds JC, Doppman JL, et al: Somatostatin receptor scintigraphy: Its sensitivity compared with that of other imaging methods in detecting primary and metastatic gastrinomas. *Ann Intern Med* 125:26–34, 1996.)

Zollinger-Ellison syndrome, and this conclusion can probably be extrapolated for carcinoid tumors and other pancreatic endocrine tumor syndromes (except insulinoma). The cost of the conventional studies combined, with equal sensitivity to SRS, is 3 times as much and necessitates more patient time, radiation exposure, and inconvenience. Further guidelines for the use of SRS in localizing pancreatic endocrine tumors are needed.

▶ This study demonstrates that SRS is the single most sensitive method for localizing primary gastrinomas and assessing tumor extent in patients with Zollinger-Ellison syndrome. Further, SRS has been shown to detect either a primary tumor or liver metastasis in 80% to 100% of patients with various pancreatic endocrine tumors but a smaller percentage (61%) in patients with insulinoma.[1]

That SRS was more sensitive than any combination of 4 tests—ultrasonography, CT scanning, MRI, and angiography—has important implications for cost-effective case finding. As the authors emphasize in their discussion, the above combined studies cost at least 3 times as much as SRS and involve more time, more radiation exposure, and more inconvenience for the patient. The authors also suggest that if SRS results are negative for the primary tumor and/or metastatic liver disease, additional imaging studies do not seem justified.

N.J. Greenberger, M.D.

Reference

1. Krenning EP, Korrekkeboom DS, Bakka WH, et al: Somatostatin receptor scintigraphy with [^{111}In-DTPA-Phe] and [1^{123}-Tyr^3] octreotide: The Rotterdam experience with more than 1,000 patients. *Eur J Nucl Med.* 20:716, 1993.

Value of Somatostatin Receptor Scintigraphy: A Prospective Study in Gastrinoma of Its Effect on Clinical Management

Termanini B, Gibril F, Reynolds JC, et al (Natl Inst of Diabetes and Digestive and Kidney Diseases, Bethesda, Md; NIH, Bethesda, Md)
Gastroenterology 112:335–347, 1997   2–18

Background.—The ability of somatostatin receptor scintigraphy (SRS) to localize neuroendocrine tumors has been demonstrated. However, this and other tumor localization methods can be time-consuming, costly, and inconvenient for the patient. Whether SRS changes clinical management in patients with Zollinger-Ellison syndrome was investigated.

Methods.—One hundred twenty-two consecutive patients underwent conventional imaging studies before SRS. Treatment plans, initially based on the findings on conventional imaging studies, were re-evaluated after SRS was performed.

Findings.—Somatostatin receptor scintigraphy was superior to any one of the other imaging modalities. Overall, the treatment plans were changed for 47% of the patients. The main reasons for changing plans were primary tumor localization and clarification of equivocal localization findings from conventional studies. The findings of SRS were equally useful in patients with and without metastatic liver disease.

Conclusions.—Somatostatin receptor scintigraphy can significantly alter management plans in patients with Zollinger-Ellison syndrome. It is a very sensitive, specific, simple, and cost-effective modality; thus, it should be considered the initial imaging modality of choice for patients with gastrinomas.

▶ The data obtained in this study provide strong support for the notion that SRS should be the initial imaging modality for patients with gastrinoma. Somatostatin receptor scintigraphy revealed important additional information not obtained by CT scanning, MRI, and other conventional localization studies in 17 (14%) of 122 patients. Importantly, SRS changed the clinical management in 57 (47%) of 122 patients. The change in clinical management was obtained in both directions. On the one hand, SRS detected disease that was not detected by other methods, both for primary localization of gastrinomas and for better delineation of the extent of metastatic disease. Conversely, SRS clarified questionable results of conventional imaging studies. It was the only modality to localize a primary tumor for surgical extirpation in 12% of the patients. Further, it was the only modality to localize liver metastasis in 4% of the patients. Somatostatin receptor scintigraphy had greater sensitivity than any conventional imaging study, and it was at least equal to or better than all conventional imaging studies combined. The authors emphasize in their conclusions that SRS may cost more than MRI or CT scanning but is less costly than selective angiography, and it certainly costs less than the combined cost of those procedures. They appropriately caution that although these results are striking, it still remains unclear whether routine use of SRS will either increase the cure rate or extend survival in patients with Zollinger-Ellison syndrome.

N.J. Greenberger, M.D.

12 Gastric Ampullary and Duodenal Neoplasm

The Risk of Stomach Cancer in Patients With Gastric or Duodenal Ulcer Disease

Hansson L-E, Nyrén O, Hsing AW, et al (Uppsala Univ, Sweden; Mora Hosp, Sweden; Natl Cancer Inst, Bethesda, Md; et al)

N Engl J Med 335:242–249, 1996

2–19

Background.—Much controversy has surrounded a purported relationship between peptic ulcer and gastric carcinoma. With the recognition of *Helicobacter pylori* as a causative factor in the development of gastric cancer and as having a strong association with duodenal and gastric ulcers, these relationships are being re-examined. Long-term follow-up was provided for a large, population-based cohort of patients hospitalized for gastric or duodenal ulcers (who did not receive surgical treatment) to assess the risk of gastric cancer.

Methods.—Patients hospitalized for gastric or duodenal ulcers between 1965 and 1983 were identified through the Swedish inpatient register. Follow-up of 57,936 patients continued until 1989 for an average of 9.1 years. The measure of relative risk was the standardized incidence ratio: the ratio of the observed number of cancers to the expected number based on incidence in the Swedish population at large.

Results.—Among 29,287 patients with gastric ulcers, the standardized incidence ratio for gastric cancer peaked in the first 3 years of follow-up and then leveled off to 1.8 (Fig 1). Among 8,646 patients with prepyloric ulcers, the standardized incidence ratio was 1.2 (nonsignificant), and among 24,456 patients with duodenal ulcers, the incidence of gastric cancer was lower than expected (standardized incidence ratio, 0.6). Overall, women showed a 40% higher relative risk of gastric cancer than did men, and patients less than 50 years old at initial hospitalization had a relative risk twice that of patients more than 70 years old.

Conclusions.—These data show that patients hospitalized with gastric ulcers have a risk of gastric cancer almost double the expected rate whereas patients hospitalized with duodenal ulcers have a 40% reduced risk of gastric cancer. Patients with duodenal ulcers have an *H. pylori* infection rate of close to 100%, whereas the corresponding age-matched

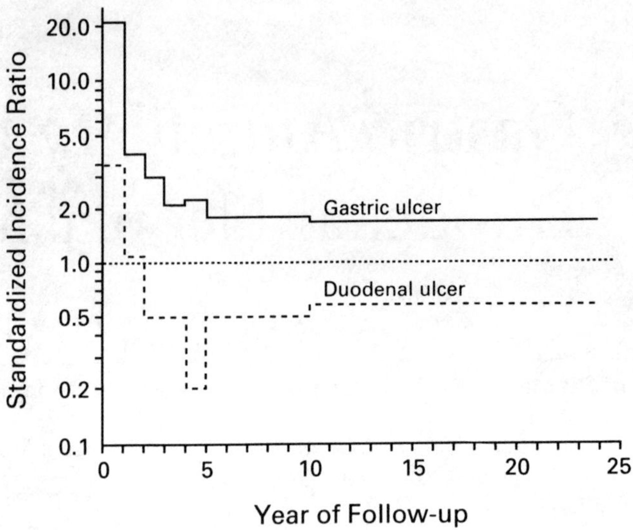

FIGURE 1.—Standardized incidence ratio for gastric cancer in patients with gastric or duodenal ulcers according to the year of follow-up. The scale for the standardized incidence ratio is logarithmic. (Reprinted by permission of *The New England Journal of Medicine* from Hansson L-E, Nyrén O, Hsing AW, et al: The risk of stomach cancer in patients with gastric or duodenal ulcer disease. *N Engl J Med* 335:242–249, Copyright 1996, Massachusetts Medical Society.)

population has an infection rate of 40%–60%. Gastric cancer probably has etiologic factors in common with gastric ulcer, whereas the carcinogenic effect of *H. pylori* may be modified by some processes occurring in patients with duodenal ulcers.

▶ This population-based long-term study of patients hospitalized for gastric ulcers found a risk of gastric cancer almost *twice* the expected rate. By contrast, among patients with duodenal ulcer there was a significant 40% *reduction* in risk. The putative link between gastric ulcer and gastric cancer is believed to be atrophic gastritis induced by *Helicobacter pylori.* The factor or factors associated with duodenal ulcer that protect against gastric cancer are unknown, but some modification of *H. pylori's* carcinogenic effects is a reasonable working hypothesis.

N.J. Greenberger, M.D.

Malignant Transformation of Benign Epithelial Gastric Polyps
Orlowska J, Jarosz D, Pachlewski J, et al (Med Ctr of Postgraduate Education, Warsaw)
Am J Gastroenterol 90:2152–2159, 1995

2–20

Background.—Benign epithelial gastric polyps (BEGPs) are uncommon lesions that sometimes undergo malignant transformation. However, the natural course of these lesions and the histologic changes involved remain unclear. The natural history of the transformation from BEGP to carcinoma was studied as part of a comparison of the malignant potential of hyperplastic polyps and adenomas.

Methods.—A total of 811 BEGPs detected by esophagogastroscopy in 432 patients were examined. The histologic diagnosis on endoscopic biopsy or polypectomy specimens, according to the World Health Organization classification, was hyperplastic polyp in 751 cases and adenoma in 60. Elster's classification was used to further categorize the hyperplastic lesions into polypoid foveolar hyperplasia (FH), 268 lesions; and typical hyperplastic polyps (HPs), 483 lesions. Signs of focal malignancy at the initial evaluation or malignant transformation during follow-up were sought. An average of nearly 3 years' follow-up was available for 96 patients with 220 BEGPs.

Results.—Focal carcinoma was found in 2% of HPs and 10% of adenomas, according to Elster's classification. In addition, 7% of patients with HPs and 13% of those with adenoma had carcinoma at another location in the stomach. Five of 131 HPs exhibited histologic signs of transformation during follow-up: focal intestinal metaplasia in 2 and focal dysplasia and focal carcinoma in 1 each. Focal carcinoma developed in 1 of 23 adenomas during follow-up. Of 58 patients with HPs, 2 had separate gastric carcinomas develop outside the polyps. There were no instances of focal carcinoma, either initially or during follow-up, among the patients with FH. Two possible sequences of events seemed to occur in the natural history of BEGPs: from erosion to FH, HP, and adenoma to focal and/or polypoid carcinoma, or directly from adenoma to carcinoma.

Conclusions.—Malignant transformation can occur in gastric HPs, as it can in adenomas. In contrast, FH appears to be always benign. The authors propose that FH should be classified separately from HPs. All patients with gastric HPs or adenoma must undergo polypectomy to exclude gastric carcinoma.

▶ The authors took advantage of a long-term follow-up of 432 patients with benign gastric polyps by esophagogastroscopy and biopsy or polypectomy to inform us of the malignant potential of such lesions. Polyps that histologically prove to be FH have no malignant potential. Hyperplastic polyps, on the other hand, act like adenomatous polyps in the stomach and can undergo malignant transformation. Even though the rate of transformation is low, they should be removed either transendoscopically or by laparoscopic or open gastrotomy.

F.G. Moody, M.D.

The Prognostic Value of Preoperative Serum Levels of CEA and CA19-9 in Patients With Gastric Cancer

Kodera Y, Yamamura Y, Torii A, et al (Aichi Cancer Ctr, Nagoya, Japan)
Am J Gastroenterol 91:49–53, 1996   2–21

Introduction.—In some experimental models, the tumor markers carcinoembryonic antigen (CEA) and CA19-9 are known as adhesion molecules. If these markers are involved in metastasis, an increase in serum levels could be a poor prognostic sign. Patients with gastric cancer were studied to determine the prognostic relevance of preoperative serum CEA and CA19-9 levels.

Methods.—Serum CEA and CA19-9 levels were measured in 663 patients with gastric cancer before laparotomy. Univariate analysis was performed to look for correlations between these levels and various clinicopathologic factors. Multivariate analysis was performed to see whether CEA and CA19-9 levels were significant prognostic factors.

Results.—Seventeen percent of the patients had elevated serum CEA levels, and 16% had elevated CA19-9 levels. An elevated CEA measurement was correlated with patient sex; with hepatic, peritoneal, and nodal metastases; and with tumor depth. It was not well correlated with the tumor histologic type however. An elevated CA19-9 level was correlated with the types of metastases and with tumor depth and size. Among patients undergoing R0 resection, the prognosis was significantly different for those with and those without an elevated CA19-9 level. The prognosis was always poor for patients undergoing noncurative operations, regardless of their tumor marker status. The serum CA19-9 level was a better prognostic factor than the serum CEA level.

Conclusions.—In patients with gastric cancer, an elevated serum CA19-9 level appears to be a significant indicator of malignant potential. By comparison, an elevated CEA level does not seem to carry such a poor prognosis. These tumor markers are currently of little clinical value, however, because little can be done to influence the outcome of recurrent gastric cancer.

▶ Tumor markers have been of little value thus far in the management of gastric cancer. This report from Nagoya, Japan, however, adds a new twist—when CEA and CA19-9 are positive, they may, because of their biological activity as adhesion molecules, indicate the extent or dissemination of the disease. The authors' evidence is that these molecules are present in the bloodstream in higher concentrations in the presence of liver and peritoneal metastases. They are fully aware of the "chicken and egg" trap and admit that CEA and CA19-9 as tumor markers is only an idea (one that I must admit never entered my mind until I read this article).

F.G. Moody, M.D.

Surgical Aspects of Patients With Adenocarcinoma of the Stomach Operated on for Cure

Söreide JA, van Heerden JA, Burgart LJ, et al (Mayo Clinic and Found, Rochester, Minn)
Arch Surg 131:481–487, 1996   2–22

Objective.—Even with the availability of upper gastrointestinal endoscopy, only half of patients with gastric adenocarcinoma will have potentially curable disease when the diagnosis is made. Survival is better in Japan than in the Western world, where there is ongoing debate about the optimal extent of gastric resection and the roles of regional lymphadenectomy, splenectomy, and adjuvant therapy. An experience with "curative" resection for gastric adenocarcinoma was presented.

Methods.—The study included 187 patients treated from 1979 to 1988, representing 64% of patients with adenocarcinoma occurring distal to the gastroesophageal junction. Those with tumors in the area of the gastroesophageal junction were not included. All patients underwent surgery with curative intent, i.e., with no evidence of distant metastases or apparent residual tumor. The patients were 66 men and 64 women, with a median age of 68 years. Fifty-six percent of patients were in American Society of Anesthesiologists (ASA) physical status 3 or greater, and 44% were in Eastern Cooperative Oncology Group status 2 or greater. The immediate- and long-term operative results were reviewed, and factors influencing morbidity, mortality, and survival were analyzed.

Results.—Seventy-eight percent of patients underwent subtotal gastrectomy, and 22% had total gastrectomy. Five percent of patients had extended lymph node dissections. Three percent of patients received adjuvant chemotherapy and 2% had radiotherapy. Postoperative morbidity was 27% and postoperative mortality was 4%. The complication rate may have been affected by synchronous splenectomy and type of gastric resection, but these factors did not influence postoperative mortality.

The median follow-up was 47 months overall and 9 years in patients who were still living. Overall survival rates were 48% at 5 years and 32% at 10 years. Factors significantly associated with survival on univariate analysis included age, ASA classification, disease stage, tumor diameter, serosal extension, lymph node metastases, and type of resection. The independent factors identified by Cox multivariate analysis were serosal extension and lymph node metastases.

Conclusions.—With standard radical surgery, 50% of patients with gastric cancer will survive for 5 years. This result is achieved even though these patients tend to be older and to have comorbid conditions. Total gastrectomy, splenectomy, and extended lymph node dissection are of unproven efficacy and may even lead to increased morbidity and mortality.

Until their value is proved in controlled, prospective studies, these techniques should not be used routinely.

▶ I always enjoy reading reports from the Mayo Clinic; this one is no exception. The authors carefully define the study population and their methods of analysis. The completeness and length of follow-up is impressive. What it clearly tells us is that gastric cancer treated surgically at the Mayo Clinic has a 5-year survival rate of 48% and a 10-year survival rate of 32%, rates much lower than these reported from Japan. Of note is that the patients were relatively old (68 years) and their lesions quite advanced (56% with nodal metastases and in 48%, the tumor extended through the serosa). Possibly more patients would have been salvaged by the more frequent use of radical node dissection. The authors do not comment on this issue but do make the point that they may have understaged the patient population because of the relatively few nodes associated with their specimens. They make a point of their relatively high survival rates, best in the Western world, but it is important to remember that they describe a carefully selected group of patients from their overall experience. Be sure you read the discussion of the presentation of their paper.

F.G. Moody, M.D.

Clinical Significance of Occult Micrometastasis in Lymph Nodes From Patients With Early Gastric Cancer Who Died of Recurrence
Maehara Y, Oshiro T, Endo K, et al (Kyushu Univ, Fukuoka, Japan; Natl Kyushu Cancer Ctr, Fukuoka, Japan)
Surgery 119:397–402, 1996   2–23

Background.—Some patients die of gastric cancer recurrence even after curative resection of early disease. Such patients may have occult micrometastases in perigastric lymph nodes at the time of their initial diagnosis. Lymph nodes dissected from early gastric cancer lesions were stained after surgery with a monoclonal antibody against cytokeratin, an essential component of the cytoskeleton of epithelial cells.

Methods.—Immunocytochemical methods and an antiserum to epithelial membrane antigen were used to investigate the possible presence of tumor cells in 420 dissected lymph nodes from 34 patients with node-negative early gastric cancer who died from disease recurrence. The monoclonal antibody CAM 5.2 can recognize the cytokeratin polypeptides that usually occur in epithelial cells. The clinicopathologic features and prognosis of patients with cytokeratin-positive cells in the lymph nodes were determined.

Findings.—Cytokeratin-positive cells at the time of primary surgery were present in 3.6% of the nodes in 23.5% of the patients. Cytokeratin positivity was unassociated with various clinicopathologic variables. In 8 cytokeratin-positive patients, histological stage was upstaged from I to II in 3 patients, to III in 4 patients, and to IV in 1 patient. Hematogenous

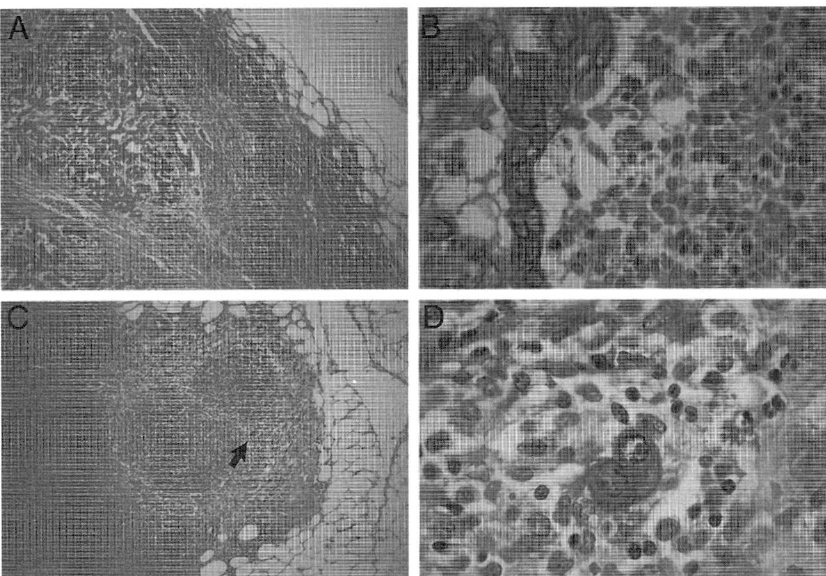

FIGURE 1.—Microphotograph of metastases in lymph node shows cytokeratin staining of perigastric lymph node with evident metastasis by use of hematoxylin-eosin staining. Perigastric lymph node has a number of cytokeratin-positive tumor cells, with low-power (original magnification, ×100) (**A**) and high-power photomicrograph (original magnification, ×800) (**B**). Perigastric lymph node has a small cluster of cytokeratin-positive tumor cells but not for hematoxylin-eosin staining, with low-power (*arrow* for tumor cells: original magnification, ×100) (**C**) and high-power photomicrograph (original magnification, ×1000) (**D**). (Courtesy of Maehara Y, Oshiro T, Endo K, et al: Clinical significance of occult micrometastasis in lymph nodes from patients with early gastric cancer who died of recurrence. *Surgery* 119:397–402, 1996.)

recurrences were common. Prognosis in these patients was poorer than in cytokeratin-negative patients (Fig 1).

Conclusions.—Immunohistochemical methods are useful to identify micrometastatic disease in lymph nodes missed in routine hematoxylin-eosin staining. Dissected nodes should undergo cytokeratin staining to precisely determine tumor stage and prognosis for patients with early gastric cancer.

▶ The authors attempt to resolve why a small percentage of patients with early gastric cancer with negative lymph node analysis die of metastatic disease. Not unexpectedly, reanalysis of hematoxylin and eosin negative nodes by utilization of cytokeratin protein detection by a specific monoclonal anatomy revealed that, in fact, metastasis had occurred in almost a quarter of patients with presumed node-negative early gastric cancer.

F.G. Moody, M.D.

Relation of Number of Positive Lymph Nodes to the Prognosis of Patients With Primary Gastric Adenocarcinoma

Wu CW, Hsieh MC, Lo SS, et al (Veterans Gen Hosp-Taipei, Taiwan; Natl Yang-Ming Univ, Taiwan)
Gut 38:525–527, 1996

2–24

Introduction.—The 2 factors acknowledged to influence survival in resectable gastric cancer are regional lymph node involvement and depth of tumor invasion. Recent studies of gastric and other cancers indicate that the number as well as the presence of positive nodes also influences prognosis. Five hundred ten patients were studied retrospectively to establish a nodal grouping category of gastric cancer as a forecaster of distant disease.

Methods.—All patients who were studied underwent curative resection for adenocarcinoma of the stomach between December 1987 and May 1994. Prognostic variables examined were age, sex, depth of cancer invasion, nodal stage, number of metastatic lymph nodes, site and size of the tumor, and Lauren's histologic classification.

Results.—The patient group had a mean age of 65 years and a male-to-female ratio of 4.7:1. Most (73%) had advanced cancers, and more than half (56.3%) had lymph node metastases. Overall, 2,811 of 17,176 lymph nodes showed metastases. Four-year survival was 91% for patients without nodal involvement vs. 39.2% for those with lymph node metastasis. In patients with a single positive node, 4-year survival was 70%. A sharp decrease in survival was noted between patients with 4 positive nodes (73%) and patients with 5 or more positive nodes (35%). A greater number of involved nodes was associated with increasingly reduced survival.

Discussion.—Multivariate analysis identified the number of positive nodes and depth of cancer invasion as independent prognostic factors in gastric cancer. Nodal grouping categories of 0, 1–4, 5–8, and 9 or greater can be used to classify nodal stage and are of greater prognostic value than node-negative and node-positive categories. Survival rates for the nodal grouping categories were 90.8% (0 positive nodes), 70.5% (1–4 positive nodes), 26.8% (5–8 positive nodes), and 12.2% ($\geq$ 9 positive nodes). Neither current nodal stage nor Lauren's histologic classification were independent variables.

▶ The 17,176 lymph nodes from 510 patients who had undergone gastric resection with radical node resection for gastric cancer reveal some interesting findings. The prognosis related to the nodal status in that none was better than 1–4 positive nodes, and the latter provided a better prognosis than 5–8, and 9 and greater. The debate continues as to whether radical removal of nodes improves prognosis or merely provides a means for predicting survival. I have been converted to the point of view that a so-called R-2 resection should be done, because it can be accomplished safely in centers where gastric cancers are now treated. Why not give the patient the benefit of the doubt and provide the oncologist with the very best information possible for evaluation of adjuvant therapeutic strategies?

F.G. Moody, M.D.

Prospective Randomized Trial Comparing Billroth I and Billroth II Procedures for Carcinoma of the Gastric Antrum
Chareton B, Landen S, Manganas D, et al (Centre Hospitalo Universitaire de Rennes, France)
J Am Coll Surg 183:190–194, 1996   2–25

Background.—Although total gastrectomy and subtotal gastrectomy have been found to be comparable in the treatment of gastric antrum carcinoma, it is still unknown whether digestive reconstruction should be done by a Billroth I (BI) gastroduodenostomy or a Billroth II (BII) gastrojejunostomy. These 2 procedures were compared prospectively in a randomized study.

Methods.—Billroth I and II procedures were performed in 30 and 32 patients, respectively. Twenty-seven percent of the tumors were stage I; 16%, stage II; 47%, stage III; and 10%, stage IV. The 2 groups were well-matched on clinicopathologic factors.

Findings.—The length of operation, amount of blood transfused, and abdominal drainage associated with the 2 procedures were comparable. However, patients undergoing BI procedures had a greater duration and volume of gastric drainage. Four fistulas developed after BI procedures and 1 after BII gastrectomy. Independent risk factors for fistula development were BI gastrectomy and a low preoperative serum albumin level. Fistula development was associated with increased length of stay in patients undergoing BI procedures. The 2 groups had similar hospital mortality.

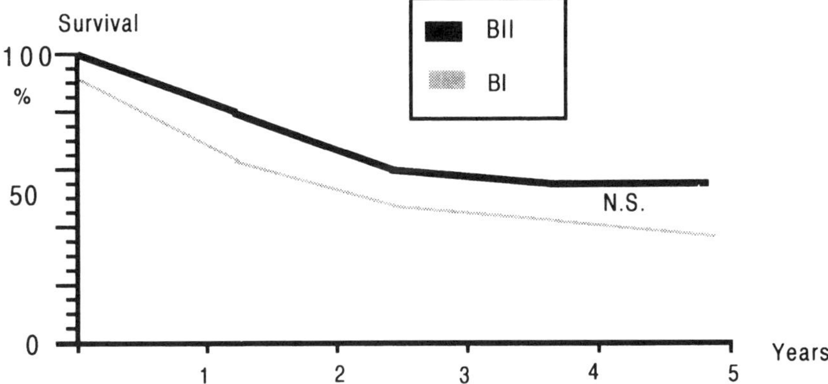

FIGURE 1.—Survival following Billroth I (*BI*) and Billroth II (*BII*) gastrectomy for carcinoma after exclusion of patients who died of unrelated causes. *Abbreviation: N.S.*, not significant. (Courtesy of Chareton B, Landen S, Manganas D, et al: Prospective randomized trial comparing Billroth I and Billroth II procedures for carcinoma of the gastric antrum. *J Am Coll Surg* 183:190–194, 1996. By permission of the *Journal of the American College of Surgeons.*)

The 5-year actuarial survival rates after BI and BII procedures were 42% and 40%, respectively. When patients who died of unrelated causes were excluded, 5-year survival rates after BI and BII were 40% and 53%, respectively (Fig 1). Long-term survival was comparable in the 2 groups for all tumor stages. Seven recurrences at the hepatic pedicle were documented in the BI, compared with 1 in the BII group. Four reoperations were required.

Conclusions.—Patients undergoing BI and BII gastrectomy for carcinoma have comparable digestive comfort and long-term survival rates. Billroth I gastrectomy carries an increased risk of fistula development and carcinoma recurrence at the hepatic pedicle.

▶ The authors establish by a randomized control trial that a BI or BII reconstruction after gastrectomy for cancer provides comparable survival and quality of life, but the BI is associated with a higher rate of fistulization. It appears that the outcome of this study will not affect the therapeutic choices of the surgeons involved, because the authors rationalize that a BII would negate access to the papilla of Vater if biliary obstruction should ensue. They have a point, but it is minor compared with the likelihood of problems with recurrence at the gastroduodenostomy. I plan to stick with the BII reconstruction.

F.G. Moody, M.D.

Long-term Follow-up After Curative Surgery for Early Gastric Lymphoma
Bartlett DL, Karpeh MS Jr, Filippa DA, et al (Mem Sloan-Kettering Cancer Ctr, New York)
Ann Surg 223:53–62, 1996   2–26

Introduction.—Early gastric lymphoma has been managed successfully by multimodality therapy, which includes surgery, chemotherapy, and radiation therapy. Currently, however, surgery tends to be limited to a role of salvage therapy after nonsurgical approaches. A retrospective review of 34 patients with stage IE and IIE-1 gastric lymphoma analyzed long-term survival after standard surgical therapy and considered whether adjuvant therapy is required after complete resection.

Methods.—The patients were treated at Memorial Sloan-Kettering Cancer Center from 1980 to 1991. All underwent curative resection and regional lymphadenectomy; 8 had adjuvant chemotherapy, 6 had adjuvant radiation therapy, and 5 received both chemotherapy and radiation. Data reviewed included clinical symptoms, pathologic staging, surgical morbidity and mortality, and survival. Follow-up (median 74 months) was available in all cases.

Results.—The mean age of the patients was 61 years; 69% were women. Weight loss averaged 6.8 pounds. The most frequently reported symptoms were vague epigastric pain (71%) and gastrointestinal bleeding (17%).

Time from onset of symptoms to treatment was 6.5 months. Preoperative staging, based on an upper gastrointestinal series, endoscopy, and CT scan, was often inaccurate; only 42% were correctly staged before resection. The average greatest dimension of tumor was 8.2 cm, and most tumors were graded as intermediate. The 4 patients who had recurrence of lymphoma after treatment all died of disease. There were 5 deaths from other causes. The overall actuarial 10-year survival rate was 88% (91% for stage IE and 82% for stage IIE-1) and no relapses occurred in the 15 patients treated with surgery alone. Patients who died of disease had a larger mean tumor size and an increased incidence of stage IIE-1 disease, factors that were not statistically significant in univariate or multivariate analysis.

Conclusion.—There is considerable controversy over how best to treat gastric lymphoma. The recent trend is to perform surgery for staging and palliation, rather than for curative intent. Primary chemotherapy and radiation therapy, however, may reduce the efficacy of treatment in stage IE or IIE-1 disease. Surgery alone is adequate for many in this patient subset, and the decision to offer adjuvant therapy should consider the presence of microscopic disease in N1 and N2 lymph nodes.

▶ This optimistic report from the Memorial Sloan-Kettering Cancer Center should leave no doubt that surgical extirpation of early gastric lymphoma is a highly effective therapy. The authors point out the essential requirements: the operation should be performed with minimal morbidity; and multimodal adjunctive therapy should be available in cases where the stage of the disease is found to be advanced at the time of surgical intervention. It is clear from the results that tumors less than 10 cm in diameter that are free of nodal extension can be cured by a radical subtotal gastrectomy with an R-2 node dissection (for staging).

F.G. Moody, M.D.

A 10-Year Experience With Japanese-type Radical Lymph Node Dissection for Gastric Cancer Outside of Japan
Jatzko GR, Lisborg PH, Denk H, et al (Hosp of Barmherzige Brüder St. Veit/Glan, Austria; Univ of Graz, Austria; Univ of Klagenfurt, Austria)
Cancer 76:1302–1312, 1995   2–27

Introduction.—The prognosis for patients with gastric cancer has improved in Japan, a country with a high incidence of the disease and a program of radical surgical treatment. The goal of surgery is complete removal of locoregional tumor with radical lymph node dissection, as defined by the Japanese Research Society for Gastric Cancer. A study of the procedure conducted in Austria, where it has been employed as early as the 1950s, examined outcome in patients with gastric cancer.

Methods.—Radical lymph node dissection was introduced at the study institution in 1984 for all patients admitted for possible resection and cure of gastric cancer. Between January 1984 and June 1994, 345 of 512 patients admitted with the disease were eligible for radical resection (R-0). The clinical, histopathologic, and surgical factors of these patients were examined by univariate and multivariate analysis for impact on long-term survival. Size, localization, and histologic classification of the tumor determined extent of resection; lymph node dissection was performed independently of type of resection. Mean follow-up for R-0 resected cases was 65.5 months. None of these patients had neoadjuvant therapy.

Results.—In the radically resected group, 215 patients had total gastrectomies and 130 had subtotal gastrectomies. The palliative resection group had 69 total and 31 subtotal gastrectomies. Overall hospital mortality was 6.8%, and ranged from 4.9% for R-0 resected patients to 13.4% for those with palliative procedures. Five- and 10-year survival rates were 40.5% and 34.4%, respectively, for all patients, 45.7% and 38.6% for patients who underwent tumor resection, and 57.7% and 44.3% for those who had curative surgery; median survival in the latter group was 96 months. Poor survival among the curative resection group was related in multivariate analysis to age greater than 65 years, previous total gastrectomy, increased number of positive lymph nodes, high pT and pN classifications, male sex, and low preoperative hemoglobin levels. Patients with more advanced tumors who underwent R-0 resection had only marginally better survival than those who underwent palliative resection.

Conclusion.—Routine lymph node dissection for patients with gastric cancer has not been widely adopted outside of Japan. The 10-year experience reported from Austria confirms the value of radical lymph node dissection with wide resection margins. Postoperative mortality was low in this series, and survival rates were similar to those reported in Japanese studies.

▶ The authors of this article from Austria show that radical lymph node dissection at the time of gastrectomy for gastric cancer is associated with a long-term survival comparable to that initially reported from Japan. The series is large enough (512 patients) to provide statistical outcomes that can be analyzed. Negative prognostic factors include age (older than 65), number of involved nodes, and some expected variables previously reported by others. Total gastrectomy also led to a worse survival rate, which suggests that more advanced tumors require a more extensive removal of the stomach.

F.G. Moody, M.D.

A Selective Therapeutic Approach to Gastric Cancer in a Large Public Hospital
Crookes PF, Incarbone R, Peters JH, et al (Univ of Southern California, Los Angeles)
Am J Surg 170:602–605, 1995   2–28

Background.—Countries with a high incidence of gastric cancer, such as Japan, have developed screening programs and followed an aggressive surgical approach to this tumor. The relevance of such methods to the United States, which has fewer patients with gastric carcinoma, is uncertain. A large public hospital in California was used to examine the role of curative resection in the patient population.

Methods.—Included in the retrospective study were patients with gastric cancer treated between July 1988 and August 1993 at the Los Angeles County/University of Southern California Medical Center, a hospital that serves a population with a high percentage of immigrants from Asia and South America. The patient group consisted of 125 men and 79 women with a median age of 56 years. Preoperative staging by CT and endoscopic US showed stage IV disease present in 59%. During the first 4 years of the study period, R1 resections were routinely performed; after August 1992, most patients had R2 resections, and those with high gastric tumors had R3 resections. Partial or subtotal esophagectomy was performed when the lower esophagus was involved. Chemotherapy was given to some patients eligible for curative resection.

Results.—The majority of patients were of Hispanic (54%) or Asian (33%) origin. Resection, performed in 98 patients, was for cure in 66 and for palliation in 32; 34 patients had total and 63 had subtotal gastrectomy. Forty of 66 patients who underwent curative resection were given neoadjuvant chemotherapy. The rate of surgical complications was similar for those who underwent curative or palliative surgery and for those who did or did not receive chemotherapy. The serious postoperative intra-abdominal infections occurred in patients whose resection included splenectomy. Survival was significantly improved in curative versus palliative resection and was improved in palliative surgery versus nonsurgical therapy.

Conclusion.—Most patients with gastric cancer who were seen at the study institution had advanced disease, which suggests the value of screening in high-risk populations. Despite late stage disease, curative surgery undertaken in selected patients may yield worthwhile survival. The benefits of neoadjuvant chemotherapy have yet to be determined.

▶ The surgeons at the Los Angeles General Hospital report their experience with gastric cancer in a large, urban, county hospital population. As you might imagine, they had to deal with quite a different stage of the disease than has been reported on so extensively by the Japanese. Three questions were asked in the discussion of this article at the 47th Annual Meeting to the Southwestern Surgical Congress that are relevant to the management of gastric cancer in the United States: (1), Would screening be of value? (2),

Should we be more deliberate in our staging? (3), Because we see so few patients with this disease, who should treat them?

The answers were as follows: (1), Screening would not be cost effective. (2), Careful preoperative and intraoperative staging helps to appropriately categorize each patient in a study, but may not have any practical value. (3), Patients with gastric cancers should probably be referred to centers that treat this disease on a regular basis. I personally do not believe that the latter would improve the care or outcome of the disease, but it might provide a way for the surgeons in the Untied States to learn more about the disease and thereby improve its treatment. Clearly, high risk populations should be endoscoped even with the mildest symptoms of dyspepsia.

F.G. Moody, M.D.

Incidence and Treatment of Periampullary Duodenal Cancer in the U.S. Veteran Patient Population
Sexe RB, Wade TP, Virgo KS, et al (St Louis Univ, Mo)
Cancer 77:251–254, 1996   2–29

Background.—Primary adenocarcinoma of the duodenum is very rare, but the duodenum is the most common site of adenocarcinoma of the small intestine. Adenocarcinoma is also the most common malignancy of the duodenum. To date, there have been fewer than 1,000 cases reported since this lesion was first described in 1746. Because its symptoms are often benign and vague, it often goes unrecognized until late in the course of the disease. Reports have often included patients whose histories were found from decades of hospital records making results confusing. Optimal treatment and prognosis are unclear. The outcome of curative resection and palliative treatment of primary periampullary duodenal adenocarcinoma in veterans was examined.

Methods.—Records of patients with periampullary duodenal adenocarcinoma were obtained from all hospitals of the Department of Veterans Affairs during a period of 4 years. Patients were grouped according to the most aggressive treatment they received: resection, operative bypass, or percutaneous or endoscopic biliary intubation. Survival was calculated and compared.

Results.—Of 2,185 periampullary cancers, only 85 were duodenal. Resection was performed in 34 patients with a 30-day mortality of 6%, bypass was performed in 44 patients with a 30-day mortality of 18%, and biliary intubation was performed in 7 patients with a 30-day mortality of 0%. All groups had a mean survival rate of more than 1 year. The mean survival rates significantly increased in patients who had resection (Fig 1). After resection, the projected 5-year survival rate was 23%. After resection of 9 stage I–II cancers, the mean survival rate was 668 days; this survival rate was similar after 5 resections of cancers with nodal or other metastases. In 13 patients who received palliative treatment, the survival rate and cancer stage did not correlate.

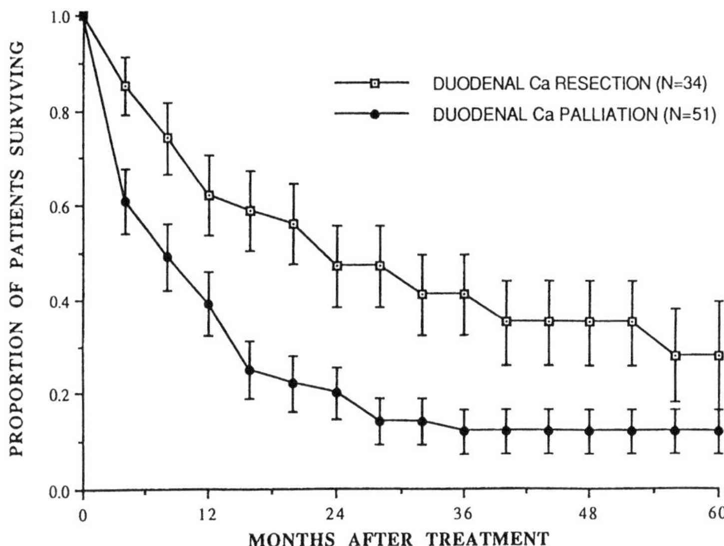

FIGURE 1.—Projected patient survival after resection as compared with that after palliative procedures for duodenal cancer. A record of death was available in 88% of the palliated patients, whereas 32% of resected patients did not have a mortality record by December 31, 1994. (Courtesy of Sexe RB, Wade TP, Virgo KS, et al: Incidence and treatment of periampullary duodenal cancer in the United States veteran patient population. *Cancer* 77:251–254, 1996. Copyright © 1996. Reprinted by permission of Wiley-Liss, Inc., a division of John Wiley & Sons, Inc.)

Conclusions.—The survival rate was higher in patients who underwent resection. In patients with low risk and without distant metastases, resection of duodenal adenocarcinoma is recommended. This is the second largest series of duodenal cancers.

▶ Periampullary duodenal cancer is such a rare disease that few physicians will encounter a case in their lifetimes. I have only encountered several that I have been able to resect during a 30-year period of treating periampullary neoplasms of diverse etiologies. Those of us in this field like to have them referred early, if possible, because the survival as seen here in the Veterans Affairs experience is relatively good after Whipple resection. It is a curiosity that the incidence of small-bowel cancers is so low considering the proliferative nature of its epithelium. Maybe these cells have within their DNA the secret as to why they behave so well, whereas only a few millimeters away, their cousins in the pancreatic duct act in such an insolent fashion as we age.

F.G. Moody, M.D.

13 Acute Upper Gastrointestinal Hemorrhage

Selection of Patients for Early Discharge or Outpatient Care After Acute Upper Gastrointestinal Haemorrhage
Rockall TA, For the National Audit of Acute Upper Gastrointestinal Haemorrhage Logan RFA, Devlin HB, et al (Royal College of Surgeons of England, London; Queen's Med Centre, Nottingham, England; St George's Hosp, London)
Lancet 347:1138–1140, 1996
2–30

Introduction.—Patients with acute upper gastrointestinal hemorrhage are usually hospitalized so that they can be monitored for further bleeding. Many of these patients, however, are at very low risk of further hemorrhage and mortality. A risk scoring system was described that could achieve considerable cost savings by identifying those patients who might safely be discharged early or managed on an outpatient basis.

Patients and Methods.—In a prospective audit of the management and outcome of 4,201 cases from 74 hospitals, 2,531 patients were identified who were admitted as emergencies with acute upper gastrointestinal hemorrhage and who subsequently underwent diagnostic endoscopy. Patients were categorized for risk according to a validated numerical scoring system. Five components were scored: age, comorbidity, shock, diagnosis, and stigmata of recent hemorrhage. The maximum possible score, indicating a very high risk of further bleeding, was 11.

Results.—Scores of 0–2 were assigned to 744 (29.4%) patients. Only 32 (4.3%) patients in this category had rebleeding and only 1 (0.1%) died; these patients had a median hospital stay of 4 days. The risk of further hemorrhage and of death increased with higher risk scores (Table 2), as did duration of hospital stay. Among patients with risk score categories of 5 or less, there was a definite trend of increasing length of hospital stay with increasing time between admission and diagnostic endoscopy.

Conclusion.—The scoring system combined with clinical judgment should help to identify a large proportion of patients with acute upper

TABLE 2.—Observed Rebleeding and Mortality by Risk Score

| | Total number of patients (% of total) | Rebleeding* | Number of cases | | Total deaths |
			Deaths without rebleeding†	Deaths with rebleeding‡	
Score					
0	143 (5–6%)	7 (4.9%)	0	0	0
1	278 (11.0%)	9 (3.2%)	0	0	0
2	323 (12.8%)	16 (5.0%)	1 (0.3%)	0	1 (0.3%)
3	402 (15.9%)	49 (12.2%)	4 (1.1%)	4 (10.0%)	8 (2.0%)
4	450 (17.8%)	62 (13.8%)	10 (2.6%)	9 (14.5%)	19 (4.2%)
5	367 (14.5%)	62 (16.9%)	16 (5.2%)	13 (21.0%)	29 (7.9%)
6	238 (9.4%)	70 (29.4%)	16 (9.5%)	20 (28.6%)	36 (15.1%)
7	202 (8.0%)	80 (39.6%)	12 (9.8%)	28 (35.0%)	40 (19.8%)
*8	128 (5.1%)	61 (47.7%)	18 (26.9%)	32 (52.5%)	50 (39.1%)
Total	2531	416 (16.4%)	77 (3.6%)	106 (25.5%)	183 (7.2%)

*Percent of total within score category;

†Deaths with no rebleeding as a percent of all patients with no rebleeding within score category.

‡Deaths with rebleeding as a percent of all patients with no rebleeding within score category.

(Courtesy of Rockall TA, for the National Audit of Acute Upper Gastrointestinal Haemorrhage: Selection of patients for early discharge or outpatient care after acute upper gastrointestinal hemorrhage. *Lancet* 347:1138–1140, 1996. Copyright by The Lancet Ltd., 1996.)

gastrointestinal hemorrhage who have a low risk of rebleeding or death. Considerable resource savings can be safely achieved with early discharge or outpatient management of approximately one fourth of patients with acute upper gastrointestinal hemorrhage. Endoscopic examination is necessary for a definitive diagnosis, and time from admission to endoscopy clearly influences duration of hospital stay.

▶ Two additional studies have quantified the risk of outpatient evaluation in patients with acute gastrointestinal bleeding. Geller et al.[1] used a logistic regression analysis to assess more than 20 important clinical variables to quantify the risk of outpatient evaluation in patients with acute gastrointestinal bleeding. These authors were particularly interested in identifying the patient at low risk of continued or recurrent bleeding. It was found that absence of 8 variables permitted identification of the patient at low risk for continued gastrointestinal bleeding: age, hypotension, orthostasis, melena, anticoagulant use, and concurrent cardiac, hepatic, or renal disease. Zuckerman and his colleagues[2] evaluated 5 criteria as predictors of outcome of gastrointestinal bleeding applied to patients presenting in the emergency department. The criteria that they used are easily remembered by the pneumonic BLEED, in which **B** stands for ongoing bleeding, **L** stands for low systolic blood pressure, **E** stands for elevated prothrombin time, **E** stands for erratic mental status, and **D** stands for comorbid diseases. These criteria identified high-risk patients who required surgery. The authors also suggest that the BLEED criteria may be helpful in determining which patients do not need emergency endoscopy. BLEED also has the advantage of being used as an outcome predictor for both upper and lower gastrointestinal bleeding.

N.J. Greenberger, M.D.

References

1. Geller A, Wans KK, Stark ME, et al: Quantifying risks of outpatient evaluation in patients with acute gastrointestinal bleeding: Identifying the low-risk patient. *Gastroenterology* 110:19A, 1996.
2. Zuckerman GK, Kollef MH, O'Brien JD: A GI bleeding clinical outcome prediction tool (BLEED) applied in the emergency room compared to endoscopic stigmata of bleeding. *Gastroenterology* 110:307A, 1996.

Care of Patients With Upper Gastrointestinal Hemorrhage in Academic Medical Centers: A Community-based Comparison

Cooper GS, Chak A, Harper DL, et al (Case Western Reserve Univ, Cleveland, Ohio; Cleveland Health Quality Choice and the Quality Information Management Corp, Ohio; Univ of Chicago)
Gastroenterology 111:385–390, 1996   2–31

Background.—Academic medical centers are commonly seen as inefficient institutions that overuse technology. However, there is little empirical evidence of this. Treatment and outcomes of patients with upper gastrointestinal (GI) hemorrhage admitted to major teaching hospitals and other hospitals in a large metropolitan area were compared.

Methods.—Data were obtained on 3,801 consecutive eligible patients admitted to 5 major teaching hospitals and 25 other hospitals between 1991 and 1993. Validated multivariate models were used to determine severity of illness on admission (Table 1).

Findings.—The rates of upper endoscopy were 82.9% among the 1,004 patients discharged from fellowship hospitals and 85.6% among the 2,797 patients discharged from other hospitals. Use of other procedures was comparable. Although patients in fellowship hospitals tended to have more severe illness, their length of hospitalization was somewhat shorter, even after risk adjustment. Death rates between types of hospitals were similar. Patients admitted to fellowship hospitals were somewhat less likely to undergo transfusion (Table 2).

Conclusion.—Compared with community hospitals, teaching hospitals do not appear to provide inefficient care or to overuse costly treatments for patients with upper GI bleeding. These findings are important in the current era of health care reform, in which the viability of academic centers and fellowship training is threatened.

▶ There is not only a perception, there are also widely stated views among purchasers of health care services that academic health centers are inefficient and overuse medical technologies. This interesting study has examined this issue by comparing in-hospital mortality, length of stay, and use of upper GI endoscopy in patients admitted to academic health centers ("fellowship hospitals") with those of patients admitted to other community hospitals. The key findings were that (1) rates of upper GI endoscopy were actually somewhat *lower* among the 1,004 patients discharged from aca-

TABLE 1.—Demographic and Clinical Characteristics of Patients With Upper Gastrointestinal Hemorrhage Admitted to Hospitals With and Without Gastroenterology Fellowships

Characteristic	Fellowship hospitals (n = 1004)	Nonfellowship hospitals (n = 2797)
Mean age ± SD (*yr*)*	61.7 ± 17.8	67.1 ± 16.6
White persons (%)*	54.4	86.2
Male persons (%)	56.5	53.1
Health insurance*		
Private (%)	27.7	27.8
Medicare (%)	46.9	62.8
Medicaid/uninsured/self pay (%)	25.4	9.4
Comorbid conditions		
Ischemic heart disease* (%)	20.5	29.3
Diabetes mellitus* (%)	21.4	16.2
Chronic obstructive lung disease*		
(%)	11.1	15.5
Prior stroke (%)	9.4	10.6
Cirrhosis† (%)	7.6	4.9
Malignancy† (%)	8.3	5.7
End-stage renal disease* (%)	5.3	1.0
Primary diagnosis*		
Gastric ulcer (%)	34.7	39.0
Duodenal ulcer (%)	22.0	27.9
Gastritis (%)	13.8	13.3
Hematemesis (%)	12.9	6.0
Mallory-Weiss tear (%)	6.7	4.2
Peptic ulcer, unspecified (%)	2.4	4.5
Esophageal varices (%)	3.4	2.2
Angiodysplasia (%)	2.4	0.8
Duodenitis (%)	0.9	0.9
Gastrojejunal ulcer (%)	0.8	1.2
Mean admission hematocrit (%)	27.6 ± 7.6	27.9 ± 7.6
Mean predicted risk of death (%)‡	3.5 ± 7.8	3.0 ± 6.5

Note: Differences were determined by logistic or linear regression analyses.
*The difference between patients in fellowship and nonfellowship hospitals is significant (*P* < 0.001).
†The difference between patients in fellowship and nonfellowship hospitals is significant (*P* < 0.01).
‡The difference between patients in fellowship and nonfellowship hospitals is significant (*P* < 0.05).
(Courtesy of Cooper GS, Chak A, Harper DL, et al: Care of patients with upper gastrointestinal hemorrhage in academic medical centers: A community-based comparison. *Gastroenterology* 111:385–390, 1996.)

demic health centers compared with 2,797 patients discharged from community hospitals; (2) length of stay was shorter for patients admitted to fellowship hospitals; and (3) patients admitted to teaching hospitals were less likely to undergo transfusion (Table 2).

It is pertinent to emphasize that these favorable results in patients admitted to fellowship hospitals were accomplished in the face of higher severity of illness. Note in Table 1 the high percentage of patients with cirrhosis, malignancy, and end-stage renal disease admitted to fellowship hospitals. Not surprisingly, there was also nearly a threefold difference in Medicare/uninsured/self-pay patients admitted to fellowship hospitals.

More empirical data on the relative quality and efficiency of academic medical centers are clearly needed, both on a regional and a national basis.

N.J. Greenberger, M.D.

TABLE 2.—Differences in Length of Stay, Use of Blood Transfusion, and In-Hospital Mortality Between Patients Admitted to Hospitals With and Without Gastroenterology Fellowships

Outcome measure*	Odds ratio or percent difference (95% confidence interval)	*P* value
Length of stay	−14% (−18% to −9%)	< 0.0001
Blood transfusion	0.74 (0.61 to 0.91)	< 0.0001
In-hospital mortality	1.26 (0.80 to 2.00)	> 0.30

Note: Differences were determined by logistic or linear regression analyses.

*All analyses controlled for admission severity of illness; blood transfusion analysis further adjusted for admission hematocrit, age, and the presence of ischemic heart disease and chronic obstructive lung disease. For transfusion and mortality, differences reflect multivariable odds ratios for the risk in fellowship relative to nonfellowship hospitals. For length of stay, the difference reflects the percent difference in length of stay in fellowship compared with nonfellowship hospitals.

(Courtesy of Cooper GS, Chak A, Harper DL, et al: Care of patients with upper gastrointestinal hemorrhage in academic medical centers: A community-based comparison. *Gastroenterology* 111:385–390, 1996.)

14 Miscellaneous

Electrogastrography in Intestinal Pseudo-obstruction

Electrogastrography in Chronic Intestinal Pseudoobstruction

Debinski HS, Ahmed S, Milla PJ, et al (St Mark's Hosp, London; Hosp for Sick Children, London)
Dig Dis Sci 41:1292–1297, 1996   2–32

Purpose.—The rare disorder chronic intestinal pseudo-obstruction (CIP) causes gut dilation and dysfunction with no mechanical obstruction. Various types of visceral myopathy and neuropathy have been described. Although transit tests, radiologic studies, and manometry are helpful diagnostic aids, precise pathologic diagnosis requires histologic examination. It would help to have some noninvasive means of establishing the diagnosis. Surface electrogastrography (EGG) was evaluated as a noninvasive diagnostic test for CIP.

Methods.—The study included 14 adult patients with confirmed CIP, as well as 14 age- and sex-matched controls. The pathologic diagnosis in the CIP group was visceral myopathy (M) in 7 patients, neuropathy (N) in 4 patients, and undifferentiated (U) in 3 patients. Each patient underwent surface EGG, with 30 min recordings of gastric electrical control activity in the fasting and fed states (Fig 1). The recordings were made using 4 pairs of Ag-AgCl bipolar skin electrodes. After the signals were amplified and digitalized, a running spectral analysis was performed. Computer-assisted analysis was used to determine the dominant frequency and power of spectrum.

Results.—All but 1 of the CPM patients had dysrhythmias, mainly with low-frequency activities of less than 2 cpm. Five patients, including all of those in subgroup N, had tachygastria—defined as an electrical control activity frequency greater than 5 cycles/min—and a normal amplitude response to food. Six patients, including 5 of those in subgroup M, had irregular continuous activity with no dominant frequency or bradyarrhythmia, along with a diminished electrical response activity (ERA) to food (Fig 3). Two patients had mixed abnormalities, and 1 had normal activity with a clear dominant frequency of 3 cycles/min.

Conclusions.—Electrogastrography may be a useful noninvasive technique for the diagnosis of chronic intestinal pseudo-obstruction. It is sensitive and specific in showing evidence of dysrhythmia in CIP patients

Normal

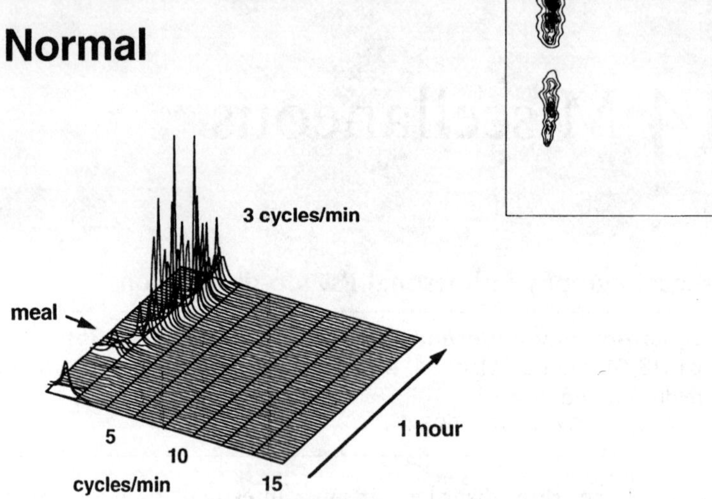

FIGURE 1.—Graphical representation of the electrogastrography of a healthy control subject. There is a small amount of 3 cpm activity prior to the meal. After the meal the frequency remains the same but the amplitude is markedly increased. On the left is a pseudo three-dimensional recreation of the electrogastrographic activity with time. On the upper right is a horizontal "slice" representation that gives a topographical guide to the height of the recorded electrical activity, as well as its frequency. (Courtesy of Debinski HS, Ahmed S, Milla PJ, et al: Electrogastrography in chronic intestinal pseudoobstruction. *Dig Dis Sci* 41:1292–1297, 1996, Plenum Publishing Corporation.)

and is able to differentiate between patients with visceral neuropathy vs. myopathy as their primary pathology. In addition to its diagnostic value, EGG could be useful in studying disturbances of electrical control activity in CIP.

Visceral Myopathy

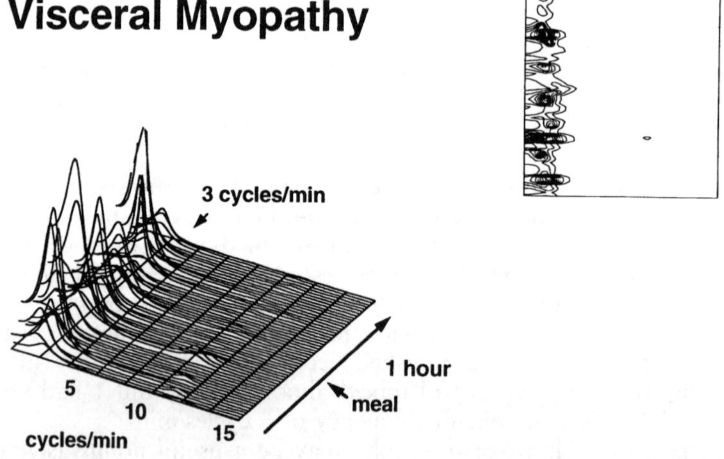

FIGURE 3.—Electrogastrographic representation from a patient with histologically proven visceral myopathy. The dominant frequency is less than 3 cpm, is irregular, and there is poor response to food. (Courtesy of Debinski HS, Ahmed S, Milla PJ, et al: Electrogastrography in chronic intestinal pseudoobstruction. *Dig Dis Sci* 41:1292–1297, 1996, Plenum Publishing Corporation.)

▶ Chronic intestinal pseudo-obstruction is 1 of the more nagging forms of abnormal gastrointestinal motility, inasmuch as it is almost impossible to diagnose and nearly impossible to treat. As can be seen in Figures 1 and 3, the EGG reveals profound differences between the normal when compared to that observed in a patient with a visceral myopathy. Tachygastria appears to be the predominant characteristic associated with a visceral myopathy; whereas bradygastria is more common in patients with a visceral neuropathy. These patients tend to make surgeons look bad no matter how simple the problem may appear at the operating table. It is important to recognize that they have a dysmotility prior to an operative intervention.

F.G. Moody, M.D.

Approach to Banded Gastroplasty in Morbid Obesity

Conversion of Failed or Complicated Vertical Banded Gastroplasty to Gastric Bypass in Morbid Obesity
Sugerman HJ, Kellum JM Jr, DeMaria EJ, et al (Virginia Commonwealth Univ, Richmond)
Am J Surg 171:263–269, 1996   2–33

Introduction.—A number of randomized, prospective trials confirmed that morbidly obese patients achieve significantly better weight loss after Roux-en-Y gastric bypass (GBP) than after vertical banded gastroplasty (VBG). There are also more complications with VBG, including gastroesophageal (GE) reflux, staple line disruption, and anastomotic leaks. The patients reported here underwent conversion from VBG to GBP and were followed to assess weight loss and resolution of complications.

Methods.—The 58 participants in the study either failed to have adequate weight loss (15) or experienced complications after VBG (43, including 23 with stomal stenosis and 15 with staple line disruption). Conversion to GBP was performed at an average of 3.2 years after VBG. In the GBP procedure, a 45-cm jejunal Roux-en-Y anastomosis was constructed, brought retrocolic, and anastomosed to the proximal gastric pouch. Superobese patients treated since 1991 have undergone a long-limb GBP with a 150-cm Roux limb. Patients were instructed to take an H_2 blocker for 3 months after surgery and a multivitamin, plus additional vitamin B_{12} and calcium, daily for life. Women who still menstruated also took ferrous sulfate tablets daily until menopause.

Results.—None of the patients died as a result of the conversion procedure, but 2 required prolonged hospitalization because of extensive morbidity. Other procedure-related complications were managed successfully. All patients with preconversion nausea, vomiting, GE reflux, or gastric ulcers had these problems resolved by GBP. After 1 year of follow-up, the entire group of patients had significant additional weight loss from a mean of 36% to 67%. The 15 patients who were "sweets eaters," a group that tends to have particularly poor weight loss outcome, increased their mean weight loss from 20% to 70%. Patients who were able to be contacted for 5 years or longer continued to maintain a reasonably constant weight and normal hemoglobin, calcium, and vitamin B_{12} levels.

Conclusion.—Conversion of a failed VBG to GBP was successful in these morbidly obese patients. It allowed them to increase and maintain a significant weight loss, and the complications associated with vertical gastroplasty procedures were resolved. At the study institution, GBP has become the primary surgical procedure for such patients.

▶ Sugerman and his associates in Richmond have successfully salvaged 58 patients from the vagaries of a VGB that was used to treat their chronic morbid obesity. There was no morbidity, but complications of a serious nature were not infrequent. Those who do reoperative surgery of this type can appreciate the complexity of a small pouch conversion as a secondary procedure. Not only is the stomach folded back on itself as mentioned, but the anterior aspect of the staple line and the band is adhered to the left lateral segment (segments 2 and 3) of the liver, and the empty space at the upper extent of the lesser sac is obliterated. Clearly, it is better to perform a small pouch gastric bypass the first time around.

F.G. Moody, M.D.

Cisapride in Postgastrectomy Duodenogastric Reflux

Placebo-controlled Trial of Cisapride in Postgastrectomy Patients With Duodenogastroesophageal Reflux
Vaezi MF, Sears R, Richter JE (Univ of Alabama, Birmingham; Cleveland Clinic Found, Ohio)
Dig Dis Sci 41:754–763, 1996   2–34

Background.—Duodenogastroesophageal reflux (DGER) is the abnormal retrograde flow of duodenal contents through the pylorus into the stomach, with subsequent reflux into the esophagus. Patients are especially predisposed to DGER after gastrectomy. Medical treatment of this condition after gastrectomy is not very effective. The efficacy of cisapride in DGER was investigated.

Methods.—Ten patients with chronic symptoms after partial gastrectomy were assigned randomly to 4 weeks of placebo or to cisapride, 20 mg 4 times a day, in a double-blind crossover design. Responses were assessed by ambulatory esophageal bilirubin monitoring. Patients with significant improvements continued to take cisapride for another 4 months.

Findings.—Cisapride significantly reduced DGER compared with placebo. Seventy percent of patients who took cisapride and only 10% who took placebo showed improvement. Mean monthly scores for abdominal pain, regurgitation, and belching were significantly better in the cisapride group. These improvements persisted after 4 months of treatment.

Conclusions.—Cisapride significantly decreases DGER in patients with this condition after gastrectomy, and results in short- and long-term symptomatic improvement. Cisapride is the first successful medical treatment for this condition.

▶ The results of this controlled trial of the use of cisapride to relieve the unpleasant side effects associated with reflux of gastrointestinal secretions into the esophagus after gastrectomy are impressive. The authors are correct to emphasize how this entity compromises the lives of patients who have it. Fortunately, it afflicts only a small number of patients after gastric surgery. This study suggests that patients at risk have an underlying dysmotility of their gastrointestinal tracts.

F.G. Moody, M.D.

Methylmalonic Acid and Homocysteine Levels After Gastric Surgery

Elevated Methylmalonic Acid and Total Homocysteine Levels Show High Prevalence of Vitamin B$_{12}$ Deficiency After Gastric Surgery
Sumner AE, Chin MM, Abrahm JL, et al (Hahnemann Univ, Philadelphia; Philadelphia College of Pharmacy and Science; Children's Hosp of Philadelphia; et al)
Ann Intern Med 124:469–476, 1996   2–35

Introduction.—There is an increased risk of vitamin B$_{12}$ (cobalamin) deficiency developing in individuals who have had gastric surgery and in some patients with Alzheimer's disease, amyotrophic lateral sclerosis, spinal cord compression, and diabetic or alcoholic peripheral neuropathy. Patients with untreated vitamin B$_{12}$ deficiency are at risk for elevated total homocysteine levels, which can lead to carotid artery stenosis, coronary artery disease, and peripheral vascular disease. The prevalence of vitamin B$_{12}$ deficiency was determined in patients who have had gastric surgery.

Methods.—In 61 patients who had gastric surgery and in 107 controls who did not have gastric surgery, the serum levels of vitamin B$_{12}$, folate, methylmalonic acid, and total homocysteine were measured before and after treatment, which consisted of daily IM injections of 1,000 µg of vitamin B$_{12}$ for 5 days, followed by monthly injection. Treatment also consisted of giving folic acid orally, 1 mg/day. The indications for surgery were peptic ulcer disease, obesity, gastric cancer, and gastric lymphoma, and surgery had been performed a median of 20 years before the study was conducted.

Results.—Vitamin B$_{12}$ deficiency was found in 19 patients (31%) who had surgery and in 2 controls (2%). Elevated total homocysteine levels were found in 12 (63%) of the patients who had vitamin B$_{12}$ deficiency. Methylmalonic acid and total homocysteine levels decreased substantially in all patients with vitamin B$_{12}$ deficiency who received treatment (15 of 21) (Fig 2). This had confirmed the deficiency before the treatment.

Conclusion.—There is a high prevalence of vitamin B$_{12}$ deficiency in patients who have had gastric surgery. The development of cardiovascular, hematologic, and neurologic abnormalities may be prevented by prompt recognition and treatment of the deficiency with resultant normalization of elevated total homocysteine and methylmalonic acid levels. In patients

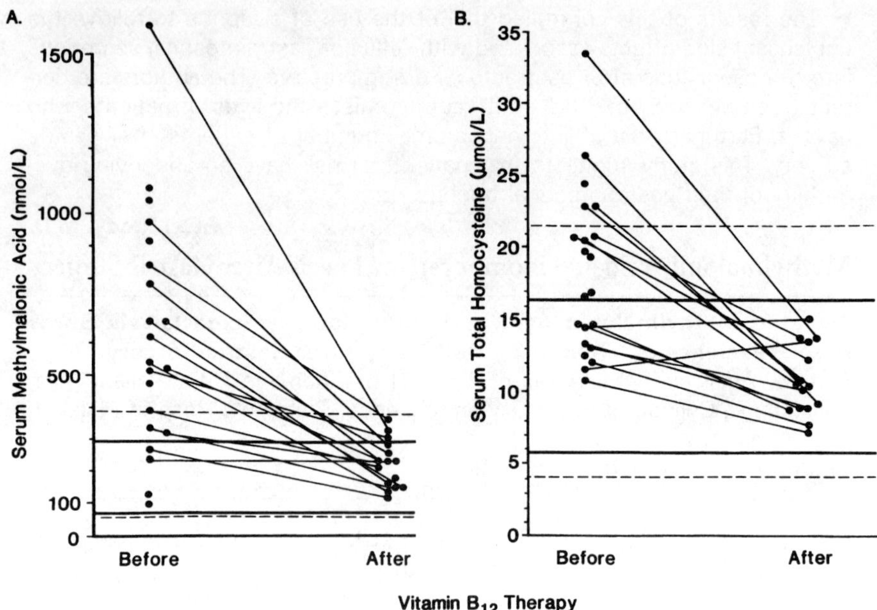

FIGURE 2.—**A**, serum methylmalonic acid levels before and after treatment. The serum methylmalonic acid levels are shown for the 19 vitamin B_{12}–deficient patients (who had gastric surgery) and the 2 vitamin B_{12}–deficient controls (who had not had surgery). Results after parenteral vitamin B_{12} therapy are shown for the 15 participants available for treatment. The *solid lines* represent the normal range, calculated as the mean ±SD after log normalization to correct for skewing toward higher values as previously reported. The *dashed line* represents the mean ± 3 SD. **B**, total serum homocysteine levels before and after treatment. The total serum homocysteine levels are shown for the same participants described in panel **A**. (Courtesy of Sumner AE, Chin MM, Abraham JL, et al: Elevated methylmalonic acid and total homocysteine levels show high prevalence of vitamin B_{12} deficiency after gastric surgery. *Ann Intern Med* 124:469–476, 1996.)

who have had gastric surgery and have serum vitamin B_{12} levels less than 221 pmol/L, frequent screening and vitamin B_{12} replacement therapy are recommended.

▶ Previous studies probably underestimated the prevalence of vitamin B_{12} deficiency in patients who had undergone gastric surgery largely because the diagnosis was based on the presence of megaloblastic anemia. The data obtained by Sumner et al, which used the 3 parameters of low levels of serum vitamin B_{12}, serum methylmalonic acid, and serum homocysteine, indicate that the prevalence of vitamin B_{12} deficiency in patients who have had gastric surgery is much higher than previously appreciated. Note that vitamin B_{12} deficiency was confirmed in 31% of the patients with previous gastric surgery as compared with 2% of the controls of similar age and race. This figure was even higher (36%) in patients 65–83 years of age.

From a practical point of view, it could be argued that all patients who have undergone subtotal gastric resection should just receive 1,000 µg of vitamin B_{12} every 3 months. This will suffice to maintain their vitamin B_{12} stores.

N.J. Greenberger, M.D.

PART THREE

SMALL INTESTINE

Introduction

This section contains 3 articles regarding celiac sprue. The first details the determination of antiendomysial antibodies, which is a highly sensitive and specific test for the diagnosis of celiac sprue. Furthermore, this test can be used to monitor the response to treatment. A classic study indicating that antiendomysial antibodies are actually produced by the mucosa of patients with celiac sprue lends further support that immunologic alterations are important in the pathogenesis of this disease. A third article documents that patients with celiac sprue not infrequently have occult gastrointestinal bleeding and that such bleeding is more likely to occur in patients with poorly controlled disease. The fatty acid binding protein is emerging as an important test to diagnose mesenteric vascular ischemia. Other topics covered include detailed expositions on primary lymphoma, malignant melanoma, lanreotide treatment of carcinoid syndrome, and small bowel transplantation.

Norton J. Greenberger, M.D.

15 Radiologic and Imaging Considerations

Conventional Radiography and Ultrasonography in the Diagnosis of Small-Bowel Obstruction and Strangulation
Czechowski J (Danderyd Hosp, Stockholm)
Acta Radiol 37:186–189, 1996   3–1

Purpose.—Plain radiographs are widely used in the assessment of possible intestinal obstruction or strangulation in patients with an "acute abdomen." They are not very diagnostically efficient, however. Ultrasonography permits assessment of morphology along with motility of the bowel loops; it can also reveal conditions other than obstruction. Ultrasonography was compared with plain radiography for the diagnosis of intestinal obstruction and strangulation.

Methods.—Ninety-six patients (51 women and 45 men; mean age, 39 years) with acute abdominal pain, most of whom had previous abdominal surgery, were studied. Patients with typical signs of appendicitis and cholecystitis were excluded. All patients underwent conventional abdominal radiography and ultrasonography. The ultrasound examinations were performed with a 5.0- or 7.5-MHz linear transducer, focusing on the findings of distention, paralysis, intramural thickening, and extraluminal fluid.

Results.—Simple mechanical obstruction was diagnosed in 9 patients and intestinal strangulation in 10 patients. Ultrasound examination was positive in 91% of the patients with small bowel strangulation, whereas conventional radiography was positive in only 30% (Figs 1 and 2). The correct diagnosis of simple obstruction was made by ultrasonography in 89% of the patients and by radiography in 78%.

Conclusions.—Ultrasonography has greater diagnostic efficiency than abdominal radiography in patients with suspected small-bowel obstruction and, especially, strangulation. Even when obstruction is not present, ultrasound can aid in making other diagnoses. Ultrasonography should be

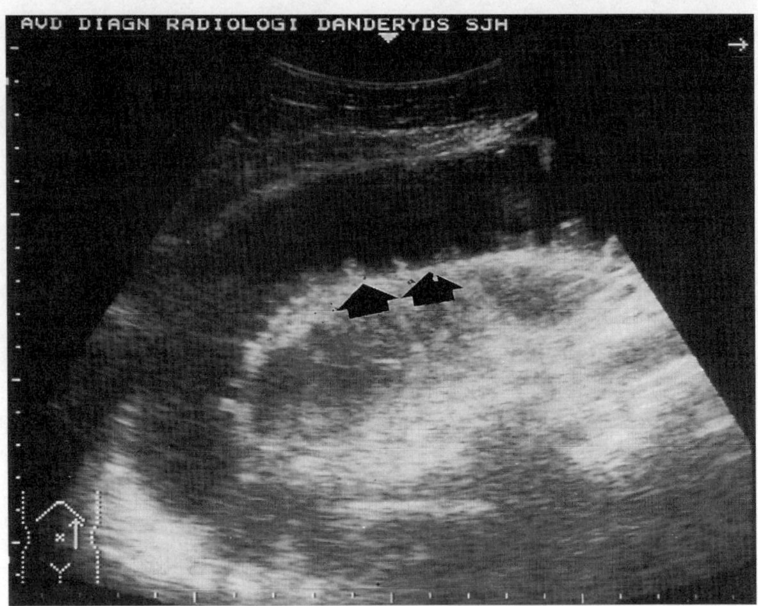

FIGURE 1.—A 59-year-old woman with gastric pain. Ultrasonography revealed an incarcerated herniation of the small-bowel close loops. Appearance of valvulae conniventes (*arrows*) permits identification of the jejunum. At surgery, strangulation was found. (Courtesy of Czechowski J: Conventional Radiography and Ultrasonography in the Diagnosis of Small Bowel Obstruction and Strangulation. *Acta Radiol* 37:186–189, 1996.)

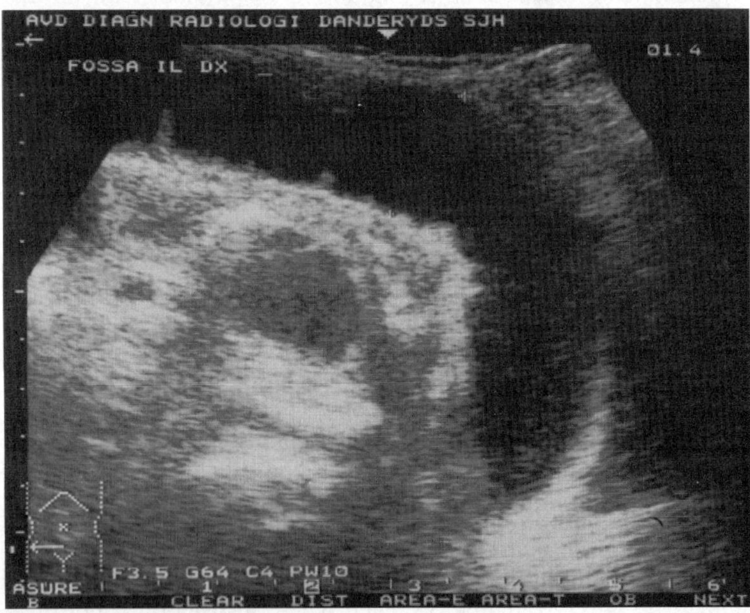

FIGURE 2.—A 67-year-old woman with 4-hour history of intermittent abdominal pain and vomiting. Abdominal radiography showed no sign of obstruction. Ultrasonography revealed a distended small-bowel loop with absence of peristalsis and wall thickening. Somewhat rare plicae conniventes permit identification of the ileum. Surgically confirmed strangulation. (Courtesy of Czechowski J: Conventional Radiography and Ultrasonography in the Diagnosis of Small Bowel Obstruction and Strangulation. *Acta Radiol* 37:186–189, 1996.)

added to plain radiography in evaluating patients with acute abdominal pain.

▶ That ultrasonography can be 90% predictive in diagnosing strangulation obstruction represents an important step in recognizing this complication. The application of this technology of course requires its timely availability in the emergency department. The level of experience and expertise required to obtain the level of success reported here is not mentioned. I believe that surgeons and emergency department physicians who interface with these patients on a frequent basis should become competent in abdominal ultrasonography.

F.G. Moody, M.D.

Computed Tomographic Enteroclysis: One Methodology
Bender GN, Timmons JH, Williard WC, et al (Madigan Army Med Ctr, Ft Lewis, Tacoma, Wash)
Invest Radiol 31:43–49, 1996   3–2

Introduction.—In patients with suspected small bowel obstruction (SBO) and negative plain film findings, CT can often be diagnostic; however, CT identifies fewer than half of patients with low-grade partial SBO. Enteroclysis is reported to detect all grades of partial obstruction yet provides little information about the bowel wall, mesentery, or remote findings. In a search for an ideal imaging alternative, researchers developed a combined CT enteroclysis (CT-E) methodology.

Technique.—The CT-E procedure uses a water-soluble contrast and begins with placement of a nasojejunal or an orojejunal enteroclysis tube. A single-contrast enteroclysis is performed in the fluoroscopy suite with a 10% to 15% water-soluble iodine solution given at a rate of 75–100 mL/min. The fluoroscopic examination continues until a low-grade partial obstruction is detected or until the terminal ileum is reached. Patients are then moved to CT, and the nasojejunal tube is again hooked up to the enteroclysis pump. The CT protocol now consists of a single abdominal sequence in most cases.

Patient Selection.—Patients with medical conditions that require immediate surgery or those with suspected ischemic/infarcted bowel should not undergo CT-E. Two major groups of patients are candidates for CT-E. The first group consists of patients with a history of abdominal surgery and 1 or more of the following criteria: (1) failure of decompression or decreased success after a successful clinical trial of decompression; (2) a successful nasogastric tube decompression followed by failure of subsequent feeding or fluid trials, and (3) known abdominal adhesive disease or previous SBO surgery. The second group consists of any decompressed patients with acute or chronic SBO symptoms and known or suspected abdominal masses or metastatic disease.

Results.—Forty-eight consecutive examinations were performed in patients with suspected partial SBO. The calculated dose per patient, 32 rad with traditional enteroclysis, was reduced to 27 rad for CT-E. For all grades of obstruction, sensitivity of CT-E was estimated to be 87.5% and specificity, 88.9%. Preliminary estimates of sensitivity and specificity for identifying the exact site and grade of low-grade partial SBO alone were 82.1% and 87.5%, respectively. One patient with diffuse abdominal metastatic disease and complete obstruction died after an aborted CT-E. Death resulted from vomiting and aspiration secondary to tube placement.

Discussion.—Water-soluble contrast CT-E can aid in operative or management planning for patients with partial SBO. Pitfalls are encountered, however, particularly in patients with adhesive disease and intermittent SBO secondary to torsion, those with hernias, and when multiple loops of bowel point toward a common focus in patients with a large area of abdominal adhesive disease or fibrosis.

▶ Water-soluble contrast enteroclysis in combination with CT has a site-specific sensitivity of 82% and a specificity of 88%. These are not bad numbers when one is in doubt about whether to operate on an incomplete obstruction. I still believe in operating on such patients at an early time, but there are some who would likely benefit from a more precise definition of the level and possibily cause of obstruction.

F.G. Moody, M.D.

Water-soluble Contrast Material Has No Therapeutic Effect on Postoperative Small-Bowel Obstruction: Results of a Prospective, Randomized Clinical Trial

Feigin E, Seror D, Szold A, et al (Hadassah Univ, Jerusalem; Hebrew Univ, Jerusalem)
Am J Surg 171:227–229, 1996   3–3

Background.—Although postoperative small-bowel obstruction (POSBO) is the most common type of intestinal obstruction in adults, the best treatment for it has not been established. Hyperosmotic water-soluble contrast materials are useful for diagnosis in such patients. Their value in treating POSBO, however, is debatable. The benefit of using meglumine ioxitalamate as a supplement to standard conservative therapy was investigated in a prospective, randomized clinical study.

Methods.—The study included 50 patients in whom conservative treatment was indicated. By random assignment, 25 patients underwent conservative treatment only, and 25 underwent conservative treatment plus 100 mL meglumine ioxitalamate by nasogastric tube.

Findings.—Three patients receiving contrast material and 4 in the control group needed surgery. Symptom resolution without surgery was achieved in 25.7 hours (mean) in patients receiving contrast material and in 28.7 hours (mean) in those not receiving contrast material. These differences were nonsignificant. None of the patients died. One patient in each group was found to have a strangulated bowel at surgery. However, only the patients receiving contrast material needed bowel resection. The 2 groups had similar lengths of stay in the hospital and similar complication rates. No complications were attributed to the use of the contrast material.

Conclusion.—The use of meglumine ioxitalamate appears to have no therapeutic effect in patients with POSBO. However, its judicious use is safe and helpful in patients in whom the diagnosis is not clear and could be established by imaging with a water-soluble contrast agent.

▶ The authors have missed the point from my point of view. Water-soluble contrast material is helpful in distinguishing partial small-bowel obstruction from postoperative ileus. Its use provides a radiographic view of the intestinal tract and a stimulus for peristalsis in the quiescent bowel. It was good of the authors to dispel the myth that the material has therapeutic value in small-bowel obstruction.

F.G. Moody, M.D.

16 Pathophysiologic Considerations

Effect of Intestinal Resection on Human Small Bowel Motility
Schmidt T, Pfeiffer A, Hackelsberger N, et al (Städtisches Krankenhaus München-Bogenhausen, Munich; Akademisches Lehrkrankenhaus, Munich)
Gut 38:859–863, 1996　　　　　　　　　　　　　　　　　　　　　　3–4

Introduction.—Little is known about changes in human small-bowel motility after intestinal resection, and animal studies have yielded conflicting results. Two groups of patients were investigated after intestinal resection by 24-hour manometry to characterize the changes in jejunal motility.

Patients and Methods.—Patients were studied a mean of 15 months after intestinal resection. The first group of 7 patients (mean age, 74 years) had a short-bowel syndrome after extensive distal small intestinal resection. In all cases an intact stomach and an intact duodenum were present and the jejunal remnant had been anastomosed to the colon. At the time of manometry, all were in a stable nutritional, fluid, and electrolyte state and were receiving oral alimentation. The second group of 6 patients (mean age, 48) underwent resection of a mean of 40 cm of the terminal ileum and the cecum with ilio–ascending colostomy. Three of these patients underwent surgery for Crohn's disease and 3 for adhesions. All were free of gastrointestinal symptoms and had a normal daily stool weight and body mass index at the time of the study. Fasting motility and the motor response to a 600-kcal solid meal were examined by 24-hour jejunal manometry, visual analysis, and a computer program.

Results.—Normal motility values were obtained from 50 healthy individuals. Jejunal motility was not changed by limited ileal resection, but after extensive distal resection patients had a significantly shorter migrating motor complex (MMC) cycle and a significantly shorter duration of the postprandial motor response than did controls. Differences in MMC cycle length between the limited and extensive resection groups were also significant (Table 5). The frequency of jejunal contractions was not affected by intestinal resection, nor were any abnormal motor patterns observed.

Discussion.—Limited ileal resection does not lead to detectable manometric changes of jejunal motility, whereas extensive distal resection of the

TABLE 5.—Parameters of Postprandial Motility in Healthy Controls, Patients With the Short-bowel Syndrome, and Patients After Partial Ileal Resection

	Controls (N=50)		Short Bowels (N=7)		Ileal Resections (N=6)
Duration of postprandial motility (min)	263 (13)	$P < 0.005$	126 (14)	$P < 0.01$	218 (12)
Contraction frequency (min^{-1})	3.1 (0.2)		2.7 (0.5)		3.0 (0.5)
Contraction amplitude (mm Hg)	23.7 (0.5)		24.5 (0.9)		24.0 (0.7)

Note: Values are means (SEM), *t* test.
(Courtesy of Schmidt T, Pfeiffer A, Hackelsberger N, et al: Effect of intestinal resection on human small bowel motility. *Gut* 38:859–863, 1996.)

small intestine alters fasting and postprandial motility in the intestinal remnant. The malabsorption and diarrhea that occur in short-bowel syndrome may result in part from shortening of digestive motility and increased frequency of MMC cycling.

▶ Resection of the small bowel results in mucosal adaptive changes and altered absorption of various nutrients. However, there is relatively little information on changes in small-bowel motility after extensive ileal resection. This provocative study has demonstrated that *limited resection* of the terminal ileum (30–60 cm) and cecum with ileo–ascending colostomy did not result in changes in MMCs during the waking and sleep state. By contrast, after extensive distal resection leaving a small-bowel remnant of 30–100 cm of jejunum, patients showed significantly shorter MMC cycle length, especially phase II. Interestingly, intestinal resection had no influence on jejunal contraction frequency and amplitude.

The more rapid cycling of luminal contents after extensive ileal resection could be an important factor in the pathogenesis of both diarrhea and malabsorption. Therapeutic agents that reduce MMC cycling and thus slow digestive motility could be a welcome addition to treatment regimens for short-bowel syndrome. Such a compound currently under study is the antimuscarinic compound trospium chloride.[1]

N.J. Greenberger, M.D.

Reference

1. Schmidt T, Widmer R, Pfeiffer A, et al: Effect of the quaternary ammonium compound trospium chloride on 24 hour jejunal motility in healthy subjects. *Gut* 35:27–33, 1994.

Effects of Somatostatin on Luminal Transit and Absorption of Nutrients in the Proximal Gut of Minipigs
Eisenbraun J, Ehrlein H-J (Univ of Hohenheim, Stuttgart, Germany)
Dig Dis Sci 41:894–901, 1996

3–5

Background.—Different animal and human studies of the effects of the gastrointestinal hormone somatostatin have had conflicting results regarding the intestinal absorption of nutrients. None of these studies has taken into account the potential influences of motility and luminal transit. The interrelationships between luminal transit and nutrient absorption were studied in a jejunal segment of minipigs.

Methods.—With the use of general anesthesia, 2 cannulas were implanted into the proximal jejunum in 5 minipigs, and a tube was inserted into the jejunum to define a 150-cm intestinal test segment. The pigs were fasted for 14 hours. Then the test segment was perfused with an elemental diet for 45 minutes, after which the pigs were fed a test meal of 1,000 mL along with somatostatin. Somatostatin was infused for 60 minutes at doses of 0.5, 1.25, 2.5, and 5 µg/kg/hr. Effluents were collected from both cannulas at 15-minute intervals throughout the experiment until 30 minutes after the somatostatin infusion was stopped. Transit time was determined by including Cu-EDTA as a marker in the perfusions. Flow rate and nutrient absorption were also calculated.

Results.—The flow rate was decreased and the transit time increased by increasing doses of somatostatin, with significant changes after doses of somatostatin exceeding 1.25 µg/kg/hr. Somatostatin infusion enhanced the absolute and percentage absorption of carbohydrate, protein, and energy in an exponential fashion, and of fat in a linear fashion. These changes became significant with somatostatin doses exceeding 2.5 µg/kg/hr. The changes in nutrient absorption were smaller than the changes in flow rate and transit time. However, there were linear relationships between the changes in flow rate, in transit time, and in nutrient absorption.

Conclusions.—The flow and transit of luminal contents contribute to nutrient absorption and must be considered in studies of absorption. Although exogenous somatostatin may have a direct inhibitory effect on absorption, this effect is probably compensated by the reduced luminal transit time, thus having a minimal effect on nutrient absorption, except for the absorption of fat.

▶ The common usage of somatostatin in the treatment of pancreatic and gastrointestinal fistulas makes the issue of its effects on 2 important aspects of gut function, transit and absorption, worthy of study. As is reported here, there is a dose-dependent decrease in transit in response to exogenous somatostatin that is compensated for in part by an increase in absorption. This work done in minipigs may have relevance to the human situation. As the authors point out in their discussion, the effects of somatostatin on transit and absorption may have a net effect that would be negligible with regard to the handling of nutrients except in the occasional patient who may have steatorrhea from the decreased bile and pancreatic secretion delivery to the gut.

F.G. Moody, M.D.

Octreotide Diminishes Luminal Nutrient Transport Activity, Which Is Reversed by Epidermal Growth Factor
Seydel AS, Miller JH, Sarac TP, et al (Univ of Rochester, NY)
Am J Surg 171:267–271, 1996

3–6

Background.—Short bowel syndrome (SBS) usually is treated with total parenteral nutrition (TPN), but long-term TPN is costly and can lead to hepatic dysfunction, sepsis, and death. For patients to wean successfully from TPN, adaptation of the small bowel to massive resection is required. The small bowel must enlarge its surface area and increase its capacity to transport nutrients to compensate for decreased length. Octreotide (SMS), a somatostatin analogue used to decrease output in SBS, may inhibit small bowel adaptation by blocking secretion of epidermal growth factor (EGF). The effects of SMS and EGF on nutrient transport in SBS were examined in an experimental study.

Methods.—Twenty male New Zealand White rabbits underwent a 70% midjejunoileal resection. One week later, the animals were administered subcutaneous infusions of saline or EGF (1.5 µg/kg/hr) and injections of saline or SMS (500 µg) twice daily. There were 5 rabbits in each of 4 study groups (EGF/saline, saline/saline, saline/SMS, and EGF/SMS). After 7 days of infusion, the animals were sacrificed, intestinal brush-border membrane vesicles were prepared, and nutrient transport was measured.

Results.—The rabbits given continuous saline and SMS injections showed significantly reduced amino acid and glucose uptake. This effect was confirmed by kinetics to be secondary to a reduction in functional carriers in the brush-border membrane, without alteration in carrier affinity. Co-infusion of EGF ameliorated this effect for all amino acids and glucose studied. Nutrient transport was upregulated 26% when the entire group was analyzed, but this effect of EGF alone did not reach statistical significance for each individual.

Discussion.—Changes in both morphology and physiology are necessary for efficient adaptation after massive resection of the small bowel. Whereas SMS is detrimental to small bowel adaptation, EGF reverses this effect. Patients who require SMS to sustain hydration may benefit from co-infusion of EGF.

▶ I appreciate studies such as this that point out a problem with existing therapies and then provide a solution. Octreotide (somatostatin) is useful in controlling gastrointestinal secretions in a variety of circumstances, but it also interferes with essential brush-border enzyme activities. Fortunately, EGF ameliorates this effect (in the rabbit). But is this also true in the clinical situation? I would guess that we will hear more about this issue in the future, because octreotide is now in common use in patients with pancreatic and gastrointestinal fistulas.

F.G. Moody, M.D.

Gastroschisis Increases Small Bowel Nitric Oxide Synthase Activity
Bealer JF, Graf J, Bruch SW, et al (Univ of California, San Francisco)
J Pediatr Surg 31:1043–1046, 1996   3–7

Introduction.—Gastroschisis, a congenital defect of the anterior abdominal wall, results in severe intestinal dysfunction. Recent studies suggest that the link between the intestinal damage that occurs and subsequent intestinal dysfunction is nitric oxide (NO), a neurotransmitter that is vital to normal bowel function and is produced by the enzyme NO synthase. A fetal rabbit model was used to investigate the role of NO synthase in gastroschisis-induced bowel dysfunction.

Methods.—New Zealand White fetuses of 22 to 23 days' gestation were removed from the uterus for evisceration of the intestines. One week later, these fetuses and control littermates without gastroschisis were delivered by cesarean section. The small intestine of each fetus was removed and prepared for determination of NO synthase activity, measured by the ^{3}H-arginine-to-^{3}H-citrulline conversion assay. The assay was able to identify 4 distinct isoforms of NO synthase activity on the basis of the activity's location (soluble or particulate) and its dependence on calcium as a cofactor (dependent or independent).

Results.—The small bowel of fetal rabbits with experimental gastroschisis was found to have a total NO synthase activity 2.5 times greater than that of the littermate controls. Three of the 4 measured NO synthase isoforms were significantly increased in the experimental animals: the calcium-dependent activity of the soluble fraction and both the calcium-dependent and calcium-independent activities of the particulate fractions. The site of increased NO synthase activity was localized to the small bowel epithelium and neurons. When a histologic staining technique (NADPH-diaphorase) was used to explore the mechanism of the increase in NO synthase activity, no quantitative increase was observed in the small bowel NO synthase of rabbits with gastroschisis. Control and experimental specimens were similar in the total amount and distribution of NO synthase.

Conclusion.—The increased NO synthase in rabbits with gastroschisis appears to be the result of accelerated enzyme kinetics and may be a contributing cause of the malabsorption and intestinal dysmotility that characterize the disorder. Thus, gastroschisis-induced hypoperistalsis may result from increased intestinal smooth-muscle relaxation mediated by excess NO.

▶ This experimental study caught my fancy, and I wanted to share it with our readers. The results of this study in which gastroschisis is produced in fetal rabbits, demonstrate increased NO activity in the affected fetuses after delivery by cesarean section a week later. This was associated with upregulation of 3 of the 4 known isoforms of NO synthase. Now, what does this have to do with gastroschisis in humans? The authors speculate that this increase in NO production may be responsible for the dysmotility that these infants experience. Not a bad idea, because NO is a potent antagonist to smooth-muscle contraction.

F.G. Moody, M.D.

17 Celiac Sprue

Gluten-sensitive Disease With Mild Enteropathy
Picarelli A, Maiuri L, Mazzilli MC, et al (Univ La Sapienza, Rome; Children's Hosp Pausilipon, Naples, Italy; Univ Federico II, Naples, Italy; et al)
Gastroenterology 111:608–616, 1996   3–8

Introduction.—Permanent intolerance of the small intestine to gluten is the definition of celiac disease. Strongly associated with HLA class II antigens, celiac disease is diagnosed by the presence of villus atrophy with crypt hyperplasia on a gluten-containing diet. The celiac-like intestinal antibody pattern has been used to identify latent celiac disease. Ten patients with suggestive symptoms of celiac disease and with serum antiendomysium antibodies are described.

Methods.—Ten patients with suggestive celiac disease were examined: 6 had chronic diarrhea and steatorrhea and 4 had relapsing hypocalcemic tetany, chronic hepatitis, recurrent aphthous stomatitis, and osteoporosis. HLA typing and immunohistochemical detection of mucosal immune activation were performed. Mucosal immune activation was also tested by in vitro challenge with gliadin digest; fecal fat, nitrogen, and water were determined from 24-hour stool collections; and serum antigliadin and antiendomysium antibodies were quantified by immunosorbent assay. Theses values were compared with those of surgical biopsy specimens from controls who had intestinal resection for biliary tract disease, gastric cancer, gastric ulcer, or pancreatic disease.

Results.—On a gluten-containing diet, mucosal immune activation was detected in the presence of normal mucosal architecture and normal γ/δ^+ intraepithelial lymphocyte counts (Table 2). Multiple biopsy specimens showed 1 sample with severe villous atrophy in 3 of 6 patients. The immunomorphological and clinical features were found to be gluten dependent. Mucosal immune activation was elicited in vitro with gliadin, and the typical HLA typing of celiac disease was seen in only 4 patients.

Conclusion.—In patients with serum antiendomysium antibodies, normal intestinal mucosa and HLA typing not commonly associated with celiac disease, gluten-sensitive celiac-like symptoms may occur. Multiple biopsies should be performed on these patients, and there should be an accurate search for signs of immunologic activation. A trial with a gluten-free diet should be encouraged to detect gluten dependency in the presence of mucosal immune activation. The diagnosis of gluten-sensitive enterop-

TABLE 2.—HLA Typing and Histologic and Laboratory Findings

			Morphology										
			IEL (CD3$^+$ Cells/ 100 Enterocytes)		γ/δ^+ Cells (Per Millimeter Epithelium)		Antigliadin Antibodies			Stools (g/24 h)			Xylose (% of Ingested Xylose)
	HLA type												
Patient	DR	DQ	Normal Diet	Gluten-free Diet	Normal Diet	Gluten-free Diet	IgA*	IgG*	IgE*	Fat†	Nitrogen‡	Water§	Urinary Excretion‖
1	5,7	A1*0201/0501 B1*0201/0301	27	21	1.8	1.3	1.18	0.93	0.57	5.68	7.09	248	17.05
2	1,2	A1*0101/0201 B1*0501/0502	28	24	0.9	1.4	0.84	0.71	0.6	5.36	7.86	252.7	22.9
3	5,6	A1*0103/0501 B1*0301/0603	52	27	2.6	3.1	0.91	0.4	0.4	2.21	7.87	280	15.7
4	4	A1*0302 B1*0301/0402	46	23	2.8	3.1	0.6	0.54	0.6	5.56	9.78	335	51.58
5	2,6	A1*0102/0102 B1*0502/0604	49	23	2.8	3.1	1.13	0.7	0.66	11.84	12.68	604	10.1
6	1,6	A1*0101/0102 B1*0501/0604	32	25	1.9	2.3	1.0	0.73	0.4	1.61	2.25	79.9	32.98
7	6,7	A1*0102/0201 B1*0201/0604	26	29	1.7	1.5	1.94	0.78	0.49	2.28	7.11	316	16.5
8	5,7	A1*0201/0501 B1*0201/0301	47	22	1.4	1.3	1.24	0.92	0.23	8.9	10.9	584	ND
9	5,6	A1*0103/0501 B1*0601/0301	23	21	0.8	1.1	0.71	0.56	0.25	8.5	11.3	602	ND*
10	5	A1*0501 B1*0301	26	20	1.1	1.3	0.63	0.47	0.31	4.1	7.1	80.3	5.24

Note: In patients 2, 3, and 8, multiple biopsy specimens showed 1 fragment with villous atrophy and the others with normal morphology; in other samples, all the mucosal fragments were morphologically normal.
*Optical density: the values express the ratio between patient's optical density and the control's optical density ± 3 SD (normal values: IgC < 1; IgA < 0.8; and IgE < 0.7).
†Normal values, 2.3; SD, 1.23.
‡Normal values, 3.3; SD, 1.67.
§Normal values, 125.8; SD, 70.1.
‖Urinary xylose excretion; normal values, >25%.
Abbreviation: IEL, intraepithelial lymphocytes.
(Courtesy of Picarelli A, Maiuri L, Mazzilli MC, et al: Gluten-sensitive disease with mild enteropathy. *Gastroenterology* 111:608–616, 1996.)

athy may be supported by the in vitro immunologic response of small intestinal mucosa to gliadin.

▶ This report underscores the fact that celiac sprue is a disorder with a wide spectrum of clinical manifestations. This study describes 10 patients with suggestive symptoms of celiac sprue, positive tests for antiendomysial antibodies, and histologically normal small-bowel specimens. However, immunocytochemical analysis of these biopsy samples showed signs of immunologic activation when exposed to gliadin peptides, similar to the findings in patients with overt celiac sprue.

The increased use of antiendomysial antibody testing to screen for celiac sprue has uncovered many patients with latent disease. Celiac sprue appears to be more common in patients with insulin-dependent diabetes mellitus. In one representative series,[1] 3 of 47 such patients (6.4%) had subclinical or latent celiac sprue.

Neurologic manifestations of celiac sprue include cerebellar ataxia, peripheral neuropathy, myelopathy, myopathy, seizures, and dementia. Two recent reports[2, 3] remind us that these neurologic abnormalities can occur without obvious gastrointestinal manifestations suggestive of celiac sprue.

N.J. Greenberger, M.D.

References

1. Rensch MJ, Merenech JA, Liebermann M, et al: Gluten-sensitive enteropathy in patients with insulin-dependent diabetes mellitus. *Ann Intern Med* 124:564–567, 1996.
2. Berensdorf D, Moses P, Reeves A: A man with weight loss, ataxia, and confusion for three months. *Lancet* 34:448, 1996.
3. Hadjivassiliou M, Gibson A, Davies-Jones GAB: Does gluten sensitivity play a part in neurological illness. *Lancet* 347:369–371, 1996.

Production of Antiendomysial Antibodies After In-vitro Gliadin Challenge of Small Intestine Biopsy Samples From Patients With Coeliac Disease
Picarelli A, Maiuri L, Frate A, et al (Univ LaSapienza Rome; Children's Hosp Pausilipon, Naples, Italy; Univ Federico II, Naples, Italy; et al)
Lancet 348:1065–1067, 1996   3–9

Objectives.—Whether the small intestine is the site of antiendomysial antibody production in patients with celiac disease was investigated, and whether a gliadin challenge can induce the release of these antibodies was determined.

Background.—Celiac disease is a common gastroenterologic illness caused by ingestion of gliadin in genetically predisposed individuals. It is believed that this disease is immunologically mediated and that gliadin induces various events that result in tissue damage. The presence of gliadin-specific T cells in the mucosa of patients with celiac disease and the

TABLE 1.—Production of Antiendomysial Antibodies by In-Vitro Cultured Intestinal Explants From Patients With Celiac Disease and Controls

Culture condition	Untreated CD patients, EMA positive	Treated CD patients, EMA positive	Controls, EMA positive
Medium	16/16*	0/23	0/18†
Gliadin	16/16*	17/23‡	0/18

*95% confidence interval, corrected for continuity = 0.969, 1.031.
†95% confidence interval, corrected for continuity = 0.027, 0.027.
‡$P = 0.002967$, $\chi^2 = 8.8$ vs. cultures with medium alone.
Abbreviations: CD, celiac disease; *EMA*, antiendomysial antibodies.
(Courtesy of Picarelli A, Maiuri L, Frate A, et al: Production of antiendomysial antibodies after in vitro gliadin challenge of small intestine biopsy samples from patients with coeliac disease. *Lancet* 348:1065–1067. Copyright 1996, The Lancet Ltd.)

presence of antigliadin antibodies support the hypothesis that gliadin induces activation of the immune system. Studies have shown that antibodies against gliadin are present in most patients with celiac disease, and are often found in patients who do not have this disease. Tests for antiendomysial antibodies are an excellent screening tool for celiac disease because their sensitivity and specificity are almost 100%. It is not known whether antiendomysial antibodies are produced in the small intestine or in another site.

Methods.—Biopsy specimens were obtained from 39 patients with celiac disease, 23 of whom had been treated, and from 18 control patients. Specimens were cultured for 24 or 48 hours with gliadin, another alimentary antigen, or medium. Enzyme-linked immunoassay was used to detect antiendomysial antibodies, and immunofluorescence was used to detect antibodies against gliadin.

Results.—In the specimens from the 18 controls, no antiendomysial antibodies were detected, whereas in specimens from all 16 untreated patients with celiac disease, antiendomysial antibodies were detected. Antiendomysial antibodies were not detected in specimens that were cultured in medium only from the 23 treated patients with celiac disease, but antiendomysial antibodies were detected in 17 of the 23 specimens from treated patients that were cultured in gliadin.

Discussion.—These findings indicate that the mucosa of untreated patients with celiac disease is a site of antiendomysial antibody production because these antibodies were present in all samples from untreated patients with celiac disease. Antibodies against gliadin IgA and IgG were not detected in all the specimens from untreated patients with celiac disease before the gliadin challenge. This provides further evidence that antiendomysial antibodies are more specific for celiac disease than antibodies against gliadin. The most interesting finding was that in 17 of the 23 treated patients with celiac disease, a 24-hour gliadin challenge resulted in production of antiendomysial antibodies (Table 1). The antiendomysial antibody antigen may be the pathogenetic antigen, although gliadin is the environmental etiologic factor in celiac disease. If reactivity to gliadin is not confined to patients with celiac disease, whereas production of antiendomysial antibodies is confined to these patients, then the real antigen that causes celiac disease may be the antiendomysial antibody antigen, not gliadin. In genetically predisposed individuals, gliadin causes an immuno-logic recognition of the antiendomysial antibody antigen. If this antigen is important in celiac disease, the understanding of the pathologic process of this illness will need to be revised.

▶ Autoimmune mechanisms are believed to be operative in the pathogenesis of celiac sprue. If untreated, celiac sprue ingested gluten triggers the production of certain IgA class serum antibodies called R_1 type reticulin, endomysial and antigliadin antibodies. Antiendomysial antibodies (EMA) have emerged as an important test for both screening and follow-up of patients with celiac sprue. Antiendomysial antibodies have a nearly 100% specificity and sensitivity for identifying patients with active as well as latent celiac sprue. This important study of Picarelli, et al. indicates that EMA can be considered autoantibodies and provides strong support for the concept that autoimmune mechanisms are operative in celiac sprue. Picarelli, et al. have demonstrated in an organ culture system that on gluten challenge EMA are produced by mucosal biopsy specimens from untreated patients with celiac sprue. This is the first direct evidence that EMA are actually produced in the small intestinal mucosa. A further striking finding was the demonstration that the intestinal mucosa from treated patients with celiac sprue did not spontaneously produce EMA but did so on gliadin challenge. The authors propose that although gliadin is an important etiologic factor in celiac sprue, the EMA antigen may represent the pathogenetic antigen. This is a classic study.

N.J. Greenberger, M.D.

The Prevalence of Occult Gastrointestinal Bleeding in Celiac Sprue

Fine KD (Baylor Univ, Dallas)
N Engl J Med 334:1163–1167, 1996   3–10

Purpose.—Patients with celiac sprue commonly have iron deficiency, which has been blamed on malabsorption of dietary iron or iron loss from the intestinal mucosa. Gastrointestinal bleeding has also been mentioned as a possible source of iron deficiency, but few studies have examined this possibility. The prevalence of gastrointestinal bleeding among patients with celiac sprue was studied.

Methods.—Thirty-six patients with small intestine biopsy specimens showing changes consistent with celiac sprue were studied; 28 patients had total villous atrophy and 8 had partial villous atrophy. A Hemoccult test was performed on a 48- or 72-hour stool collection to detect fecal occult blood. Several control groups were studied as well, including normal individuals, before and after laxative-induced diarrhea; patients with microscopic colitis; patients with pancreatic steatorrhea; and patients with treated celiac sprue who had normal findings on intestinal biopsy speci-

TABLE 1.—Fecal Weight, Fecal Fat, and Hemoccult-test Positivity in the Control Groups and in Patients With Villous Atrophy

Group of Subjects	No. of Stool Specimens*	Fecal Weight†	Fecal Fat†	No. (%) of Hemoccult-positive Subjects	P Value‡	
		grams per day				
Control group						
Normal subjects (n = 18)						
With normal stools	18	133 ± 55	—§	1 (6)		
With induced diarrhea	50	361 ± 156	—§	3 (6)		
Patients with idiopathic secretory diarrhea (n = 17)	17	627 ± 252	6 ± 4	0 (0)		
Patients with microscopic colitis (n = 63)	63	537 ± 341	5 ± 3	5 (8)		
Patients with pancreatic insufficiency (n = 23)	23	562 ± 412	43 ± 34	1 (4)		
Patients with previously treated celiac sprue and normal small-intestinal histology (n = 7)	7	188 ± 89	3 ± 2	0 (0)		
All control subjects (n = 128)	178	—	—	10 (6)		
Patients with villous atrophy						
Previously treated patients with celiac sprue and partial villous atrophy (n = 8)	8	499 ± 223	21 ± 17	2 (25)	0.09	5.7 (1.0–34.5)
Patients with celiac sprue and total villous atrophy (n = 17)	17	724 ± 907	21 ± 16	7 (41)	< 0.001	12.0 (3.5–41.7)
Patients with refractory sprue and total villous atrophy (n = 11)	11	1054 ± 718	29 ± 20	8 (73)	< 0.001	45.4 (10.0–200.0)
All the patients with total villous atrophy (n = 28)	28	865 ± 830	25 ± 18	15 (54)	< 0.001	20.0 (6.9–58.8)
All the patients with partial or total villous atrophy (n = 36)	36	762 ± 864	24 ± 18	17 (47)	< 0.001	15.4 (5.6–41.7)

*Number of stool specimens tested per group.

†Plus-minus values are means ± SD.

‡These values pertain to 128 independent tests in the control groups (excluding the group with induced diarrhea) by Fisher's exact test.

§Not measured.

Abbreviation: CI, confidence interval.

(Courtesy of Fine KD: The prevalence of occult gastrointestinal bleeding in celiac sprue. *N Engl J Med* 334:1163–1167. Copyright 1996, Massachusetts Medical Society. Reprinted by permission of *The New England Journal of Medicine*. All rights reserved.)

mens. All patients had a thorough diagnostic workup, and the patients with total villous atrophy were retested for occult fecal blood after treatment with a gluten-free diet.

Results.—The Hemoccult test detected fecal occult blood in 0% to 8% of individuals in the control groups, compared with 54% of the patients with total villous atrophy and 25% of those with partial villous atrophy. Of the 17 patients with total villous atrophy who responded to a gluten-free diet, 41% were Hemoccult-positive when retested, compared with 73% of those who did not respond to gluten withdrawal (Table 1). The patients with celiac sprue had no other lesions that might have caused gastrointestinal bleeding. The mean hemoglobin concentration was significantly lower in the Hemoccult-positive patients; there was no significant difference in serum iron levels, however.

Conclusions.—Many patients with celiac sprue will test positive for occult fecal blood. The way in which the small intestine abnormalities cause gastrointestinal blood loss is uncertain but may involve microerosions caused by chronic inflammation or compromise of the epithelial cell barrier. From a clinical standpoint, the findings suggest that Hemoccult testing should not be used to screen for cancer in patients with celiac or refractory sprue.

▶ The main finding in this study is that patients with celiac sprue often have Hemoccult-positive stools. Further, this is more likely to occur in patients with refractory sprue and villous atrophy. It is pertinent to note that none of the patients with villous atrophy had any lesions identified on upper or lower gastrointestinal endoscopic examinations that could account for gastrointestinal blood loss. Thus, the authors speculate that chronic inflammation causes microerosions that escape detection by endoscopic and radiographic measures. This notion is indirectly supported by the finding that patients with villous atrophy and Hemoccult-positive stools had significantly lower hemoglobin values compared with patients with villous atrophy and Hemoccult-negative stools (11.3 ± 2.5 g/dL vs. 12.9 ± 1.7 g/dL). As the authors point out, one of the practical applications of this study is that the Hemoccult test should not be used as a screening test for cancer in patients with celiac sprue, especially patients with refractory sprue, because of its poor predictive value.

N.J. Greenberger, M.D.

18 Mesenteric Ischemia

CT and MRI of Experimentally Induced Mesenteric Ischemia in a Porcine Model
Klein H-M, Klosterhalfen B, Kinzel S, et al (Univ of Technology, Aachen, Germany)
J Comput Assist Tomogr 20:254–261, 1996   3–11

Background.—Mesenteric ischemia is fatal in about 60% of affected patients. When immediate surgery is not needed, patients undergo a diagnostic regimen of initial plain radiography and ultrasonography, followed by angiography. The value of CT and MRI in detecting bowel wall changes in experimentally induced mesenteric ischemia was investigated.

Methods.—Eighteen female pigs were studied. A percutaneous embolization of the superior mesenteric artery was done with buthyl-2-cyamoacrylate and Lipiodol in 12 pigs. The other 6 served as the control group. Computed tomography was performed 3, 6, and 12 hours after occlusion. Incremental and spiral CT were performed before and after contrast injection. Serial CT was conducted after IV contrast injection. Magnetic resonance imaging was done with T1, T2, and proton density images in axial orientation. The slice thickness was 3 mm, and the slice gap was 1 mm. A T1-weighted GE sequence was also obtained in dynamic technique with a slice thickness of 5 mm.

Findings.—Histologic assessment of the specimen 3, 6, and 12 hours after vascular occlusion showed a mean Chiu state of 3, 4, and 5. On CT scans, the bowel wall in ischemic segments was a mean 4.7 mm thick. This was significantly different from the control group. In 80%, free intraperitoneal fluid and intramural gas were observed after 12 hours of ischemia. There was no mural enhancement in ischemic bowel segments. Normal segments and control bowel showed a mean enhancement of 34 HU. On MRI, S/N and C/N were significantly different between experimental and control groups in T1 and proton density images. The bowel wall did not show contrast enhancement in ischemic segments of all phases. Healthy segments and control bowel were significantly enhanced.

Conclusion.—The most important parameter for diagnosing mesenteric low-flow states in MRI is the missing enhancement of the ischemic bowel wall after contrast agent injection. Other parameters, such as the signal intensity on plain MR images in different sequence modalities, may be significant when compared directly with control values but are not specific in acute clinical situations.

▶ Computed tomography and MRI both reveal distinguishing characteristics of arterial mesenteric ischemia in an experimental pig simulation of the disease. I am not at all convinced that either test, even when combined, would reach the sensitivity of early laparotomy. It takes only 10 minutes or so to look into an abdomen, and it is unusual to miss the diagnosis these days if the patient is seen early by a well-trained, experienced surgeon. Possibly, the shift to primary care and the "gate keeper" mentality will make more sophisticated diagnostic techniques valuable in the future, as medicine by managers further unfolds.

F.G. Moody, M.D.

Intestinal Fatty Acid-binding Protein Is a Useful Diagnostic Marker for Mesenteric Infarction in Humans
Kanda T, Fujii H, Tani T, et al (Niigata Univ, Japan)
Gastroenterology 110:339–343, 1996

3–12

Objective.—Ischemic bowel diseases, particulary mesenteric infarction, are potentially fatal conditions. There are no clinical signs that distinguish small bowel disease from other causes of acute abdominal pain, nor are there any specific laboratory tests for bowel ischemia. Experiments in rats have suggested that intestinal fatty acid-binding protein (I-FABP) is a potentially useful serum marker of bowel ischemia. Its value in the diagnosis of ischemic diseases of the small bowel, particularly mesenteric infarction, was evaluated.

Methods.—Serum samples from 96 individuals were analyzed: 13 patients undergoing surgery for ischemic bowel disease, including 5 with mesenteric infarction and 8 with strangulated small bowel obstruction; 35 healthy controls; and 48 patients hospitalized with acute abdominal pain. Serum I-FABP levels were evaluated using an antibody-sandwich enzyme immunoassay.

Results.—All healthy individuals had a serum I-FABP level of less than 65 ng/mL. For those with acute abdominal pain, the range was less than 20–87 ng/mL, which was not significantly different from normal. The mean value in this group was 27 ng/mL. In contrast, the mean I-FABP level in the patients with ischemic bowel disease was 266 ng/mL, with a range of less than 20–1,496 ng/mL. For patients with mesenteric infarction, the I-FABP level was always greater than 100 ng/mL (Fig 2).

Conclusions.—Serum I-FABP measurement provides a useful diagnostic test for mesenteric infarction. This highly specific biochemical marker is elevated in patients with ischemic diseases of the small bowel, but low in healthy subjects and controls with acute abdominal pain. It is 100% sensitive for the diagnosis of mesenteric infarction. Further studies are being conducted.

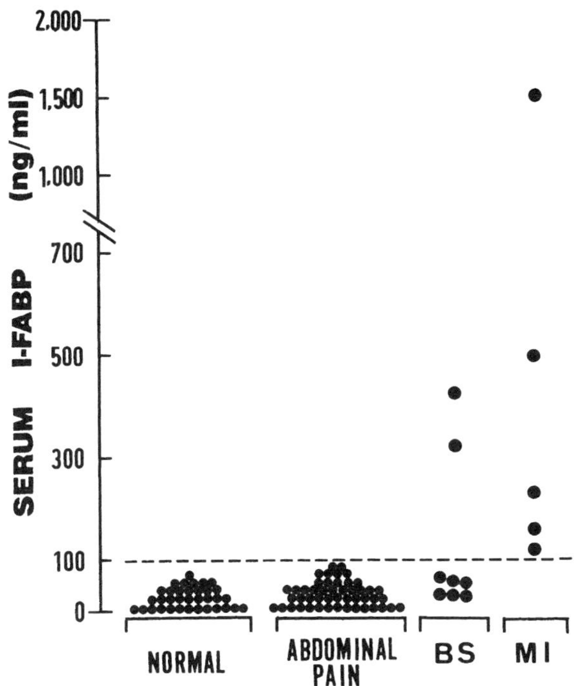

FIGURE 2.—Comparison among healthy controls (*normal; n* = 35), patients with acute abdominal pain; *n* = 48), patients with strangulation of the small bowel (*BS; n* = 8), and patients with mesenteric infarction (*MI; n* = 5). The *dashed line* indicates the tentative cutoff value (100 ng/mL) for the serum I-FABP level in enzyme immunoassay. *Abbreviation: I-FABP,* intestinal fatty acid-binding protein. (Courtesy of Kanda T, Fujii H, Tani T, et al: Intestinal fatty acid-binding protein is a useful diagnostic marker for mesenteric infarction in humans. *Gastroenterology* 110:339–343, 1996.)

▶ Ischemic bowel disease and impending mesenteric infarction are potentially lethal and often difficult to diagnose. Current laboratory tests do not provide specific biochemical markers for bowel ischemia. When hemoccult positive stools, air in the bowel wall, metabolic acidosis, and elevated transaminase levels are present, frank infarction has already occurred. Accordingly, there is a clear need for diagnostic marker for ischemic diseases of the small bowel. The study by Kanda, et al. shows that intestinal fatty acid-binding protein is a useful biochemical marker for the accurate diagnosis of mesenteric infarction.

N.J. Greenberger, M.D.

19 Small Bowel Neoplasms

Primary Lymphoma

Role of Surgery in the Management of Primary Lymphoma of the Gastrointestinal Tract

Law MM, Williams SB, Wong JH (Univ of California, Los Angeles; Sepulveda VA Med Ctr, Calif)

J Surg Oncol 61:199–204, 1996

3–13

Objective.—There is no clearly optimal approach to the management of primary lymphoma of the GI tract. Although some believe that surgery improves the outcome of patients with GI tract lymphoma, others have found that surgery offers no benefit over that of chemotherapy and/or radiotherapy. The surgical management of primary GI tract lymphoma was evaluated retrospectively.

Methods.—The review included 107 patients (mean age, 52 years) who were treated for GI tract lymphoma over a 34-year period. Surgical exploration was performed in 64 patients, of whom 35 had resection for cure. Nineteen patients received postoperative adjuvant therapy and 16 did not. "Noncurative" resection was performed in 29 patients.

Results.—The postoperative mortality rate was 8%, and the overall morbidity rate was 48%. Of 53 patients who received multiagent chemotherapy, three had perforations. The 5-year actuarial survival rate was 59% for patients who underwent curative resection alone, 51% for those who received adjuvant therapy in addition to curative resection, and 28% for those who underwent palliative or noncurative resection. Factors independently associated with survival on multivariate analysis were disease stage and curative resection.

Conclusions.—Surgery with curative intent appears to improve survival rates in patients with primary lymphoma of the GI tract. The results suggest that patients with extensive, unresectable disease should not undergo routine debulking because the risk of perforation during chemotherapy is low, and the risk of surgical morbidity and mortality is substantial.

The risks of perforation and bleeding during chemotherapy and radiation therapy may have been overstated.

▶ The optimum management protocol for primary gastric lymphoma remains poorly defined, even after this retrospective review of 107 patients treated at UCLA over a 3-year period. The authors have confirmed that the patient does better if the lesion is resectable for cure than when a noncurative resection is carried out. This appears to be self-evident. Their observation that a debulking gastrectomy probably is not indicated because of the high rate of surgical morbidity and the low incidence of postirradiation bleeding is useful and mirrors my bias in the treatment of patients with advanced disease.

F.G. Moody, M.D.

Malignant Melanoma

Malignant Melanomas in the Small Intestine: A Study of 103 Patients
Elsayed AM, Albahra M, Nzeako UC, et al (Armed Forces Inst of Pathology, Washington, DC)
Am J Gastroenterol 91:1001–1006, 1996   3–14

Background.—Malignant melanoma often metastasizes to the gastrointestinal tract, particularly the small intestine. Because primary malignancies are rare at this site, metastatic melanoma represents a large proportion of all malignancies of the small intestine. There are also cases in which these lesions occur without an antecedent primary in the skin. The demographic, chronological, and pathologic features of 103 cases of malignant melanoma in the small intestine were reviewed.

Methods.—Cases were obtained through a search of the patient database at the Armed Forces Institute of Pathology for the years 1945–1991. Records of 103 cases of malignant melanoma in the small intestine were reviewed; 77 were surgical cases and 26 were autopsies. In all autopsy cases the primary cause of death was listed as malignant melanoma of the small intestine. Data analyzed included patient race and sex, age at primary (AAP) and primary site, age at the time of small intestine involvement (AASI), age at death, and recorded diagnoses.

Results.—Patients ranged in age from 21 to 72 years; 75 were men and 28 were women. Race was recorded for 79 patients, all of whom were white. Fifty-six patients had a history of a primary malignant melanoma, and 47 had no record of a primary lesion preceding the intestinal tumor. All but 2 of the known primary melanomas were in the skin. The mean age at the time of primary was 45.6 years for surgical cases and 34.1 years for autopsy cases, a significant difference. The mean AASI was 52.2 years for surgical cases and 42.7 years for autopsy cases. Primary melanomas had preceded intestinal lesions by an average of 5.6 years for surgical cases and 2.1 years for autopsy cases. Age distribution for patients with and without known primary melanomas did not differ significantly within the surgical or autopsy groups. Regression equations were presented that allow AASI to be calculated from AAP and AAP estimated from AASI.

Conclusion.—Although a high proportion (46%) of small intestinal melanomas have no known primary, analysis of the age at diagnosis in these cases indicates that small bowel involvement is probably metastatic. There appear to be 2 subsets of primary tumor: one occurring in younger patients and characterized by rapid metastasis and early death, and another occurring in older patients that is more indolent and responsive to surgery.

▶ Although primary malignancies of the small bowel are rare, metastases from melanoma in patients with established disease are common. The Armed Forces Institute of Pathology has the capacity to track down such important pieces of information and put them into a statistical perspective such as was done in this report. Apparently it takes several years for metastatic disease to manifest its presence in the small intestine. The results of the study suggest that the presence of an unknown primary can be predicted by backtiming from the time of discovery of metastatic small bowel disease. It remains to be determined why melanoma has a predilection for the small intestine.

F.G. Moody, M.D.

Lanreotide Treatment of Carcinoid Syndrome

Treatment of the Carcinoid Syndrome With the Longacting Somatostatin Analogue Lanreotide: A Prospective Study in 39 Patients
Ruszniewski P, Ducreux M, Chayvialle J-A, et al (Hôpital Beaujon, Clichy, France; Institut Gustave Roussy, Villejuif, France; Hôpital E Herriot, Lyon, France; et al)
Gut 39:279–283, 1996   3–15

Introduction.—Depending on the site of the primary tumor, malignancy of carcinoid tumors occurs in up to 60% of patients. The most common symptoms of the carcinoid syndrome are flushing and diarrhea, which are caused by small-intestinal tumors. The hormones serotonin, bradykinin, and tachykinin are released in the general circulation. The recently developed somatostatin analogue lanreotide, an octapeptide available in slow-release form, has proved to be effective for patients with acromegaly. The efficacy and tolerability of 30-mg IM injections of lanreotide every other week for 6 months were evaluated in patients with the carcinoid syndrome.

Methods.—The prospective study included 39 patients with carcinoid syndrome who were given lanreotide, 30 mg IM every 2 weeks for 6 months. Recordings were taken of the number and intensity of flushing episodes and bowel movements, urinary 5-hydroxyindoleacetic acid concentrations, and variations in tumor mass.

Results.—In 39% of the patients, flushing episodes decreased significantly from 3 to 1 episode per day after 1 month of treatment. The number of bowel movements and discomfort related to diarrhea were significantly decreased. In 57% of the patients, urinary 5-hydroxyindoleacetic acid levels remained the same, but they decreased in 18% of the patients. Fifty-four percent of the patients had at least a 50% decrease in the number of flushing episodes, and 56% of the patients had a 50% decrease in the number of bowel movements after 6 months of treatment. There was a 50% reduction in 5-hydroxyindoleacetic acid levels in 42% of the patients treated for 6 months. None of the patients experienced any signs of regression. In 25% of the patients, lanreotide was well tolerated despite transient mild pain or erythema at the injection site. In 2 patients, biliary lithiasis appeared after 6 months of lanreotide therapy.

Conclusion.—For patients with the carcinoid syndrome, lanreotide, 30 mg IM every 2 weeks, is an effective and convenient treatment. Most patients who were previously taking octreotide preferred to continue treatment with lanreotide because of its simplification of therapy. In patients with incomplete control of symptoms of tachyphylaxis, further research should be conducted to determine the best interval between 2 consecutive injections.

▶ Somatostatin and its stable analogue octreotide inhibit the release of many gut and pancreatic peptides. Several reports have documented the effectiveness of octreotide in alleviating symptoms of flushing and diarrhea in patients with the carcinoid syndrome. However, this requires 2 to 3 subcutaneous injections of octreotide in doses ranging between 300 and 1,500 µg/day. The report by Ruszniewski et al. describes a newly developed somatostatin analogue, lanreotide, which is a slow-release form that eliminates the inconvenience of multiple daily injections. Lanreotide, given IM at a dosage of 30 mg every other week, was effective in decreasing the frequency and intensity of flushing episodes; complete resolution was observed in 40% of the patients during the first month. The effect of lanreotide on diarrhea was less pronounced, although high frequency and intensity were significantly improved; 30% of the patients had complete resolution. Lanreotide appears to be an effective and convenient treatment in patients with carcinoid syndrome.

N.J. Greenberger, M.D.

Miscellaneous

Treatment and Prognosis of Primary Malignant Small Bowel Tumors
Lambert P, Minghini A, Pincus W, et al (Eastern Virginia Med School, Norfolk)
Am Surg 62:709–715, 1996   3–16

Introduction.—Less than 2% of all malignant lesions occur in the small bowel. Nearly 75% of symptomatic small bowel tumors detected at surgery are malignant, compared to 26% of asymptomatic small bowel tumors found at autopsy. The low incidence of neoplasms in the small bowel, compared to the stomach and colon, probably results from the rapid transit time of the small bowel with its consequent reduced period of carcinogen exposure. Small bowel tumors are associated with a poor prognosis. Patients with primary malignant small bowel tumors were reviewed retrospectively to determine the effects of different clinical parameters on patient outcome.

Methods.—The charts of 53 patients with primary malignant small bowel tumors were reviewed for signs and symptoms at initial visit, history of development of other neoplasms, presence or absence of familial neoplasia syndromes, past medical history, physical examination, pertinent laboratory and diagnostic testing, preoperative diagnosis, operative procedure, postoperative complications, operative mortality, location and size of tumor, involvement of lymph nodes, histology of tumor, adjuvant chemotherapy or radiation therapy, metastatic workup, date and size of first recurrence, treatment of recurrence, date of last follow-up, and date and cause of death.

Results.—The histologic distribution of the tumors was as follows: 28 adenocarcinomas, 17 carcinoids, 4 lymphomas, 3 leiomyosarcomas, and 1 nonspecific malignant tumor. Because of vague and nonspecific signs and symptoms, only 6 of 53 patients were suspected to have a small bowel tumor at admission. After initial diagnostic workup, only 24 of 48 patients undergoing surgery were suspected of having a small bowel neoplasm. The most common surgical procedure performed was segmental resection. The duodenum was the site of 46% of the adenocarcinomas and the ileum was the site of 76% of the carcinoids. In univariate analysis, the factors determining survival included histologic type, location of tumor, and tumor stage. Patients who received chemotherapy or radiation therapy tended to have worse survival. This may have been the result of patient selection factors. In multivariate analysis, histology and tumor stage were the only significant factors affecting survival. The overall 10-year survival rate in this patient series was 44%. Patients with carcinoids and lymphomas had better 5-year survival rates than patients with adenocarcinomas or leiomyosarcomas.

Conclusions.—The survival rate in patients with primary malignant small bowel tumors is highly dependent on tumor histology and stage. These patients are at great risk for the development of malignancies at other sites.

▶ Malignant tumors that arise within the small bowel are not only relatively rare, but of a variety of cellular types. This study reaffirms what has been shown previously—that lesions in this location are difficult to diagnose early in their course. In spite of delay in diagnosis, 44% of the 53 patients studied lived for 10 years. The more frequent use of CT may assist in earlier diagnosis. Surgical extirpation is the only option for cure. Chemotherapy and radiation are ineffective.

F.G. Moody, M.D.

The Continuing Clinical Dilemma of Primary Tumors of the Small Intestine

Ciresi DL, Scholten DJ (Butterworth Hosp, Grand Rapids, Mich; Michigan State Univ, Grand Rapids)
Am Surg 61:698–702, 1995

3–17

Introduction.—Even with modern imaging techniques, it is difficult to diagnose primary tumors of the small intestine, which have often reached an advanced stage by the time treatment begins. Although these tumors are relatively rare, they account for approximately 900 cancer-related deaths per year in the United States. Differences were sought between benign and malignant tumors of the small intestine, and between symptomatic and asymptomatic tumors, in terms of their clinical presentation, diagnosis, and surgical management.

Patients and Findings.—Forty-nine patients who were treated for neoplasms of the small intestine over a 12-year period at one hospital were studied retrospectively. Most patients were aged 60 to 70. There were 32 malignant and 17 benign tumors. Acute GI bleeding was more common with benign tumors, occurring in 29% vs. 6% of the cases. Forty-seven percent of the benign tumors were asymptomatic, compared with 6% of the malignant tumors. Abdominal pain was present in 63% of the patients with malignancies, compared with 24% of those with benign tumors. Thirty-eight percent of the patients with malignant tumors had a history of weight loss, compared with none of the patients with benign tumors. The average number of diagnostic tests performed per patient was 2.3, and the symptoms were present for an average of 30 weeks before resection.

Results.—The most sensitive diagnostic techniques were upper GI endoscopy, angiography, and upper GI contrast studies. Operative treatment ranged from biopsy or excision to limited bowel resection, segmental resection with regional lymphadenectomy, and bypass procedures. Forty-one percent of the benign tumors were leiomyomas, and 53% of the malignancies were adenocarcinomas. Fifty-six percent of the patients with malignant tumors had positive lymph nodes at the time of surgery.

Conclusions.—The nonspecific clinical presentation of small intestinal tumors contributes to the difficulty of diagnosing them. Early clinical suspicion is needed to detect these tumors in patients with vague abdominal complaints. Patients may need multiple diagnostic procedures before undergoing surgery, which is the mainstay of treatment for both benign and malignant tumors of the small intestine.

▶ The take-home message is clear; small-bowel tumors, whether benign or malignant, are hard to diagnose. Benign tumors tend to bleed but are by and large asymptomatic. Malignant tumors are associated with abdominal pain and weight loss. In my experience, weight loss is the most important predictor of an organic basis for GI complaints. This is an important point to emphasize because primary care physicians may be tempted to join their patients in denying a serious reason for the patients' complaints.

F.G. Moody, M.D.

20 Small Bowel Transplantation

Small Bowel Transplantation: A Life-saving Option for Selected Patients With Intestinal Failure

Asfar S, Atkison P, Ghent C, et al (Univ Hosp, London, Ont, Canada; Children's Hosp of Western Ontario, London, Canada; Univ of Montreal)

Dig Dis Sci 41:875–883, 1996   3–18

Background.—Although home total parenteral nutrition is life-saving in patients with chronic intestinal failure, it has many disadvantages. An alternative is intestinal transplantation. With the use of tacrolimus (FK 506), a new immunosuppressant, outcomes associated with bowel transplantation have improved. One experience with 16 intestinal transplants was reviewed.

Methods and Outcomes.—The 16 patients transplanted were among 37 patients wait-listed for small bowel transplantation. The other 15 died while waiting for a donor. Immune suppression was achieved with cyclosporine in 6 patients and tacrolimus in 10. Patients receiving combined liver and small bowel grafts had lower graft rejection rates than those receiving isolated transplants. All the patients given cyclosporine died. Their median survival was 25.7 months. Two of these patients lived for more than 5 years. Patients receiving tacrolimus had fewer infections and a shorter hospital stay. Only 2 of these patients died. Median survival in this group was 13 months. Seven of 8 long-term survivors have stopped IV feedings.

Conclusion.—In patients with intestinal failure who cannot be maintained on total parenteral nutrition, small bowel transplantation is a life-saving option, allowing patients to maintain normal oral nutrition. Although the morbidity and mortality associated with this procedure are still higher than with other solid organ transplants, outcomes are improving steadily.

▶ Tacrolimus immunosuppression has done for small bowel transplantation what cyclosporine did for liver transplantation. It provides hope that transplantation will become a mainstream therapy for intestinal invalids who are at the end of their tolerance of total parenteral nutrition.

F.G. Moody, M.D.

21 Enteroscopy in Occult Bleeding

Complete Intraoperative Small-bowel Endoscopy in the Evaluation of Occult Gastrointestinal Bleeding Using the Sonde Enteroscope
Lopez MJ, Cooley JS, Petros JG, et al (Tufts Univ, Boston)
Arch Surg 131:272–277, 1996

3–19

Background.—It can be difficult, frustrating, and expensive to localize the site of chronic occult GI bleeding. In patients with chronic, slow bleeding of presumed small intestinal origin, enteroscopy is the main method of investigation. The authors have successfully detected bleeding from the small intestine using the Sonde enteroscope. A further experience with this technique is reported.

Methods.—16 consecutive patients were referred for evaluation of occult GI bleeding. In each patient, esophagogastroduodenoscopy, push enteroscopy, and colonoscopy had been unable to identify the bleeding site, and 14 patients had required 1 or more transfusions. Intraoperative enteroscopy was performed using a Sonde enteroscope with an outer diameter of 5 mm, a working length of 279 cm, and a 120-degree field of view. The enteroscopic examination was performed after exploratory laparotomy, including visualization and palpation of the stomach, duodenum, and large and small intestine. The completeness of visualization and the diagnostic accuracy of the procedure were evaluated. Complications of Sonde enteroscopy were recorded, and the patients were followed up for recurrent bleeding.

Findings.—All patients underwent enteroscopy of the entire small intestine, with the endoscope passing into the ascending colon or beyond. The cause of bleeding was detected by Sonde enteroscopy in 14 patients: 3 had ileal angiodysplasia; 6 had ileal ulcers; 2 had neoplasia; and 1 each had ileal ulcers caused by Crohn's disease, small intestinal enteropathy, and varices resulting from portal hypertension and radiation stricture. No abnormalities were detected in the other 2 patients. The identified bleeding sites were managed by small-bowel resection or oversewing. The only postoperative complications were 1 case of prolonged ileus and 1 case of small-bowel obstruction that resolved without surgery. Bleeding recurred after surgery in 2 of the patients with angiodysplasia.

Conclusions.—In patients with occult GI bleeding, intraoperative Sonde enteroscopy can safely and effectively identify bleeding sites in the small intestine. This technique permits complete visualization of the small-bowel mucosa while avoiding the trauma associated with push endoscopy. Sonde enteroscopy is the procedure of choice in patients with occult GI bleeding of presumed small intestinal origin, although its success relies on close cooperation between the surgery and gastroenterology teams.

▶ Identifying not only the site but also the level of occult GI bleeding remains problematic. Using a combined transoral and transabdominal technique for examining the small bowel, the offending lesion was found in 14 of 16 patients. The key to success was the Sonde enteroscope, an instrument of sufficient length to allow careful dissection of the lining of the entire small bowel as it is segmented by the exploring hands of the surgeon.

F.G. Moody, M.D.

22 Short Bowel Syndrome: Role of Cholecystectomy

The Role of Prophylactic Cholecystectomy in the Short-bowel Syndrome

Thompson JS (Univ of Nebraska, Omaha)

Arch Surg 131:556–560, 1996

3–20

Background.—Cholelithiasis develops in 30% to 40% of patients with the short-bowel syndrome. The factors associated with this complication and the role of prophylactic cholecystectomy in patients with short-bowel syndrome were investigated.

Methods.—Fifty consecutive patients older than 16 years of age seen during a 15-year period were included in the retrospective clinical review. All had intestinal remnants of less than 180 cm.

Findings.—Prophylactic cholecystectomy was done in 10% of the patients. Another 20% died with no evidence of gallstones within 30 days. Biliary disease developed in 31% of the remaining 35 patients at risk. Six of these patients had inflammatory complications or common bile duct stones. Biliary disease was more likely to develop in patients with intestinal remnant lengths of less than 120 cm, an absent ileocecal junction, long-term total parenteral nutrition, and Crohn's disease. Initial mortality rate among patients with mesenteric vascular disease was 50%. The incidence of biliary disease in these patients was 38%. The initial mortality rate in patients with cancer and/or irradiation was 7%. No biliary disease occurred in this group. Patients with benign conditions had a 57% incidence of cholelithiasis.

Conclusion.—The risk for cholelithiasis in patients with small-bowel syndrome is significant when the intestinal remnant length is less than 120 cm, total parenteral nutrition is needed, and the terminal ileum is resected. Patients with benign conditions expected to have a long-term survival benefit from prophylactic cholecystectomy. Such prophylaxis should also be considered in patients with mesenteric vascular disease who may have a high incidence of early biliary problems despite significantly shortened survival.

▶ This retrospective analysis of the incidence of gallstone and biliary tract disease in patients with short-bowel syndrome identifies a subpopulation of patients who would benefit from a prophylactic cholecystectomy. Length (less than 120 cm), parenteral nutrition, and lack of an ileocecal valve are the relevant risk factors.

F.G. Moody, M.D.

23 Meckel's Diverticulum

Meckel's Diverticulum in Amsterdam: Experience in 136 Patients
Bemelman WA, Hugenholtz E, Heij HA, et al (Univ of Amsterdam; Free Univ of Amsterdam; Onze Lieve Vrouwe Gasthuis, Amsterdam)
World J Surg 19:734–737, 1995   3–21

Objective.—The medical charts of 136 patients with Meckel's diverticulum were examined retrospectively to determine whether a relationship exists between symptoms of the diverticulum and ectopic tissue, patient age, and patient gender. Findings were used to develop guidelines for the management of incidentally found Meckel's diverticulum.

Patients and Methods.—The patients had been surgically treated at 5 hospitals in Amsterdam from 1970 to 1992. Patient charts were analyzed for age, gender, medical history, and whether diverticula were symptomatic or asymptomatic. The patients ranged from 0 to 83 years of age (mean 24.9 years); 82 were male and 54 were female.

Results.—Surgery was performed in 51 patients because of diverticulum-related symptoms. In the other 85 patients, Meckel's diverticula were found during laparotomy for appendicitis (58%), congenital anomaly (14%), abdominal malignancy (6%), or bowel obstruction (6%). Patients with symptomatic diverticula were significantly younger (mean 16.8 years) than those with incidentally resected diverticula (mean 29.8 years). Males outnumbered females in the symptomatic group (ratio 3:1), and males were 2 to 4 times more likely to have complications from Meckel's diverticulum. Symptoms were most often caused by obstruction from bands and torsion (39%). Perforation occurred primarily in patients 10 to 30 years of age, and obstruction in patients younger than 10 years of age. The presence of ectopic gastric tissue was associated with hemorrhage and perforation.

Conclusion.—The presence of ectopic gastric tissue, found most often in symptomatic diverticula, was a risk factor for complications in patients with Meckel's diverticulum. Resection should be undertaken in patients younger than 30 years of age who have incidentally discovered diverticula, and in older patients with suspected ectopic gastric tissue. Symptoms caused by bands or ectopic tissue occur predominantly in younger, male patients. Instead of removing diverticula with adhesive bands, the diverticula bands can simply be cut.

▶ This review of the surgical management of Meckel's diverticulum from 1 geographic area provides interesting and useful information. Most complications appear to be associated with adhesive bands or ectopic gastric mucosa within the diverticulum, and if problems are to occur, they usually do so in males before 30 years of age. I will have to think about the recommendation that all such diverticula be excised if encountered coincidental to celiotomy, because the increase in use of laparoscopy for diagnostic purposes may lead to a large number of diverticulectomies and their associated morbidity. The key is to further refine the techniques that help to identify the patients who have gastric heterotopia.

F.G. Moody, M.D.

24 Miscellaneous

Prevention of Postoperative Abdominal Adhesions by a Sodium Hyaluronate-based Bioresorbable Membrane: A Prospective, Randomized, Double-blind Multicenter Study
Becker JM, Dayton MT, Fazio VW, et al (Boston Univ; Univ Hosp, Salt Lake City, Utah; Cleveland Clinic Found, Ohio; et al)
J Am Coll Surg 183:297–306, 1996   3–22

Introduction.—Intraperitoneal adhesions occur in 67% to 93% of general surgical abdominal operations and up to 97% of open gynecologic pelvic procedures. A sodium hyaluronate and carboxymethylcellulose bioresorbable membrane (HA membrane) has been found to reduce the frequency and severity of postsurgical adhesions in several animal models. The incidence of adhesions was evaluated with and without the HA membrane in patients undergoing colectomy and ileal pouch anastomosis with diverting-loop ileostomy with a required staged second operation to close the ileostomy in a prospective, randomized, double-blind, multicenter investigation.

Methods.—A total of 183 patients with ulcerative colitis or familial polyposis from 11 centers were randomly assigned to receive or not receive the HA membrane placed under the midline incision before closure of the surgical wound. At the time of ileostomy closure 8 to 12 weeks later, laparoscopy was performed to evaluate the incidence, extent, and severity of adhesion formation to the midline incision.

Results.—Fourteen and 8 patients in the control and HA membrane groups had pre-existing adhesions, respectively. Assessable data were available for 175 of 183 patients. There was a highly significant between-group difference ($P < 0.00000000001$) in the incidence of 1 or more adhesions to the midline incision (94% in the control group versus 49% in the HA membrane group). Five of 90 patients in the control group had no evidence of adhesions, compared to 43 of 85 patients in the HA membrane group. The mean percent of involved incision length was significantly greater in the control group, compared to the HA membrane group (63% versus 23%). Fifty-two patients (58%) in the control group had dense adhesions, compared to 13 patients (15%) in the HA membrane group. There were no significant between-group differences in the incidence of adverse postoperative events.

Conclusion.—This is the first known controlled, prospective, randomized, blinded, multicenter trial conducted to evaluate comprehensively the postoperative formation and prevention of abdominal adhesions after general abdominal surgery using standardized direct peritoneal visualization. Use of the HA membrane in patients undergoing abdominal surgery may result in reduced risk associated with abdominal wall adhesions.

▶ Wow! One does not often obtain the scientific blessing of an 11–decimal-point *P* value. In fact, the results speak for themselves. The bioabsorbable membrane almost prevents adhesions to the abdominal wound. If the material is appropriately priced, it should gain wide acceptance, especially in cases such as the ones selected here, in which adhesion formation is common and can be devastating.

F.G. Moody, M.D.

PART FOUR

THE COLON

Introduction

This section contains 2 articles about infectious enterides, the first of which concerns a wide-spread outbreak of salmonella infections from ice cream. The second article details an outbreak of gastroenteritis caused by *Listeria monocytogenes*, a pathogen not commonly linked with gastrointestinal disturbances. Seven articles concern Crohn's disease and related topics. An offspring or a sibling of a patient with Crohn's disease has approximately a 10% chance of Crohn's disease developing. The disease appears at a younger age in offspring, and there is a high correlation between parent and offspring in site of disease. A provocative article on therapy of Crohn's disease with fish oil capsules will no doubt trigger intensive investigation of this treatment modality. Six articles relate to ulcerative colitis, including 2 articles regarding medical treatment with 5-aminosalicylic acid analogues. The extensive experience of the Oxford group in treating patients with severe ulcerative colitis is captured in a fine article in which clinical response to an intensive treatment regimen during 3–7 days was found to accurately identify patients who would be more likely to undergo colectomy. Fourteen articles concern colorectal cancer and other neoplasms. Three articles relate to screening. An important article compares the sensitivity of colonoscopy with barium enema; colonoscopy appears to be a more effective diagnostic modality, especially in Dukes' A–type lesions. The data obtained indicate, however, that colonoscopy still misses approximately 5% of lesions that should be detected. The risk of colorectal cancer in families of patients with polyps is clearly increased, especially if the index case has polyps diagnosed before age 60. Whereas it was formerly believed that diminutive (less than 5 mm) and small (6–10 mm) polyps detected during flexible sigmoidoscopy are unlikely to be associated with more proximal lesions, the article in this section indicates that as many as 29% of patients with diminutive or small polyps may be harboring more proximal lesions. Indeed, 4 patients with diminutive or small polyps were found to be harboring carcinomatous lesions. A provocative report details that approximately 20% of patients with acromegaly were found to have colonic polyps, although none of the patients was found to have invasive carcinoma. Other articles concern diverticular disease, bowel dysfunction, spinal cord injury, and visible rectal bleeding in a population of patients presenting to primary care physicians. The latter report was striking in that 24% of patients who reported visible rectal bleeding to their primary care physicians were found to have a serious problem.

Norton J. Greenberger, M.D.

25 Physiology and Pathophysiology

Adhesion Molecule-1 (CAM-1) and Neutrophil Adhesion

Infection of Human Intestinal Epithelial Cells With Invasive Bacteria Upregulates Apical Intercellular Adhesion Molecule-1 (ICAM-1) Expression and Neutrophil Adhesion

Huang GT-J, Eckmann L, Savidge TC, et al (Univ of California, San Diego; Babraham Inst, Cambridge, England)
J Clin Invest 98:572–583, 1996   4–1

Background.—To infect a host by way of the gastrointestinal tract, pathogenic bacteria must gain access to the mucosa by penetrating the overlying epithelial surface. These intestinal epithelial cells function as an integral part of the mucosal immune system in addition to being a physical barrier. The host responds to bacterial invasion with accumulation of neutrophils in the lamina propria and transmigration of neutrophils to the luminal side of the crypts. Little is known about the molecules expressed by epithelial cells that are involved in this process. The finding that intercellular adhesion molecule type 1 (ICAM-1) expression on human colon epithelial cells and enterocytes is upregulated in response to bacterial invasion in vivo is reported.

Findings.—Four to 9 hours after infection, ICAM-1 expression increases, apparently in response to a direct interaction between host epithelial cells and the invading bacteria. It colocalized to cells invaded by bacteria; soluble factor release by epithelial cells seemed to play only a minor role in increasing ICAM-1 expression. Expression of ICAM-1 occurred on the apical side of polarized intestinal epithelial cells, and neutrophil adhesion to these cells was increased.

Discussion.—The ICAM-1 response allows for neutrophils that have transmigrated through the epithelial cell layer to adhere to the luminal side of the epithelium and form a barrier to further invasion. The intestinal epithelial cells are thus involved in the postinfection inflammatory process at several steps: secretion of chemoattractant cytokines and cytokines that activate neutrophils and other inflammatory cells, transmigration of neutrophils from the mucosa to the intestinal lumen, and formation of a neutrophil barrier on the epithelial surface.

▶ I selected this article because it provides new insights explaining how epithelial cells are involved in several steps of the inflammatory process following bacterial invasion. Intercellular adhesion molecule type 1 in human colon epithelial cell lines and human enterocytes is upregulated in response to bacterial invasion, which in turn results in increased neutrophil adhesion to these cells and ostensibly into the intestinal lumen.

For an additional reference on mucosal factors inducing neutrophil movement in colonic mucosa see the article by Cole et al.[1]

N.J. Greenberger, M.D.

Reference

1. Cole AT, Pekington BJ, McLaughlan J, et al: Mucosal factors inducing neutrophil movement in ulcerative colitis: The role of interleukin 8 and leukotriene B_4. *Gut* 39:248–254, 1996.

Opioid Receptor in Human Colon Cancer

Identification and Characterization of ζ-Opioid Receptor in Human Colon Cancer
Hytrek SD, Smith JP, McGarrity TJ, et al (Pennsylvania State Univ, Hershey)
Am J Physiol 271:R115–R121, 1996
4–2

Introduction.—Various endogenous growth factors may play a role in the development of cancers of the gastrointestinal tract and other neoplasia. Experimental studies in nude mice have shown that [Met⁵]enkephalin, termed opioid growth factor (OGF), inhibits the growth of human colon cancer in receptor-mediated fashion. However, little is known about the opioid receptor or receptors involved in this growth regulation. Receptor binding assays were performed to identify the receptor responsible for the effects of OGF on human colon cancer xenografts.

Findings.—Ligand binding assays were performed using HT-29 human colon cancer tissues and [³H][Met⁵]enkephalin. These studies showed specific and saturable binding. On Scatchard analysis, the data suggested a single binding site with a binding affinity of 15 nmol and a binding capacity of 365 fmol/mg protein. Binding was restricted to the nuclear fraction on subcellular fractionation studies. The ligand that most effectively displaced [³H][Met⁵]enkephalin was cold [Met⁵]enkephalin. In addition, resected specimens of large-bowel adenocarcinoma showed binding to radiolabeled [Met⁵]enkephalin.

Conclusions.—Taken together, these findings suggest that the ζ-opioid receptor is the receptor responsible for the growth-regulatory effects of OGF in colon cancer. The identification of this receptor could provide important clues to the causes and pathogenesis of colon cancer. The available evidence suggests that the primary defect in HT-29 colon cancer is with the peptide rather than the receptor. Cellular and molecular studies of the ζ-receptor and OGF are needed.

▶ Human colon cancer has a receptor for [Met[5]]enkephalin (opioid growth factor OGF), a substance that inhibits the growth of human colon cancer when it has been implanted in nude mice. The authors speculate that changes in the activity of this opioid receptor could lead to profound changes in the factors that control epithelial cell growth and death within colonocytes. In fact, exogenous OGF inhibits experimental tumor growth. This sounds like a promising lead in attempts to understand and prevent or treat colon cancer.

F.G. Moody, M.D.

Gas and Abdominal Bloating

The Relation of Passage of Gas and Abdominal Bloating to Colonic Gas Production

Levitt MD, Furne J, Olsson S (Veterans Affairs Med Ctr, Minneapolis)
Ann Intern Med 124:422–424, 1996   4–3

Introduction.—It has always been difficult to determine what is considered "too much gas." The physician is generally forced to rely on the patient's assessment, which results in uninformative radiographic and endoscopic tests. Rectal gas passage and sensations of abdominal bloating were monitored in 25 healthy participants who were given 2 laxatives associated with symptoms of gaseous distress.

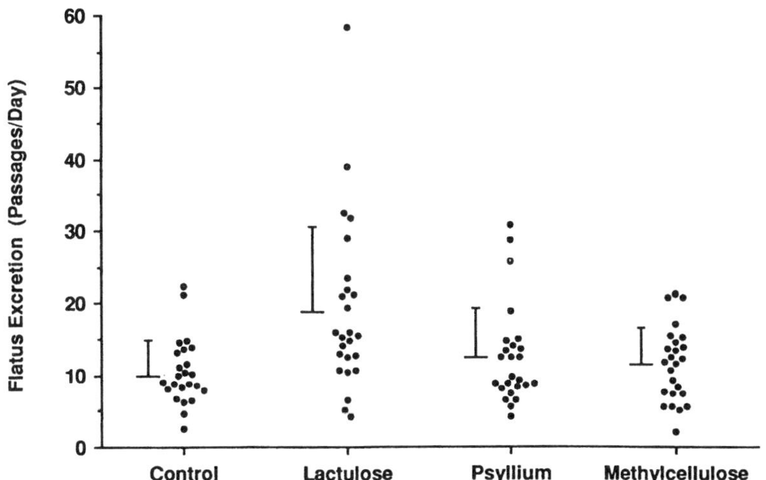

FIGURE 1.—Average daily frequency of flatus passage. The mean value plus 1 SD for all 24 participants during the 1-week control period and weeks during which the diet was supplemented with lactulose, psyllium, or methylcellulose is shown. (Courtesy of Levitt MD, Furne J, Olsson S: The relation of passage of gas and abdominal bloating to colonic gas production. *Ann Intern Med* 124:422–424, 1996.)

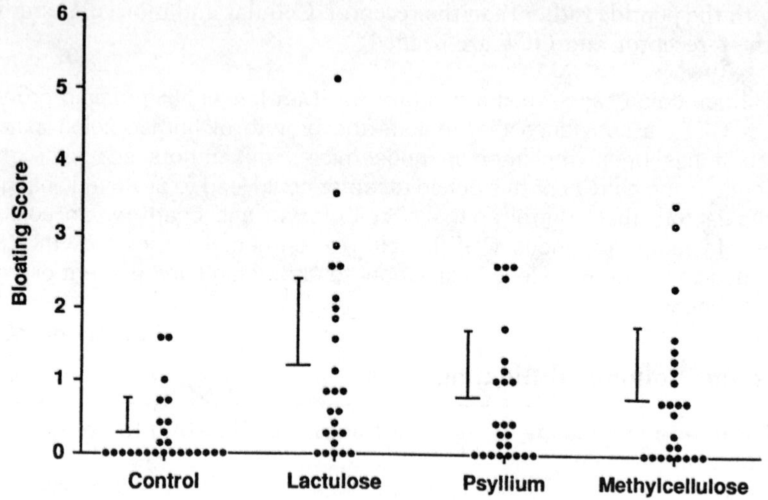

FIGURE 2.—Average daily score (sum of noon and bedtime scores) for abdominal bloating. The mean value plus 1 SD for all 25 participants during the 1-week control period and the weeks during which the diet was supplemented with lactulose, psyllium, and methylcellulose is shown. (Courtesy of Levitt MD, Furne J, Olsson S: The relation of passage of gas and abdominal bloating to colonic gas production. *Ann Intern Med* 124:422–424, 1996.)

Methods.—Twenty-five healthy participants were given either placebo, psyllium (a fermentable fiber), or methylcellulose (a nonfermentable fiber). The participants had no previous history of bowel distress, and they were tested for 2-week periods followed by a 1-week washout period. The participants recorded their flatus passage, sensations of abdominal bloating, and impressions of flatus volume. In 5 participants, the influence of the fiber preparation on breath hydrogen excretion, an indicator of hydrogen production in the colon, was recorded.

Results.—During the placebo period, participants passed gas 10 ± 5.0 times per day. While taking lactulose, the participants reported a significant increase in gas passages (19 ± 12 times per day) and increased rectal gas (Fig 1). The participants did not record an increase with the other 2 fiber preparations. After ingestion of either of the fibers, breath hydrogen excretion did not increase. While taking the fiber preparations and the lactulose, the participants reported a statistically significant increase in feelings of abdominal bloating (Fig 2). They perceived this as excessive gas in the bowel.

Conclusion.—Increased gas production is not always responsible for the symptoms commonly attributed to excess intestinal gas. Excessive rectal gas would be treated by limiting the supply of fermentable material to the colonic bacteria, whereas symptoms of bloating usually indicate irritable bowel syndrome.

▶ As Levitt and colleagues point out in the introduction to this study, few medical problems are approached in a less scientific fashion than in the common symptoms of "too much gas." This carefully done investigation demonstrates that symptoms commonly attributed to intestinal gas do not necessarily reflect increased gas production. The studies with psyllium and methylcellulose indicate that there is a *dissociation* between bloating and intestinal gas. Bloating is unrelated to excessive gas production and may respond to promotility drugs. Conversely, excessive rectal gas indicates excessive gas production, and the approach to treatment of this problem is to limit the dietary intake of fermentable carbohydrate.

N.J. Greenberger, M.D.

26 Infectious Enterides

Salmonella

A National Outbreak of *Salmonella enteritidis* Infections From Ice Cream
Hennessy TW, and the Investigation Team (Minnesota Dept of Health, Minneapolis; Centers for Disease Control and Prevention, Atlanta, Ga; Food and Drug Administration, Minneapolis; et al)
N Engl J Med 334:1281–1286, 1996   4–4

Background.—The Public Health Laboratories for the Minnesota Department of Health received a sudden increase in *Salmonella enteritidis* isolates in southeastern Minnesota in September 1994, prompting an investigation of the source.

Methods.—In a case-control study, cases were patients with confirmed *S. enteritidis* infection in September 1994 in southeastern Minnesota, and control subjects were chosen with matching for age and area of residence (by telephone exchange). When Schwan's ice cream, eaten by 73% of the cases and only 13% of the controls, was identified as the only risk factor for infection, the product was recalled. Data was then obtained from the national salmonella surveillance system at the Centers for Disease Control and Prevention on patients with *S. enteritidis* infection within 1 week of eating Schwan's ice cream. Adults in 200 randomly selected Minnesota households were interviewed in October 1994 to collect data on the recent history of diarrheal illness and the products eaten. From these data, the attack rate was calculated for eating Schwan's ice cream. To identify the source of salmonellosis in the manufacturing process, environmental samples were obtained and cultured from the ice cream plant, tanker trailers that carried ice cream premix, and the facilities producing the premix.

Results.—Consumption of Schwan's ice cream was associated with an attack rate of 6.6%. At the time of the outbreak, 87% of Schwan's ice cream was distributed outside Minnesota. Therefore, it was estimated that *S. enteritidis* gastroenteritis developed in 224,000 individuals nationwide after they ate Schwan's ice cream. There were no sources of salmonella contamination found in the ice cream plant or the facilities producing the premix. However, some of the tanker trailers transporting the premix had previously carried nonpasteurized liquid eggs. There was a dose-response relationship between the premix transported by these tanker trailers and ice cream associated with salmonella infection. These ice cream products had the highest level of *S. enteritidis.*

Conclusions.—The nationwide outbreak of *S. enteritidis* gastroenteritis was caused by consuming ice cream that was contaminated during transport of the pasteurized ice cream premix in tanker trailers that had previously transported nonpasteurized liquid eggs infected with *S. enteritidis.* It is recommended that food products not expected to be repasteurized should be transported only in dedicated containers and that surveillance of foodborne illness be increased.

▶ The estimate that *S. enteritidis* gastroenteritis developed in 224,000 individuals after they ate ice cream is mind-boggling. Further, the attack rate for consumers was estimated to be 6.6%. As the authors emphasize, foodborne diseases continue to present a major challenge to public health authorities. In carrying out basic functions such as detecting and controlling outbreaks, clinical surveillance is obviously important, and such surveillance initially requires that clinicians have a high index of suspicion, order appropriate laboratory tests, and perhaps most importantly, report positive results to appropriate public health agencies. There needs to be more dissemination of information regarding potential foodborne illnesses among the public and health care providers. This might well encourage appropriate microbiologic testing in suspected cases.

N.J. Greenberger, M.D.

Listeria Monocytogenes

An Outbreak of Gastroenteritis and Fever Due to *Listeria monocytogenes* in Milk
Dalton CB, Austin CC, Sobel J, et al (Natl Ctr for Infectious Diseases, Atlanta, Ga; Ctrs for Disease Control and Prevention, Atlanta, Ga; Illinois Dept of Public Health, Springfield; et al)
N Engl J Med 336:100–105, 1997   4–5

Background.—In 1994, an outbreak of gastroenteritis and fever occurred among attendees of a picnic in Illinois. Complaints about the taste of commercial pasteurized milk served at the picnic prompted investigations that resulted in the culture of *Listeria monocytogenes* in milk samples.

Methods.—Picnic attendees were interviewed, and surveillance for invasive listeriosis was implemented in the states receiving milk from the dairy implicated. Stool, milk, and serum samples were analyzed.

Findings.—The symptoms of 45 persons met the case definition for illness from *L. monocytogenes.* Stool cultures from 11 persons were found to contain the organism. Illness occurring in the week after the picnic was associated with chocolate milk intake. Diarrhea and fever were the most common symptoms. Four patients were admitted to the hospital. The median infection incubation period was 20 hours. Levels of antibody to listeriolysin O were increased in individuals who became ill. Isolates from stool specimens from patients who became ill after the picnic, from sterile sites in another 3 patients found by surveillance, from the milk samples, and from a tank drain at the dairy all were serotype 1/2b. These isolates were indistinguishable on multilocus enzyme electrophoresis, ribotyping, and DNA macrorestriction analysis.

Conclusions.—*L. monocytogenes* can cause gastroenteritis with fever. Sporadic cases of invasive listeriosis may be related to unrecognized outbreaks caused by contaminated food.

▶ *Listeria* infection previously has not been recognized as a primary gastrointestinal illness. Dalton and colleagues now provide clear evidence that a gastroenteritis syndrome characterized by fever, chills, diarrhea, abdominal cramps, and nausea can occur after the ingestion of food contaminated by *L. monocytogenes*. That chocolate milk was the vehicle of infection in this outbreak underscores the role of contaminated dairy products in still another food-borne infection. As I read the report, I was struck by the numerous breaks in recommended procedures for processing, packaging, and distributing the milk—in short, poor sanitation practices.

N.J. Greenberger, M.D.

27 Crohn's Disease and Related Topics

Hereditary Influences

Crohn's Disease: Concordance for Site and Clinical Type in Affected Family Members: Potential Hereditary Influences
Bayless TM, Tokayer AZ, Polito JM II, et al (Johns Hopkins Univ, Baltimore, Md; Johns Hopkins Hosp, Baltimore, Md)
Gastroenterology 111:573–579, 1996   4–6

Background.—Crohn's disease, a form of idiopathic inflammatory bowel disease, is presumed to have genetic and environmental influences. A greater understanding of the genetic heterogeneity of inflammatory bowel disease may be provided by the relationship of genetic influences between bowel location and clinical type of Crohn's disease. Familial occurrences of Crohn's disease were investigated to determine concordance of site and type.

Methods and Findings.—Seventeen percent of 554 consecutive patients with documented Crohn's disease had a family history of the disorder. Eighty-six percent of the 60 families investigated were concordant in at least 2 members for disease site. Eighty-two percent were concordant for clinical type. When family members were paired together, a greater-than-expected concordance was evident. A conditional logistic regression model indicated that concordance significantly predicted disease site and type in other affected family members.

Conclusions.—The finding that relatives had a greater-than-expected concordance for site and clinical type of Crohn's disease is consistent with the concept of multiple, distinct forms (possibly phenotypes) of this disease. Participants in genetic, pathophysiologic, and therapeutic trials should be stratified for site and type of disease, as differences in sites of involvement and clinical types may represent different diseases in the Crohn's spectrum.

▶ A large number of studies have shown a universal prevalence of inflammatory bowel disease (IBD) among relatives of patients with Crohn's disease and ulcerative colitis. Collectively these studies indicate that IBD is at least partly determined by genetic predisposition. The risk of having Crohn's disease if a patient or sibling is affected is approximately 10%. Several recent studies have evaluated familial aggregation of IBD and 3 are summarized below.

Colombel et al.[1] compared the age of onset and the clinical features of Crohn's disease between patients with familial disease and those with sporadic disease and concordance for disease location and type in 176 patients with familial Crohn's disease and 1,377 patients with sporadic nonfamilial Crohn's disease. Patients with familial Crohn's disease were characterized by (1) an early age of onset; (2) more extensive disease; and (3) more frequent involvement of both small bowel and colonic disease. In families with more than 2 affected members, 83% were concordant for disease location and 75% for disease type.

Peeters et al.[2] studied 40 patients with Crohn's disease and 800 control subjects. Probands with Crohn's disease more frequently had a positive family history than controls. Age at diagnosis was younger for offspring than parents and initial disease location was especially striking between siblings.

Lee et al. studied IBD in 67 families each with 3 or more affected relations.[3] When IBD affected successive generations, disease in parents was diagnosed at a later age than in children. In concert with other studies a significant association between smoking and Crohn's disease and nonsmoking with ulcerative colitis was found.

N.J. Greenberger, M.D.

References

1. Colombel JF, Grandbastin B, Gower-Rausscau C, et al: Clinical characteristics of Crohn's disease in 72 families. *Gastroenterology* 111:604–607, 1996.
2. Peeters M, Nevans H, Baert F, et al: Familial aggregation in Crohn's disease: Increased age-adjusted risk and concordance in clinical characteristics. *Gastroenterology* 111:597–603, 1996.
3. Lee JE, Lennard-Jass JE: Inflammatory bowel disease in 67 families each with three or more affected first-degree relatives. *Gastroenterology* 111:587–596, 1996.

Medical Treatment

Effect of an Enteric-coated Fish-oil Preparation on Relapses in Crohn's Disease
Belluzzi A, Brignola C, Campieri M, et al (Univ of Bologna, Italy; S Giovanni Battista Hosp, Turin, Italy)
N Engl J Med 334:1557–1560, 1996   4–7

Objective.—The anti-inflammatory actions of fish oil could make it useful in patients with inflammatory bowel disease and other inflammatory diseases. However, the unpleasant taste and gastrointestinal side effects of fish oil have limited its use. New enteric-coated fish oil preparations reduce side effects and increase compliance, thus making long-term fish-oil treatment feasible. Enteric-coated fish oil was tested for its ability to reduce the frequency of relapses in patients with Crohn's disease.

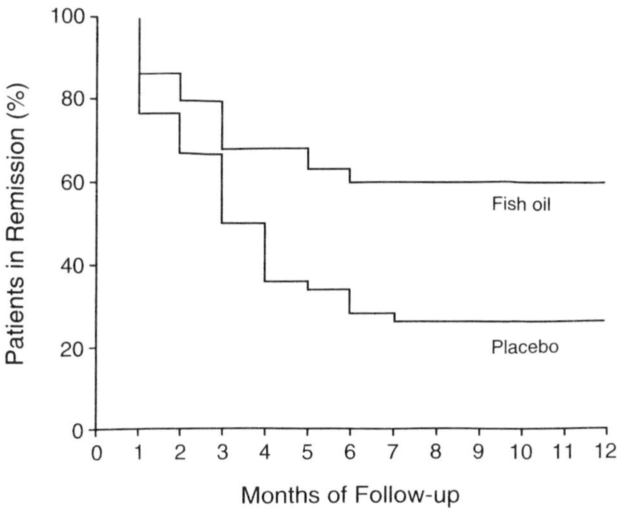

FIGURE 1.—Life-table curves showing the percentage of all randomized patients who remained in clinical remission during the 1-year treatment period. There were 39 patients in each group. *P* = 0.006 for the comparison of the 2 groups by log-rank analysis. (Courtesy of Belluzzi A, Brignola C, Campieri M, et al: Effect of an enteric-coated fish-oil preparation on relapses in Crohn's disease. *N Engl J Med* 334:1557–1560. Copyright 1996, Massachusetts Medical Society. Reprinted by permission of *The New England Journal of Medicine*. All rights reserved.)

Methods.—The double-blind, placebo-controlled trial included 78 patients with Crohn's disease who were considered at high risk for relapse. The patients were randomly assigned to receive either 9 enteric-coated fish-oil capsules per day—for a total dose of 2.7 g of n-3 fatty acids—or the same number of placebo capsules. The enteric coating was designed to resist gastric acid for at least 30 minutes, so that the capsules disintegrated in the small intestine. The 2 groups were compared for clinical relapse rate at up to 1 year.

Results.—Relapse rates were 28% in the fish-oil group vs. 69% in the placebo group; the difference was 41%, with a 95% confidence interval of 21% to 61% (Fig 1). Five patients dropped out in the fish-oil group—most because of diarrhea—compared with 2 in the placebo group (Table 2). The percentage of patients still in remission at 1 year was 59% in the fish-oil group vs. 26% in the placebo group. Fish oil was the only significant predictor of the likelihood of relapse on logistic regression analysis; the odds ratio of relapse for the placebo group was 4.2, with a 95% confidence interval of 1.6–10.7.

Conclusions.—Enteric-coated fish-oil capsules may reduce the relapse rate for high-risk patients with Crohn's disease. Further studies are needed to compare its effectiveness with that of mesalamine, the current treatment. The effectiveness of fish oil may be related to its ability to inhibit thromboxane A_2 production, which is elevated in the intestinal mucosa of patients with Crohn's disease.

TABLE 2.—Clinical Results During Treatment With Fish Oil or Placebo in Patients With Crohn's Disease in Remission

Variable	Placebo	Fish Oil
	no. (%)	
Outcome*		
Total no. of patients	39	39
Lost to follow-up	1 (3)	1 (3)
Withdrew because of diarrhea	1 (3)	4 (10)
Remained in remission	10 (26)	23 (59)
Relapse	27 (69)	11 (28)
Major symptoms in patients with relapse		
Total no. of patients	27	11
Diarrhea (>4 liquid stools/day)	23 (85)	10 (91)
Moderate or severe abdominal pain	25 (93)	10 (91)
Fever (temperature, >37.7°C)	12 (44)	3 (27)
General condition poor or very poor	27 (100)	11 (100)
Arthritis	14 (52)	6 (55)

*Because of rounding, percentages do not total 100 for the placebo group.

(Courtesy of Belluzzi A, Brignola C, Campieri M, et al: Effect of an enteric-coated fish-oil preparation on relapses in Crohn's disease. *N Engl J Med* 334:1557–1560. Copyright 1996, Massachusetts Medical Society. Reprinted by permission of *The New England Journal of Medicine*. All rights reserved.)

▶ These results indicate that a novel coated fish-oil preparation containing largely eicosapentaenoic and docosahexaenoic acids is an effective, well-tolerated treatment that prevents clinical relapse in patients with Crohn's disease in remission. Belluzi and colleagues found a remarkable reduction in the frequency of relapse; after 1 year, 59% of the patients in the fish-oil group remained in remission, compared with only 26% in the placebo group. The rationale for fish oil as a treatment for a chronic inflammatory disease such as Crohn's disease lies in its anti-inflammatory effects, which may lead to reduced production of leukotriene B, thromboxane A_2, and tumor necrosis factor.

It will be interesting to compare fish oil with other treatments that have been shown to reduce the 3-month and 1-year relapse rates in patients with Crohn's disease. Effective medications include 5-aminosalicylic acid analogues and metronidazole.[1] Trials are also underway evaluating a combination of agents. Another important consideration is cigarette smoking, which is clearly deleterious for patients with Crohn's disease. Cosnes et al.[2] demonstrated that patients who smoke, particularly women and heavy smokers, run a high risk of developing severe disease. In this regard, for female smokers the 10-year risk of requiring immunosuppressive therapy was 52% compared with 24% for nonsmokers. Further, the surgical rate increased in patients who started smoking after diagnosis and decreased significantly in patients who stopped smoking, compared with matched controls. Thus, in the substantial proportion of patients with Crohn's disease who smoke, there is a clear message to stop.

N.J. Greenberger, M.D.

References

1. Greenberger NJ, Miner PB: Is maintenance therapy effective in Crohn's disease? *Lancet* 344:900–901, 1994.
2. Cosnes T, Carbonnal F, Beaugeire L, et al: Effects of cigarette smoking on the long-term course of Crohn's disease. *Gastroenterology* 110:424–431, 1996.

Effects of Cigarette Smoking on the Long-term Course of Crohn's Disease
Cosnes J, Carbonnel F, Beaugerie L, et al (Hôpital Rothschild, Paris)
Gastroenterology 110:424–431, 1996   4–8

Introduction.—More patients with Crohn's disease smoke tobacco than does a matched control population, and smoking has been linked to recurrence of Crohn's disease after surgery, particularly in heavily smoking women. The interactions between medical therapy and smoking remain to be clarified, and the influence of cigarette smoking on the overall severity of Crohn's disease is not yet clear. To document the harmful effect of smoking, more information is needed. In 400 patients, smoking habits and the long-term course of Crohn's disease were compared.

Methods.—A review of the medical records of 400 patients whose smoking habits were recorded by direct interview was conducted. Patients with Crohn's disease who were smokers were given an explanation of the effects of smoking on therapy and were encouraged to quit. If the patients had smoked more than 7 cigarettes per week for at least 6 months, they were classified as smokers. The effects of starting and stopping cigarette smoking were analyzed by comparing the need for immunosuppressive therapy and the surgical rate before and after the change in smoking habits. Each patient was also age-matched with a control who did not smoke.

Results.—In smokers and nonsmokers, the frequency and extent of excisional surgery were not significantly different; however, more glucocorticoids and immunosuppressive drugs were required for the smokers. In women, the effect of smoking on the need for immunosuppressive drugs was dose dependent and significant, but not in men. The 10-year risk of immunosuppressive therapy for women smokers was 52% ± 11% vs. 24% ± 10% for the nonsmokers. In patients who smoked and did not take immunosuppressive drugs, the risk of surgery increased (Table 5). In 19 patients who started smoking after diagnosis, the surgical rate increased significantly during their smoking period when compared with matched controls. In 34 patients who stopped smoking, the surgical rate decreased significantly in comparison to matched controls.

Conclusion.—A high risk of disease development occurs among patients who smoke, particularly women and heavy smokers. The influence of smoking on surgical rates is neutralized by immunosuppressive therapy. The risk of surgery is lowered for those who stop smoking.

TABLE 5.—Effect of Smoking and Immunosuppressive Therapy on Excision Surgery for Crohn's Disease

Period	Patients (n)	Patient-Years	Operations (n)	Operations Per Patient-Year (n)	Relative Risk (95% CI)	P
No smoking, no immunosuppressive therapy	237	1770	123	0.069	1	
No smoking, immunosuppressive therapy	58	117	7	0.060	0.86 (0.41–1.80)	NS
Smoking, no immunosuppressive therapy	219	1476	134	0.091	1.31 (1.03–1.65)	0.025
Smoking, immunosuppressive therapy	81	252	16	0.063	0.91 (0.55–1.51)	NS

Abbreviations: CI, confidence interval; *NS*, not significant.
(Courtesy of Cosnes J, Carbonnel F, Beaugerie L, et al: Effects of cigarette smoking on the long-term course of Crohn's disease. *Gastroenterology* 110:424–431, 1996.)

▶ This study provides clear evidence that Crohn's disease patients who smoke, particularly women and heavy smokers, are at increased risk of development of severe disease. Interestingly, the risk of surgery increased significantly in patients who started smoking and decreased in patients who stopped. The data obtained also suggest that smoking blunts the therapeutic effectiveness of glucocorticoid and immunosuppressive drugs. The message seems quite clear. Patients with Crohn's disease who smoke should be urged in the strongest possible terms to stop. This recommendation is especially important in patients contemplating pregnancy. Finally, all future clinical trials of therapeutic agents in Crohn's disease will have to be controlled for smoking.

N.J. Greenberger, M.D.

Surgical Considerations

Effect of Resection Margins on the Recurrence of Crohn's Disease in the Small Bowel: A Randomized Controlled Trial

Fazio VW, Marchetti F, Church JM, et al (Cleveland Clinic Found, Ohio)
Ann Surg 224:563–573, 1996   4–9

Introduction.—Most investigations evaluating recurrence rates in Crohn's disease (CD) are limited because of their retrospective nature. Their collective conclusions are not conclusive. One of the most important issues regarding recurrence rates involves the width of surgical margins. The effect of surgical margin width on recurrence rates was evaluated in a randomized, controlled investigation.

Methods.—A total of 152 patients undergoing small-bowel resection for CD were randomly assigned 2 treatment groups: (1) patients with limited resection, with a proximal line of resection 2 cm from the limit of macroscopically diseased bowel; and (2) patients with extended resection, with a 12-cm margin of proximal clearance. Patients also were assigned to groups according to histologic findings: category 1 patients had normal margins; category 2 patients had mild, nonspecific changes; category 3 patients had changes suggestive of, but not diagnostic of, CD; and category 4 patients had changes diagnostic of CD. The recurrence rates for both groups were calculated.

Results.—Complete data were available for 131 patients. There were 75 patients in the limited resection group and 56 in the extended resection group. Of 32 patients who underwent reoperation, 29 had recurrence involving the pre-anastomotic ileum (22.1%). Of these, 10 patients with extended resection (18%) and 19 with limited resection (25%) had recurrent disease (Fig 1). Age at the time of surgery, gender, and duration of disease before first operation had no significant effect on recurrence. There was no significant correlation between recurrence and the extent of disease in the small bowel or the length of resected small bowel.

Conclusions.—Extended resection margins offer no advantage to patients with CD in decreasing cumulative recurrence rates. The presence of

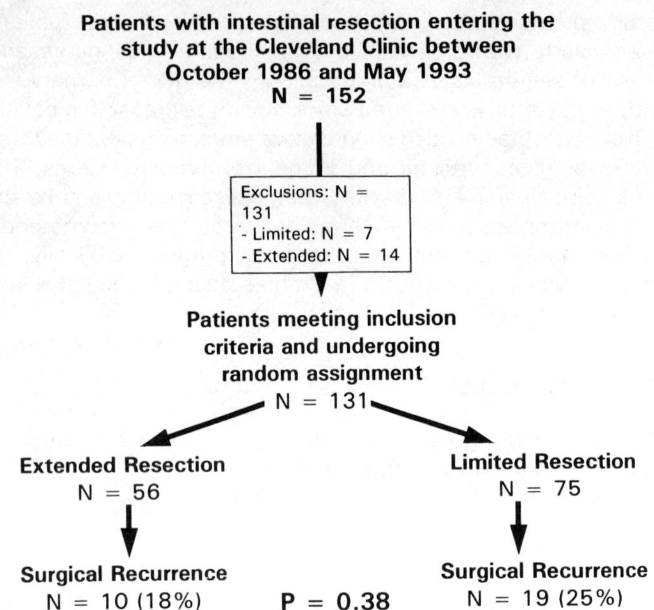

FIGURE 1.—Schematic summary of a randomized, controlled trial testing the effect of limited and extended resection margins on surgical recurrence in 131 patients with Crohn's disease. (Courtesy of Fazio VW, Marchetti F, Church JM: Effect of resection margins on the recurrence of Crohn's disease in the small bowel: A randomized controlled trial. *Ann Surg* 224:563–573, 1996.)

residual microscopic CD at resection margins was not significantly correlated with increased recurrence rates, compared to normal margins.

▶ This should be the frosting on the cake. The margin of resection from macroscopic disease does not influence the recurrence rate. The evidence for this, obtained by a randomized, controlled trial, is shown in Figure 1. Microscopic margins are not necessary; bowel conservation in this disease is.

F.G. Moody, M.D.

Resting Energy Expenditure Before and After Surgical Resection of Gut Lesions in Pediatric Crohn's Disease

Varille V, Cézard JP, de Lagausie P, et al (Hôpital Robert Debré, Paris; Hôpital Trousseau, Paris)
J Pediatr Gastroenterol Nutr 23:13–19, 1996   4–10

Introduction.—Some children with Crohn's disease (CD) continue to have a slow growth rate, despite nutritional support and optimal medical treatment. This problem may involve cytokines and an increased need for specific nutrients. Children with CD were compared for resting energy expenditure (REE) and body composition before and 1 month after surgical resection of gut lesions.

Patients and Methods.—The patient group included 8 boys and 3 girls ranging in age from 8 to 18 years. Indications for surgery were intestinal stenosis in 7 cases and insufficient control of remission by medical therapy in 4. Nine children had been treated with nonsteroidal anti-inflammatory drugs, and 7 were receiving alternate-day steroid therapy at the time of surgery. Nutritional support was provided at night in all patients. After surgery, all received the same steroid and nutritional intakes for 1 month. Eleven healthy children served as controls. Indirect calorimetry was used to measure REE; fat-free body mass (FFM) was assessed by anthropometry.

Results.—Before surgery, the age- and sex-matched controls differed from patients in mean height, mean weight as a percentage of ideal weight-for-height, mean expected height-for-age, FFM, and fat mass as a percentage of body weight; REE per kilogram of FFM was significantly higher in patients than in controls. At the second assessment, performed at a mean of 36 days after surgery, patients had protein and energy intakes that were within normal age requirements and similar to values for healthy children. Mean body weight and height did not change significantly in children with CD, but arm muscle area had increased significantly and mean protein oxidation rate was reduced. Patients showed a significant decrease in mean REE per kilogram of FFM per day and approached control values in this parameter. There was no correlation between changes in REE per kilogram of FFM per day and changes in orosomucoid serum concentrations.

Discussion.—Surgical resection of gut lesions was beneficial for children with mildly active CD. At the 2 assessment periods, nutritional intake and steroid doses were similar and the inflammatory process was under control. Thus decreases in REE and protein breakdown might be attributed to removal of the energy expenditure of the damaged gut, allowing better use of energy substrates.

▶ The finding of a decrease in REE and increase in nitrogen utilization after excision of CD bowel in children is an interesting observation. This occurred in a setting of maintaining steroids and nutritional intake at preoperative levels. Possibly, tumor necrosis factor (cachectin) or other cytokines elaborated by the diseased tissue played a role in the wasting catabolic state experienced by these youngsters before surgery, as was suggested by the authors. If that is the case, then possibly receptor blockage of the cytokines involved may be of value during the active phase of the disease.

F.G. Moody, M.D.

Ileal Pouch/Anal Anastomosis for Crohn's Disease

Panis Y, Poupard B, Nemeth J, et al (Hôpital Lariboisière, Paris)
Lancet 347:854–857, 1996   4–11

Background.—Ileal pouch/anal anastomosis is contraindicated in patients with Crohn's disease because recurrent disease often requires pouch excision and may lead to short-bowel syndrome. Therefore, patients with Crohn's disease that require coloproctectomy undergo definitive end-ileostomy. Young patients who require definitive end-ileostomy may prefer to maintain acceptable continence and defecation, if only for a few years before the disease recurs. Selected patients with Crohn's disease who require rectal resection may be candidates for ileal pouch/anal anastomosis. The short- and long-term results after ileal pouch/anal anastomosis in patients with Crohn's disease and in patients with ulcerative colitis were compared.

Methods.—Ileal pouch/anal anastomosis was done in 31 patients (mean age, 36 years) with Crohn's disease but with no evidence of anoperineal or small-bowel disease. Results were compared with results of the same procedure in patients with ulcerative colitis. Follow-up was 59 months.

Results.—The postoperative complication rate was similar for both groups of patients. The following complications were noted in 6 patients with Crohn's disease between 9 months and 6 years postoperatively: pouch-perineal fistulas, pouch-vaginal fistula, and extrasphincteric abscess. Two patients had recurrence of Crohn's disease on the reservoir. At 5 years, stool frequency, continence, gas/stool discrimination, leak or need for protective pads, and sexual activity were similar for both groups of patients.

Conclusions.—Ileal pouch/anal anastomosis is a viable alternative to definitive end-ileostomy in selected patients with Crohn's disease without anoperineal or ileal involvement. In this study, all of the patients with Crohn's disease were stoma-free and had not developed short-bowel syndrome after 5 years.

▶ I thought that it was about time for me to rewrite my lecture on the role of ileal-anal pouch anastomosis in the surgical treatment of Crohn's colitis. Until I read this paper, my position on this was: don't do it. The authors discuss which patients are candidates for this procedure; they are those who have no perianal or ileal involvement. But even with these strict selection criteria, almost 1 in 5 patients had complications related specifically to the operation, and 2 of these required takedown of their pouch. Sounds like a high risk group, even under the best of circumstances.

F.G. Moody, M.D.

Laparoscopic Surgery in the Management of Inflammatory Bowel Disease
Reissman P, Salky BA, Pfeifer J, et al (Cleveland Clinic Florida, Fort Lauderdale; Mount Sinai Med Ctr, New York)
Am J Surg 171:47–51, 1996   4–12

Background.—The safety, cost effectiveness, and increased morbidity related to the learning curve of laparoscopic surgery for treating gastrointestinal disorders are unclear. New instrumentation, patient demand, and surgeon experience have resulted in the feasibility of laparoscopic techniques for more complex gastrointestinal surgical procedures. Laparoscopy may have a role in inflammatory bowel disease. The outcome of laparoscopic procedures for inflammatory bowel disease was evaluated.

Methods.—Laparoscopic or laparoscopic-assisted procedures were performed in 72 patients between 20 and 79 years with inflammatory bowel disease. Diagnoses included terminal ileitis, mucosal ulcerative colitis, Crohn's colitis, severe perianal Crohn's disease, and duodenal Crohn's disease.

Results.—Procedures included total abdominal colectomy, ileocolic resection, and diverting loop ileostomy. There were 16 complications in 13 patients, but only 3 patients required laparotomy for these complications. In 10% of patients, laparoscopic procedures were converted to laparotomy. The mean length of operation was almost 3 hours. The mean hospital stay was 6.5 days. Total colectomy was associated with higher morbidity and a longer hospital stay when compared with ileocolic resection.

Conclusions.—Laparoscopic surgery in patients with inflammatory bowel disorders was feasible, safe, and versatile. Laparoscopic total abdominal colectomy was associated with higher morbidity and much longer operating time and should not be performed routinely. Several technical tips for the management of Crohn's disease are also discussed.

▶ The surgeons at the Cleveland Clinic in Ft. Lauderdale describe a favorable experience with laparoscopically assisted small-and large-bowel resection for the complications of inflammatory bowel disease. Total colectomy was associated with a relatively high morbidity. In fact, the operating times and hospital lengths of stay did not appear to be much different than those experienced with an open approach. The Cleveland Clinic has the volume if the northern and southern components work together to do a randomized, controlled trial of the standard open approach to the laparoscopic-assisted technique to establish cost effectiveness, safety, and efficacy.

F.G. Moody, M.D.

28 Ulcerative Colitis

Medical Treatment

Oral Budesonide Versus Prednisolone in Patients With Active Extensive and Left-sided Ulcerative Colitis

Löfberg R, Danielsson Å, Suhr O, et al (Huddinge Univ, Stockholm; Univ Hosp, Umeå, Sweden; Univ Hosp, Lund, Sweden; et al)
Gastroenterology 110:1713–1718, 1996   4–13

Introduction.—Because budesonide has a high affinity for the glucocorticosteroid receptor, it is a highly potent glucocorticosteroid that is readily absorbed and rapidly degraded to metabolites with low glucocorticosteroid activity during first passage through the liver. Systemic glucocorticosteroids have undesired systemic side effects, and it would be valuable to have glucocorticosteroids with high topical activity and a high rate of metabolism. In the treatment of active extensive and left-sided ulcerative colitis, the efficacy of an oral formulation of budesonide, optimized to release the drug throughout the colon, was evaluated and compared with a standard regimen of oral prednisolone. An evaluation was also done on the safety and tolerability of budesonide along with the impact on endogenous plasma cortisol production.

Methods.—Thirty-four patients were given 10 mg budesonide and 38 patients were given 40 mg prednisolone every day during a 9-week, randomized, double-blind controlled trial. Assessments were made of endoscopic improvement and the effect on endogenous plasma cortisol.

Results.—In both groups, the mean endoscopic scores improved significantly and similarly. The study had 5 withdrawals from the budesonide group and 7 from the prednisolone group because of deterioration in the patients' condition. In the prednisolone group, morning plasma cortisol levels were suppressed. At entry, these levels were 440 nmol/L, at 2 weeks they were 116 nmol/L, and at 4 weeks they were 195 nmol/L. In the budesonide group, the morning plasma control levels were not changed.

Conclusion.—For the treatment of active ulcerative colitis, oral administration of the glucocorticosteroid budesonide has an effect similar to that of prednisolone, but without suppression of plasma cortisol levels. There could be suboptimal release of budesonide in the distal region of the colon, because endoscopic and histologic improvement in this area was in favor

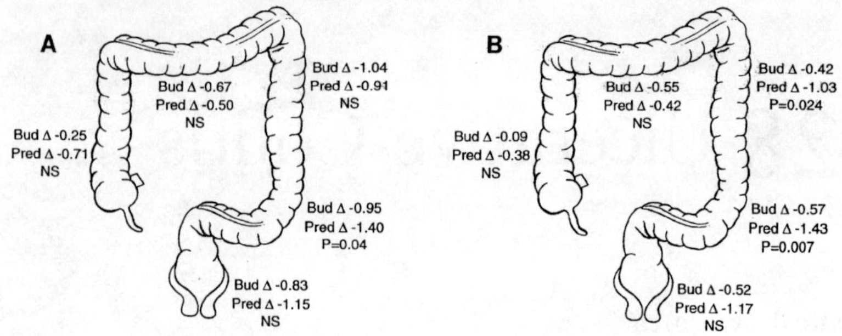

FIGURE 2.—Mean colonoscopic (A) and histopathologic activity (B) scores in each of the 5 colorectal segments at entry and after 4 weeks of treatment with either budesonide (*Bud*) or prednisolone (*Pred*) expressed as Δ values. Colonoscopy scored between 0 and 3, and histopathology scored between 1 and 5. (Courtesy of Löfberg R, Danielsson Å, Suhr O, et al: Oral budesonide versus prednisolone in patients with active extensive and left-sided ulcerative colitis. *Gastroenterology* 110:1713–1718, 1996.)

of prednisolone (Fig 2). Further evaluations are necessary for improved formulations of budesonide.

▶ There is heightened interest in budesonide, which is a highly potent glucocorticoid that is rapidly degraded to metabolites resulting in low systemic bioavailability. Previous studies have demonstrated that budesonide in enema form is as effective as conventional prednisone or mesalamine retention enemas in active distal ulcerative colitis. The study by Löfberg and colleagues now demonstrates that an oral controlled-release formulation of budesonide at an initial dose of 10 mg/day gives overall treatment results approaching that of prednisone administered at an initial dose of 40 mg/day. Importantly, budesonide capsules in the doses and formulation used in this trial did not affect plasma cortisol levels. The authors point out the 2 reasons for this: (1) high first-pass metabolism of the drug and (2) incomplete release of budesonide, particularly in the distal portion of the colon. The latter finding has triggered additional studies using an improved formulation of budesonide. The drug appears to be an important addition to regimens for treating active ulcerative colitis.

N.J. Greenberger. M.D.

An Oral Preparation of Mesalamine as Long-term Maintenance Therapy for Ulcerative Colitis: A Randomized, Placebo-controlled Trial

Hanauer SB, Sninsky CA, Robinson M, et al (Univ of Chicago Hosp; Univ of Florida, Gainesville; Univ of Oklahoma, Oklahoma City; et al)
Ann Intern Med 124:204–211, 1996   4–14

Objective.—Although sulfasalazine is the drug of choice for treating mild-to-moderate ulcerative colitis and to maintain remission, it has a substantial incidence of side effects and idiosyncratic reactions mainly as a result of the sulfapyridine carrier molecule. Other methods of delivering the active molecule, mesalamine, have been studied, including coating the

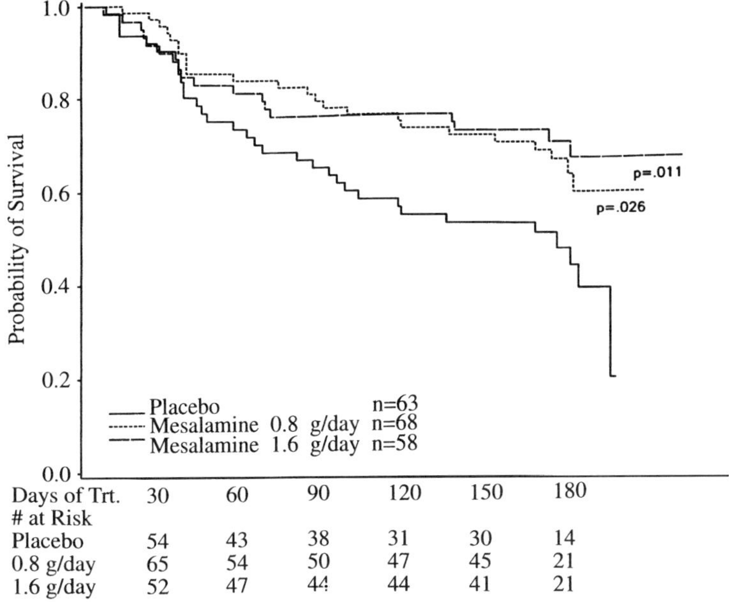

# at Risk	30	60	90	120	150	180
Placebo	54	43	38	31	30	14
0.8 g/day	65	54	50	47	45	21
1.6 g/day	52	47	44	44	41	21

FIGURE 1.—Percentage of patients with ulcerative colitis who remained in remission during treatment with placebo; with mesalamine, 0.8 g/day; or with mesalamine, 1.6 g/day. *P* values are for comparisons between treatment and placebo. (Courtesy of Hanauer SB, Sninsky CA, Robinson M, et al: An oral preparation of mesalamine as long-term maintenance therapy for ulcerative colitis: A randomized, placebo-controlled trial. *Ann Intern Med* 124:204–211, 1996).

drug to preventing the adverse effects of stomach acid. The safety and efficacy of a pH-sensitive, polymer-coated oral formulation of mesalamine in maintaining remission in patients with ulcerative colitis was studied in a multicenter, double-blind, placebo-controlled, randomized clinical trial.

Methods.—A total of 264 patients with ulcerative colitis (146 males), aged 18 to 75 years, received either 0.8 g/day, 1.6 g/day, or placebo, administered as 4 tablets a day. Tablets were coated with a pH-sensitive resin that breaks down only at a pH of 7 or higher. Patients received endoscopic examinations at baseline, and at 1, 3, and 6 months. Findings were graded on a 0-to-3 scale, with 0 representing normal or mild granularity and other mild symptoms, 2 for marked erythema or granularity, and 3 representing spontaneous bleeding and ulcerations. Efficacy was measured as treatment outcome. Safety was evaluated at each visit, and adverse events were documented.

Results.—Failure to meet study criteria and protocol violations resulted in the exclusion of 75 patients. The percentage of treatment successes in the low dose (*n* = 68) and high dose (*n* = 58) groups were 58.8% and 65.5%, significantly more than in the placebo (*n* = 63) group with 37%. Similarly, in the intent-to-treat group, significantly more low and high dose patients, 63.3% and 70.1%, were considered treatment successes than in the placebo group, at 48.3%. Age, sex, and race did not affect the analyses. In the intent-to-treat analysis, the high dose group but not the low dose group had a significantly longer time to relapse when compared with the placebo group (Fig 1). Adverse events were reported 81 times by placebo-treated patients, 72 times by patients in the low dose group, and 106 times in the high dose group. Most adverse events were mild to moderate and included headache, flu syndrome, diarrhea, rhinitis, and abdominal pain.

Conclusion.—Coated mesalamine at daily doses of 0.8 g and 1.6 g was well tolerated and was significantly more effective than placebo in maintaining remission in patients with ulcerative colitis.

▶ Accumulating evidence indicates that mesalamine is effective in maintaining remission in patients with quiescent ulcerative colitis. In earlier trials, mesalamine was used in doses of 1.2 to 2.4 g/day to induce remissions, and at doses of 0.8 g and 1.6 g/day to maintain remission. It is not generally appreciated that considerably higher doses of mesalamine may be necessary for both induction as well as maintenance of remission. In this regard, doses as high as 4.8 g/day to induce remission and of 3.6–4 g/day have been used to maintain remission. The medication has a good safety profile, and in the above report by the Mesalamine Study Group, adverse events were reported with approximately equal frequency in the placebo group and in the group receiving mesalamine.

N.J. Greenberger, M.D.

Predicting Outcome in Severe Attacks

Predicting Outcome in Severe Ulcerative Colitis
Travis SPL, Farrant JM, Ricketts C, et al (John Radcliffe Hosp, Oxford, England; Univ of Plymouth, England)
Gut 38:905–910, 1996   4–15

Purpose.—Early colectomy greatly reduces the mortality of severe ulcerative colitis. The introduction of cyclosporine and other medical treatments carries a risk of inappropriately delaying colectomy. There is currently no way to predict which patients with severe ulcerative colitis will not respond to intensive medical therapy and therefore require colectomy. Patterns of change in inflammatory markers were among the factors analyzed in an attempt to predict the need for surgery.

Methods.—The prospective study included 51 consecutive episodes of severe colitis in 49 patients. Each episode was treated with IV and rectal hydrocortisone; in addition, 14 were treated with cyclosporine. A complete response was defined as 3 or fewer stools on day 7, without visible blood. An incomplete response was defined as more than 3 stools or visible blood on day 7, but no colectomy. Thirty-six different clinical, laboratory, and radiographic variables were evaluated for their ability to predict the need for surgery. Patient outcomes were evaluated after 1 year of follow-up.

Results.—A complete response was obtained in 41% of episodes and an incomplete response in 29%. The remaining 29% of episodes required colectomy. The only factors capable of distinguishing between outcomes were stool frequency and C-reactive protein (CRP) level during the first 5 days of the episode. This was so on both per-episode and per-patient analysis. Using these 2 factors, it was possible to predict that colectomy would be required in 85% of patients who had more than 8 stools on day 3 or who had 3 to 8 stools along with a CRP level of greater than 45 mg/L. Colectomy was avoided in 4 of 14 patients treated with cyclosporine; however, 2 of these patients had continued symptoms. Patients with a complete response to intensive medical therapy stayed in remission for a median of 9 months and had just a 5% chance of colectomy. For patients with an incomplete response, the chance of continuous symptoms during the same time was 60%, and the chance of colectomy was 40%.

Conclusions.—Among patients with severe ulcerative colitis, those who have frequent stools or an elevated CRP level after 3 days of intensive medical therapy are likely to require colectomy during that admission. Patients who still have more than 3 stools per day or visible blood after 1 week of treatment are likely to have continuous symptoms or to require colectomy in the subsequent months. Although there is an urgent need for better medical treatment of severe ulcerative colitis, the role of cyclosporine in the management of this disease remains to be determined.

▶ Despite advances in the management of severe ulcerative colitis, it remains difficult to predict at an early stage which patients will respond poorly to medical treatment and require colectomy. This study from the Oxford group, which has a vast experience with severe ulcerative colitis, provides some useful guidelines. All 49 patients (51 total episodes) received the following intensive medical therapy for ulcerative colitis: correction of fluid, electrolyte, and hemoglobin abnormalties; IV hydrocortisone 100 mg every 6 hours; rectal hydrocortisone 100 mg twice daily; and oral fluids or parenteral nutrition to malnourished patients. This treatment was continued for 5–7 days until it was clear that the patients had responded or colectomy was needed. Twenty or more patients had a complete response, 14 required colectomy, and 14 had an incomplete response. Incomplete responses required further treatment with IV cyclosporine at a dosage of 3 mg/kg/day for up to 6 days. Only 4 of 14 patients receiving cyclosporine avoided colectomy, so in most patients who received cyclosporine, colectomy was merely delayed. A complete response with less than 3 stools per day without visible blood occurred in 21 patients. Two simple parameters predicted with 85% accuracy the patients who would need colectomy during the same admission: more than 8 bowel motions on day 3 or 3–8 bowel motions with a CRP level of greater than 45 mg/L. After a week of treatment, patients who had more than 3 stools per day or visible blood in the stool had a 60% chance of continuous symptoms and a 40% chance of colectomy in the following months.

N.J. Greenberger, M.D.

Surgical Considerations Including Pouchitis

Pouchitis Following Pelvic Pouch Operation for Ulcerative Colitis: Incidence, Cumulative Risk, and Risk Factors
Ståhlberg D, Gullberg K, Liljeqvist L, et al (Huddinge Univ, Sweden)
Dis Colon Rectum 39:1012–1018, 1996   4–16

Background.—In patients with ulcerative colitis (UC) who undergo restorative proctocolectomy, pouchitis—a nonspecific inflammation of the ileal mucosa of the pelvic pouch—is a major complication. The symptoms and course of pouchitis are similar to those of UC itself. There are no agreed-on diagnostic criteria for pouchitis, and there have been few studies of the risk factors. The incidence of and risk factors for pouchitis in patients undergoing pelvic pouch operation for UC were studied.

Methods.—The prospective study included 149 patients undergoing colectomy, restorative pelvic pouch, and ileoanal anastomosis for UC at 1 Swedish hospital. There were 89 men and 60 women, median age 34 years at the time of colectomy. The patients were followed up for pouchitis, diagnosed by the symptoms and endoscopic findings of inflammation. A pouchitis scoring system was devised, and each case was classified as mild or severe. Risk factors were analyzed using uniformly collected data.

Results.—The patients were followed up for a median of 54 months. The cumulative risk of pouchitis increased from 21% at 6 months to 26% at 12 months and 39% at 48 months. The cumulative risk of severe pouchitis was 9% at 6 months, 11% at 12 months, and 14% at 48 months. The overall risk was 51% at 48 months. Pouchitis was most frequent, with an occurrence rate of 23%, in the first 6 months after closure of the loop ileostomy. The incidence dropped to 11% in the next 6 months and only 3% after that. About 22% of patients required long-term metronidazole for chronic symptoms, and 9% had severe chronic pouchitis. Two patients had to have surgical removal of the pouch and ileostomy. Pouchitis was more likely in patients with extracolonic manifestation and early onset of UC. Ex-smokers had a lower rate of pouchitis.

Conclusions.—In patients undergoing pelvic pouch operation for UC, the complication of pouchitis is most likely to occur in the first 6 postoperative months. Although cumulative risk drops off after 2 years, by 4 years more than half of patients have at least mild pouchitis. Pouchitis becomes severe and chronic in less than 10% of patients, but only about 1% require pouch removal.

▶ This report on pouchitis after ileoanal reconstruction for UC from Huddinge Hospital in Sweden provides useful information, not the least of which is that smoking seemed protective. It is also of interest that if it does not occur within a year, then its occurrence is unlikely. Patients with early onset of their disease and those with extracolonic manifestations were especially at risk. Could it be that these individuals did not have the protective benefits of smoking?

F.G. Moody, M.D.

Prospective Controlled Trial of Duplicated (J) Versus Quadruplicated (W) Pelvic Ileal Reservoirs in Restorative Proctocolectomy for Ulcerative Colitis
Johnston D, Williamson MER, Lewis WG, et al (Gen Infirmary, Leeds, England)
Gut 39:242–247, 1996   4–17

Background.—Although the pelvic ileal reservoir has long been used in the treatment of ulcerative colitis, there is still no consensus about the best design to use. At the study institution, the quadruplicated (W) reservoir appears to provide a lower bowel frequency than the duplicated (J) reservoir. However, a randomized clinical trial found no significant difference. It has been suggested that bowel frequency is inversely proportional to reservoir capacity. The effects of reservoir design and the length of ileum used in its construction on the functional outcomes of restorative proctocolectomy were studied.

Methods.—The study included 60 patients operated on for ulcerative colitis. They were randomly allocated to receive a J reservoir made with 30 or 40 cm of ileum or a W reservoir made with 20 or 40 cm of ileum. Anorectal function tests were performed in the laboratory before surgery in all patients and 1 year postoperatively in 50 patients. Clinical assessments of outcome were made at 1 year in 57 patients.

Results.—All patients evaluated had good anal continence and could defer defecation for longer than 15 minutes. Eight patients had minor mucous leakage. The median bowel frequency per 24 hours was 5 in both groups. Neither was there any significant difference in bowel frequency between patients with the smaller and larger reservoirs. Bowel frequency was lowest—4 per 24 hours—in the patients with W reservoirs made with 40 cm of ileum. This difference was not significant, however. These reservoirs also had greater capacity and compliance than the other types of reservoirs, but again the difference was not significant.

Conclusions.—The outcomes of restorative proctocolectomy are similar for patients with duplicated and quadruplicated reservoirs. Using 30 vs. 40 cm of ileum to construct the reservoir does not seem to make any difference either. A 30-cm J ileal reservoir, which is easily constructed using linear stapling instruments, gives results just as good as a 40-cm W reservoir, which takes a long time to suture by hand.

▶ Johnson and his associates demonstrate in a randomized control trial that the duplicated J-pouch provides as good a functioning reservoir following ileoanal reconstruction after total proctocolectomy as the larger quadruplicated pouch. They, therefore, recommend the simpler procedure (J-pouch), which can easily be fashioned with contemporary stapling techniques.

F.G. Moody, M.D.

Morbidity of Subtotal Colectomy in Patients With Severe Ulcerative Colitis Unresponsive to Cyclosporin

Fleshner PR, Michelassi F, Rubin M, et al (Cedars-Sinai Med Ctr, Los Angeles; Univ of Chicago)
Dis Colon Rectum 38:1241–1245, 1995   4–18

Background.—Patients with severe ulcerative colitis who do not respond to steroids have traditionally undergone colectomy. Early results have shown that colectomy can usually be avoided by treating these patients with cyclosporine. The effect of preoperative cyclosporine on morbidity and mortality after colectomy was investigated in patients with severe ulcerative colitis.

Methods.—The medical records were reviewed of 14 patients with severe ulcerative colitis who did not respond to treatment with cyclosporine and who underwent subtotal colectomy. Various intraoperative and postoperative features were examined, including the method of rectal stump closure, the use of transanal stump drainage, and the length of hospital stay.

Results.—Postoperative complications including ileus, deep-vein thrombosis, wound infection, and partial dehiscence of the rectal stump, were noted in 8 patients. The average hospital stay was 8.8 days. There were no deaths.

Conclusions.—Cyclosporine did not adversely affect morbidity or mortality in patients with severe ulcerative colitis who underwent a subtotal colectomy. The exact role of cyclosporine in the management of patients with inflammatory bowel disease is unclear. Cyclosporine may affect T-cell activation and proliferation at the systemic or intestinal level in these patients.

▶ It is useful to know that when cyclosporine therapy fails it does not jeopardize the outcome after subtotal colectomy for ulcerative colitis. The dramatic response obtained with cyclosporine in patients with severe, acute forms of the disease makes it likely that surgeons will be seeing an increasing number of such patients.

F.G. Moody, M.D.

29 The Appendix

Laparoscopic vs. Open Appendectomy

Laparoscopic Versus Open Appendectomy: Prospective Randomized Trial
Hansen JB, Smithers BM, Schache D, et al (Princess Alexandra Hosp, Brisbane, Queensland, Australia; Univ of Queensland, Brisbane, Australia)
World J Surg 20:17–21, 1996   4–19

Background.—There have been many large studies of laparoscopic appendectomy. Comparative studies of laparoscopic and open appendectomy have supported the laparoscopic method. Laparoscopic and traditional appendectomy using a muscle-splitting approach in the right iliac fossa were compared in a prospective, randomized trial.

Methods.—One hundred fifty-one patients were randomly assigned to undergo laparoscopic or open appendectomy. There were no differences between groups, including classification of appendicitis. Operating time, analgesia, complications, hospital stay, return to normal activity, and cost were recorded.

Results.—Patients who had laparoscopic surgery had longer operating time, had fewer wound infections, needed less analgesia, and returned to normal activity sooner than patients who had open appendectomy. The morbidity and hospital stay were similar for both groups.

Conclusions.—Laparoscopic appendectomy is safe and offers some advantages to patients. One technique is not recommended more than the other. Both patient and surgeon should determine which technique is best for them.

▶ I imagine that this will be the last word needed on the relative advantages of open vs. laparoscopic appendectomy. If you want to have lower postoperative morbidity and get back to work sooner, select a laparoscopic surgeon. However, you will do just about as well with a surgeon who recommends a standard approach. The world does not need another randomized trial on this topic.

F.G. Moody, M.D.

30 Colorectal Cancer and Other Neoplasms

Screening–Randomized Trials

A Comparison of Fecal Occult-blood Tests for Colorectal-Cancer Screening

Allison JE, Tekawa IS, Ransom LJ, et al (Kaiser Permanente Med Ctr, Oakland, Calif; Kaiser Permanente Med Care Program, Oakland Calif)
N Engl J Med 334:155–159, 1996   4–20

Background.—Hemoccult II is a widely used guaiac test for the detection of fecal occult blood. However, it is not very sensitive in detecting colorectal neoplasms in asymptomatic patients at average risk. Other tests, such as Hemoccult II Sensa—a more sensitive guaiac test—and HemeSelect—an immunochemical test for human hemoglobin—have been introduced to improve on the performance of Hemoccult II. However, their performance characteristics are unknown. These 3 tests were evaluated for their sensitivity, specificity, and predictive value in colorectal cancer screening.

Methods.—All 3 tests were mailed to a large, racially diverse sample of people 50 years of age or older who were scheduled for personal health appraisals. The sample was considered to be at average risk for colorectal cancer. The patients were followed up for 2 years for the occurrence of colorectal neoplasms, defined as carcinoma or a polyp measuring 1 cm in diameter or greater. Each test's performance was evaluated, including the use of HemeSelect to confirm a positive Hemoccult II Sensa result.

Results.—Eight thousand one hundred four patients returned at least 1 interpretable sample, representing 76% of eligible patients. Two-year follow-up was complete in 96% of this group: 142 proved to have neoplasms, including 107 with benign polyps and 35 with carcinoma. Hemoccult II's sensitivity in detecting carcinoma was only 37%, compared with 67% for the combination of Hemoccult II Sensa and HemeSelect, 69% with HemeSelect alone, and 79% with Hemoccult II Sensa alone. Specificity values were 87% for Hemoccult II Sensa, 94% with HemeSelect, 97% with the combination test, and 98% with Hemoccult II (Table 2). More colorectal neoplasms were detected with HemeSelect, alone or with Hemoccult II

TABLE 2.—Performance Characteristics of Fecal Occult-blood Tests

Test and Finding*	Sensitivity	Specificity	Positive Predictive Value
	percent (95% confidence interval)		
Hemoccult II			
Carcinoma	37.1 (19.7–54.6)	97.7 (97.3–98.0)	6.6 (3.7–11.2)
Polyp ≥1 cm	30.8 (21.6–40.1)	98.1 (97.7–98.4)	16.7 (11.9–22.8)
Combined	32.4 (24.3–40.4)	98.1 (97.7–98.4)	23.2 (17.7–29.9)
Hemoccult II Sensa			
Carcinoma	79.4 (64.3–94.5)	86.7 (85.9–87.4)	2.5 (1.7–3.7)
Polyp ≥1 cm	68.6 (59.2–77.9)	87.5 (86.7–88.2)	6.7 (5.3–8.4)
Combined	71.2 (63.3–79.1)	87.5 (86.7–88.2)	9.2 (7.6–11.2)
HemeSelect			
Carcinoma	68.8 (51.1–86.4)	94.4 (93.8–94.9)	5.0 (3.2–7.6)
Polyp ≥1 cm	66.7 (57.0–76.3)	95.2 (94.7–95.7)	15.5 (12.3–19.3)
Combined	67.2 (58.8–75.5)	95.2 (94.7–95.7)	20.5 (16.8–24.6)
Combination			
Carcinoma	65.6 (47.6–83.6)	97.3 (96.9–97.6)	9.0 (5.8–13.6)
Polyp ≥1 cm	50.0 (39.8–60.2)	97.9 (97.6–98.2)	21.9 (16.9–27.9)
Combined	53.7 (44.9–62.5)	97.9 (97.6–98.2)	30.9 (25.1–37.3)

*The calculations for polyps did not include patients with carcinoma.
(Courtesy of Allison JE, Tekawa IS, Ransom LJ: A comparison of fecal occult-blood tests for colorectal-cancer screening. *N Engl J Med* 334:155–159, 1996.)

Sensa, than with Hemoccult II. At the same time, the number of colonoscopies required increased only slightly.

Conclusions.—The newer fecal occult blood tests for colorectal cancer screening appear to be superior to Hemoccult II screening. Using the HemeSelect test to confirm a positive Hemoccult II Sensa result takes advantage of the high sensitivity of Hemoccult II Sensa while improving on its sensitivity. This combination of tests, along with flexible sigmoidoscopy for patients in whom only Hemoccult II Sensa is positive, will detect most cases of colon polyps and cancer.

▶ This study provides evidence supporting the concept that a combination of tests in which HemeSelect is used to confirm positive Hemoccult II Sensa tests improves on results of hemoccult screening in patients for colorectal cancer. However, even under optimal circumstances, using the currently available tests, one third of colorectal carcinomas or polyps larger than 1 cm will not be detected. Accordingly, it would seem reasonable to ensure that patients older than 50 years of age undergo flexible sigmoidoscopy at least once every 10 years, and preferably, every 5 years.

N.J. Greenberger, M.D.

Randomised Study of Screening for Colorectal Cancer With Faecal-occult-blood Test

Kronborg O, Fenger C, Olsen J, et al (Odense Univ, Denmark; Aarhus Univ, Denmark)

Lancet 348:1467–1471, 1996
4–21

Introduction.—Reports indicate that participation in fecal–occult-blood (FOB) screening tests is associated with reduced colorectal cancer (CRC) mortality rates. Over a 10-year period, deaths from CRC after biennial screening by FOB were compared with deaths from CRC in a similar, unscreened population.

Methods.—There were 140,000 people aged 45–75 years living in Funen, Denmark in 1985. Before this population was randomized, individuals were excluded if they had known CRC or precursor adenomas or had participated in a pilot investigation. Eligible residents were randomized to be asked to participate in biennial FOB screening or were not informed regarding the screening and continued to use health-care facilities as usual (controls). Hemoccult-II blood tests were sent to screening-group participants but not to controls. Participants who completed the first screening round were invited to participate in subsequent screening. Five rounds of screening were offered in a 10-year period. Participants with positive Hemoccult-II cultures were offered full examination with colonoscopy. Death from CRC was the primary end point.

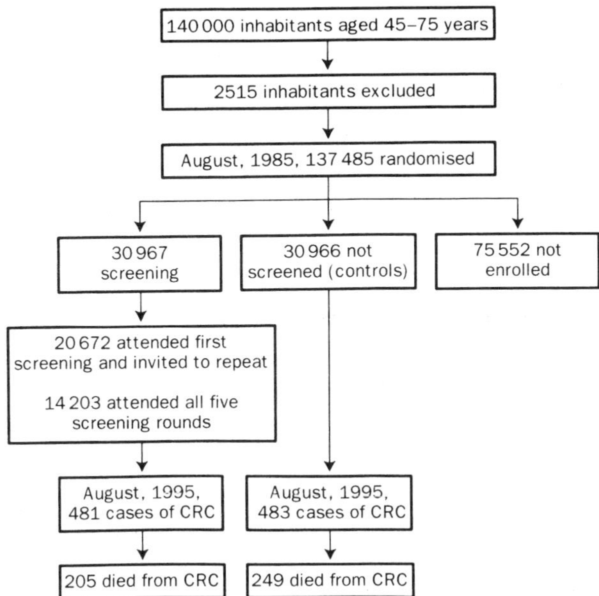

FIGURE 1.—Study profile. (Courtesy of Kronborg O, Fenger C, Olsen J, et al: Randomised study of screening for colorectal cancer with faecal-occult-blood test. *Lancet* 348:1467–1471. Copyright 1996 by The Lancet Ltd.)

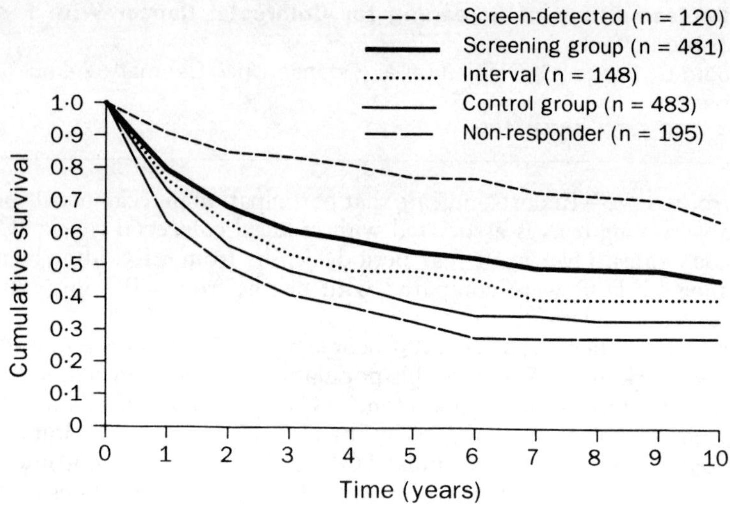

FIGURE 3.—Cumulative survival in screening (by subgroups) and control groups. Subgroup of patients who died or had colorectal cancer diagnosed between randomization and first invitation are omitted. (Courtesy of Kronborg O, Fenger C, Olsen J, et al: Randomized study of screening for colorectal cancer with faecal-occult-blood test. *Lancet* 348:1467–1471. Copyright 1996 by The Lancet Ltd.)

Results.—A total of 20,672 of 30,967 people (67%) in the screening group participated in the first round and were invited for further screening (Fig 1). Over the 10-year trial period, 481 participants in screening groups and 483 unscreened controls were given a diagnosis of CRC. In the screening and controls groups, respectively, there were 205 and 249 CRC deaths. The survival rate for screen-detected CRC was significantly higher, compared with unscreened controls (Fig 3). Nonresponders had lower survival rates than controls.

Conclusion.—The CRC mortality rate was lower for the screening group, compared with controls. Biennial screening using FOB testing can reduce mortality from CRC.

Randomised Controlled Trial of Faecal-occult-blood Screening for Colorectal Cancer

Hardcastle JD, Chamberlain JO, Robinson MHE, et al (Univ Hosp, Nottingham, England; Inst of Cancer Research, Sutton, England)
Lancet 348:1472–1477, 1996

4–22

Introduction.—There has been little reduction in colorectal cancer (CRC) mortality during the past 30 years, but earlier detection might increase long-term survival rates. At present, only about 10% of the patients have tumor confined to the bowel wall and approximately 25% have metastatic disease at diagnosis. A randomized controlled trial evaluated the effect of biennial fecal–occult-blood (FOB) screening on CRC mortality.

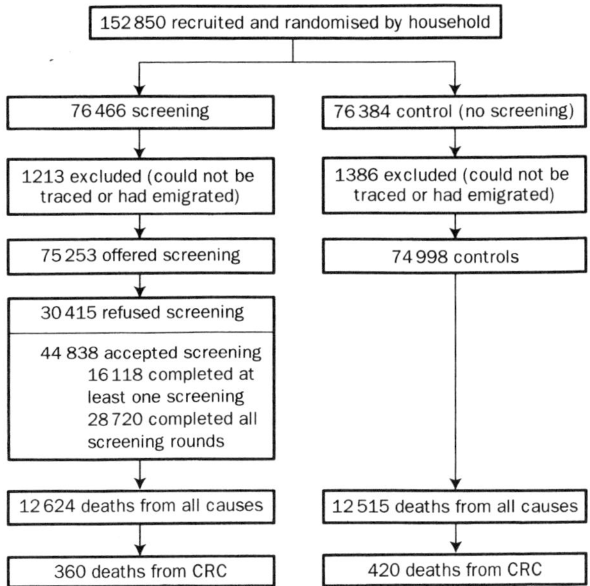

FIGURE 1.—Trial profile. (Courtesy of Hardcastle JD, Chamberlain JO, Robinson MHE, et al: Randomised controlled trial of faecal–occult-blood screening for colorectal cancer. *Lancet* 348:1472–1477, 1996. Copyright by The Lancet Ltd.)

Methods.—During a 10-year period (1981–1991), 152,850 individuals living in the Nottingham, England, area and aged 45–74 were recruited for the study. Participants were randomized (Fig 1) to FOB screening or to no screening. The controls were not informed of the study and received no interventions. Screening group members received a Hemoccult FOB test kit with instructions from their family doctor. Those with negative results at the first screening and those with positive results but found free of neoplasia at colonoscopy were invited to continue biennial screenings. All participants were monitored until June 1995.

Results.—Only 1.7% of the participants could not be traced and were excluded from analysis. Median follow-up was 7.8 years. The screening and control groups were well matched in age and sex distribution. Screening group members were offered 3 to 6 FOB tests depending on their entry date. At least 1 screening was completed by 59.6%, and 38.2% completed all FOB tests they were offered; 40.4%, however, did not complete any test. Screening group participants had a total of 893 cancers diagnosed, 20% of which were stage A. Most (44.8%) of the cancers occurred in nonresponders, 26.4% were detected by FOB screening, and 27.9% were found after a negative FOB test. The control group had 856 cases of cancer; 11% were stage A. Although the incidence of cancer was similar in the screening and control groups (1.49 and 1.44 per 1,000 person-years), cumulative CRC mortality was reduced by 15% in the screening group (Fig 3). Participants who accepted the first FOB test had a 39% reduction in CRC mortality when compared with controls. The predictive value for

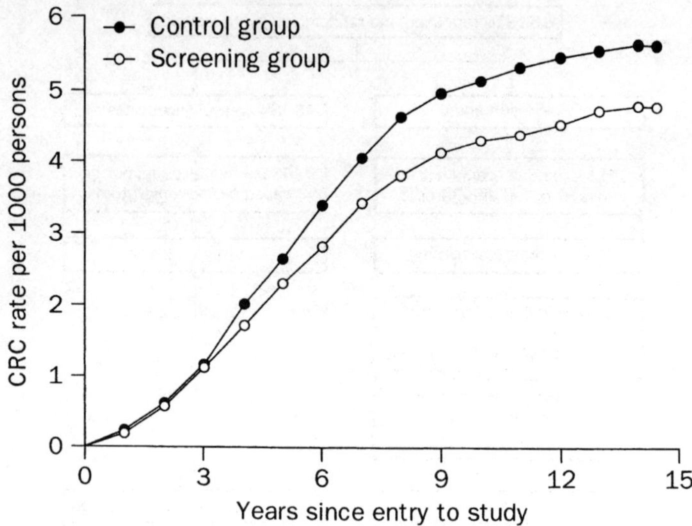

FIGURE 3.—Cumulative mortality from colorectal cancer (*CRC*). (Courtesy of Hardcastle JD, Chamberlain JO, Robinson MHE, et al: Randomised controlled trial of faecal–occult-blood screening for colorectal cancer. *Lancet* 348:1472–1477, 1996. Copyright by The Lancet Ltd.)

cancer after a positive FOB test was 9.9% at the first screening, 11.9% when rescreening was completed within 27 months, and 13.3% when rescreening took place after 27 months.

Discussion.—Compliance with the screening test was generally good and might be improved with participant education. The reduction in the rate of advanced CRC and significant reduction in CRC mortality support the use of widespread FOB screening tests.

▶ It is estimated that colorectal carcinoma will develop in approximately 6% of Americans, and currently, 160,000 new cases are diagnosed each year. There is now evidence from 3 randomized controlled trials, i.e., Abstracts 4–21 and 4–22 and a previously publicized study,[1] that screening average-risk individuals for colorectal cancer with FOB tests can reduce mortality from colorectal cancer. While it seems clear that such screening clearly prevents death and adds years of life, several important questions arise.

1. *How sensitive is FOB screening?* The positive predictive value of a positive FOB test for the detection of colorectal cancer ranged from 17% with the first screening round to 9% in the third screening round on the Funen study. The predictive value of a positive test for the detection of large adenomas ranged from 32% at the first round to 21% at the final round. Similar results in the studies suggest a cancer detection rate of only 25%, and as expected, positive tests are much more likely to be positive in individuals older than 75 years. Clearly, there now is a need for more sensitive tests without lowering specificity. Furthermore, case-control studies have indicated that sigmoidos-

copy every 5–10 years after age 50 can reduce mortality from colorectal cancer by 60%.

2. *Balance between sensitivity and specificity.* The use of more sensitive but less specific tests employing rehydrated FOB resulted in a greater reduction in mortality in the screened group but at a much higher colonoscopic examination rate, i.e., 28% to 38% in the Minnesota study as compared with 4% in the Funen and Nottingham studies. Further, it has been estimated that up to one third of the reduction in mortality in the Minnesota study was accounted for by false positive FOB tests.

3. *Compliance.* In the Funen study, only 46% of the paticipants completed all tests offered, and in the Nottingham study, only 38% did. If more extensive screening is to be offered, it will not be effective unless physicians educate and encourage patients.

4. *Cost-effectiveness.* Liebermann and Sleisenger[2] cite data indicating that the cost of screening at $10,000–$30,000 per year of added life is comparable to other accepted treatments but the cost for each prevented death is substantial, i.e., $200,000. It has been estimated that each 2% increase in false positive FOB tests could raise the evaluation costs by up to $1 billion if all such individuals underwent colonoscopy at current reimbursement rates.

5. *Screening and surveillance in the future.* It should be possible in the next 4 years to identify subjects at marked risk for colorectal cancer by utilizing new tests based on genetic alterations. In the interim, FOB testing and flexible sigmoidoscopy have both proved effective in reducing mortality from colorectal cancer and should be employed in all individuals older than 50 years of age.

N.J. Greenberger, M.D.

References

1. Mandel JS, Band JH, Church TK, et al: Reducing mortality from colorectal cancer by screening for fecal occult blood. *N Eng J Med* 328:1365–1371, 1993.
2. Liebermann DA, Sleisenger MH: It is time to recommend screening for colorectal cancer. *Lancet* 348:1463–1464, 1996.

Sensitivity Colonoscopy vs. Barium Enema

Relative Sensitivity of Colonoscopy and Barium Enema for Detection of Colorectal Cancer in Clinical Practice
Rex DK, Rahmani EY, Haseman JH, et al (Indiana Univ, Indianapolis)
Gastroenterology 112:17–23, 1997   4–23

Background.—The relative sensitivities of barium enema and colonoscopy in the diagnosis of colorectal cancer have not been established. The performances of each were investigated in clinical practice.

Methods and Findings.—The medical records of 2,193 consecutive patients with colorectal cancer in 20 central Indiana hospitals were reviewed.

TABLE 4.—Distribution of Dukes' Classes Among Cases Detected by
Barium Enema and Colonoscopy

Dukes' class	Barium enema (%)	Colonoscopy (%)
A	56 (9.8)*	209 (24.9)
B	256 (44.6)	320 (38.2)
C	168 (29.3)	202 (24.1)
D	94 (16.4)	106 (12.7)
Total	574	837

Note: 22 barium enema cases and 57 colonoscopy cases with unknown Dukes' classes were not included.
*Number of cases and percentage with given Dukes' class.
(Courtesy of Rex DK, Rahmani EY, Haseman JH, et al: Relative sensitivity of colonoscopy and barium enema for detection of colorectal cancer in clinical practice. *Gastroenterology* 112:17–23, 1997.)

For diagnosing colorectal cancer, colonoscopy had a sensitivity of 95% and barium enema had a sensitivity of 82.9%. The odds ratio for a missed cancer by barium enema was 3.93 compared with colonoscopy. The sensitivities of double-contrast and single-contrast barium enemas were 85.2% and 81.8%, respectively. The performance of barium enema was not better in the right than in the left colon. Cancers detected by colonoscopy were more likely to be Dukes' class A than were those detected by barium enema. The sensitivity of colonoscopy done by gastroenterologists was 97.3%, compared with 87% for colonoscopy done by nongastroenterologists, yielding a 5.36 odds ratio for a missed cancer by a nongastroenterologist compared with that by a gastroenterologist (Table 4).

Conclusions.—Hospital quality assurance committees and third-party payers need to review the sensitivities of barium enema and colonoscopy as performed by the practitioners in their institutions. When sensitivity is significantly less than the standard of the gastroenterologists evaluated here, corrective measures are warranted.

▶ The key finding in this study is that the "miss" rate for early cancer on a prior diagnostic examination was 5% for colonoscopy and 17% for the barium enema x-ray examination. However, as Waye[1] points out in an accompanying editorial, the vast difference in the ability of colonoscopy to detect colorectal cancer at an early stage was in patients with Dukes' A lesions. If Dukes' A stage lesions are excluded from the analysis, the detection rates for Dukes' stage B, C, and D lesions are comparable for barium enema and colonoscopy. Colonoscopy performed by gastroenterologists was more sensitive (97.7%) for cancer than colonoscopy by nongastroenterologists, with an odds ratio of 5.36 for a missed cancer by a nongastroenterologist.

The miss rate of 3% for gastroenterologists and 5% overall for early colorectal cancer was addressed by Rex and colleagues in a comparison paper.[2] Two consecutive same-day colonoscopies were performed on 183 patients. The overall miss rate for adenomas was 24%, with the expected result that the highest miss rate was 27% for small adenomas of 5 mm or less, decreasing to 13% for adenomas of 6–9 mm and to 6% for adenomas of 10 mm or greater. Rex and colleagues conclude that, although colonoscopy is the gold standard for colorectal polyp detection, it is imperfect even when meticulously performed. Further, they suggest the need for improvement in colonoscopy technology.

N.J. Greenberger, M.D.

References

1. Waye JD: What is a gold standard for colon polyps? *Gastroenterology* 112:292–293, 1997.
2. Rex DK, Cutler CS, Lemmel GT, et al: Colonoscopic miss rate of adenomas determined by back-to-back colonoscopies. *Gastroenterology* 112:24–28, 1997.

Risk of Colorectal Cancer in Families of Patients With Polyps

Risk of Colorectal Cancer in the Families of Patients With Adenomatous Polyps
Winawer SJ, and the National Polyp Study Workgroup (Mem Sloan-Kettering Cancer Ctr, New York; Boston City Hosp; Veterans Affairs Med Ctr, Minn; et al)
N Engl J Med 334:82–87, 1996   4–24

Objective.—There appears to be a sequence from adenoma to adenocarcinoma in colorectal cancer, suggesting that family members of patients with colorectal adenomas may also be at increased risk of colorectal cancer. Because adenomatous polyps are such a common finding, it is important to understand the nature of this risk. The colorectal cancer risk of family members of patients with colorectal adenomatous polyps was assessed, along with the patient and polyp factors associated with this risk.

Methods.—The analysis included a random sample of patients from the National Polyp Study who had newly diagnosed adenomatous polyps. Of this sample, 1,199 provided information on their parents' and siblings' histories of colorectal cancer in an interview. The family members' cancer risk was assessed in terms of the characteristics of the patients with adenoma and compared with that of the patients' spouses, who served as a control group. Families with incomplete information and patients referred for colonoscopy solely on the basis of a history of colorectal cancer were excluded from the study.

Results.—The final analysis included 1,031 patients with adenomas, along with 1,865 parents, 2,381 siblings, and 1,411 spouses. Compared with the spouse controls, relative risk of colorectal cancer among the parents and siblings was 1.78, after adjustment for year of birth and sex. This risk rose to 2.59 for siblings of patients in whom adenoma was diagnosed before the age of 60 years, compared with the siblings of patients in whom this diagnosis occurred at an older age and after adjustment for year of birth, sex, and parental history of colorectal cancer (Fig 1). As the patient's age at diagnosis of adenoma increased, the siblings'

Siblings of Patients with Adenomas
A
Cumulative Incidence (%)
15
10
5
0
40 45 50 55 60 65 70 75 80 85
Age of Sibling (yr)

Parents of Patients with Adenomas
B
Cumulative Incidence (%)
15
10
5
0
40 45 50 55 60 65 70 75 80 85
Age of Parent (yr)
Age of Patient at Diagnosis (yr)
<50
50-59
≥60
Spouse

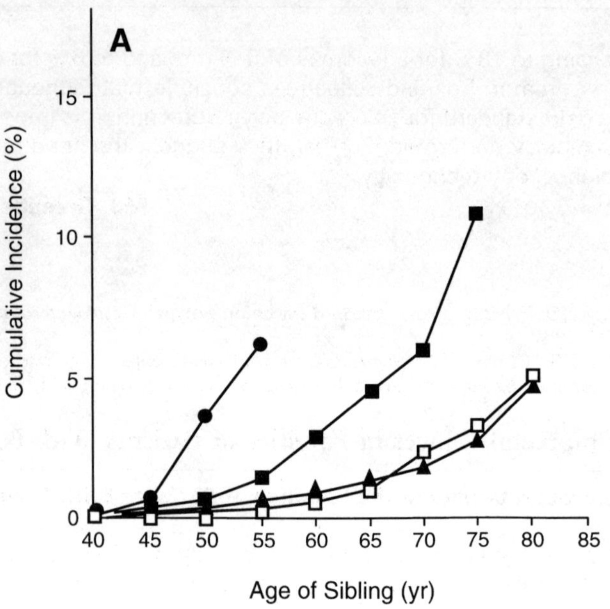

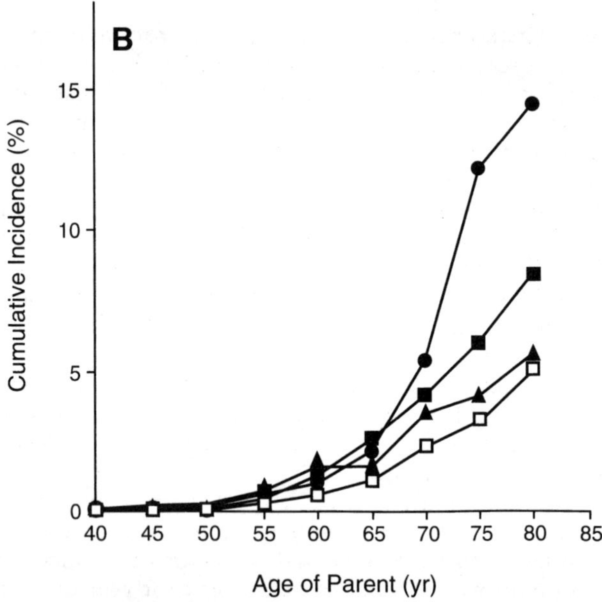

(Continued)

FIGURE 1 (cont.)

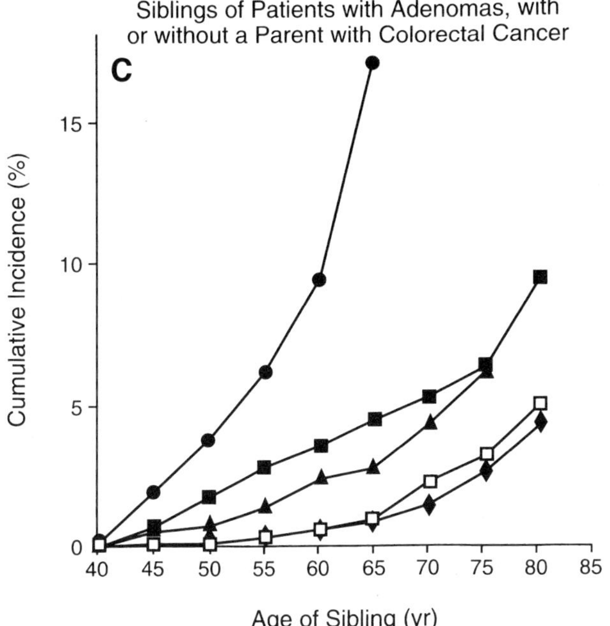

FIGURE 1.—Cumulative incidence of colorectal cancer in the family members of patients with adenomas. A shows the cumulative incidence of colorectal cancer in the siblings of patients with adenomas, according the the patients' ages at the time of diagnosis of the adenomas (younger than 50 years, 50–59, or 60 years old and older). B shows the cumulative incidence in the parents of patients with adenomas, according to the patients' ages at the time of diagnosis (younger than 50 years, 50–59, or 60 years old and older). C shows the cumulative incidence in the siblings of patients with adenomas, according to the patients' ages at the time of diagnosis (younger than 60 or 60 years old and older) and whether a parent had had colorectal cancer. In all 3 panels, the incidence among the spouse controls is shown for purposes of comparison. (Courtesy of Winawer SJ, and the National Polyp Study Workgroup: Risk of colorectal cancer in the families of patients with adenomatous polyps. *N Engl J Med* 334:82–87, 1996.)

colorectal cancer risk increased. Relative risk was 3.25 for siblings of patients who had a parent with colorectal cancer, compared to those with no such parental history and after adjustment for year of birth, sex, and patient's age at diagnosis.

Conclusions.—Colorectal cancer risk appears to be increased for siblings and parents of patients in whom adenomatous polyps have been diagnosed. The risk is even greater for both siblings and parents of patients whose adenoma is diagnosed before the age of 60 years and for siblings when a parent has a history of colorectal cancer. Colonoscopic screening programs could permit identification and removal of premalignant adenomas and thus help to reduce the incidence of colorectal cancer in families.

▶ This study more clearly defines the risk of colorectal cancer in the families of patients with colorectal cancer. In this regard, it has been demonstrated that siblings and parents of patients with adenomatous polyps had an increased risk of colorectal cancer, as compared with the risk among spouse controls in whom rates of colorectal cancer were similar to those in the general population. Further, the risk is greater if an adenoma is diagnosed before the age of 60 or when a parent has had colorectal cancer. Individuals in such families should enter into a surveillance program after age 40 and undergo colonoscopic examinations at least at 5-year intervals. If polyps with advanced pathologic features are discovered and treated, the interval may well have to be 3 years. Although this seems reasonable, the cost-effectiveness of this approach needs to be further evaluated.

N.J. Greenberger, M.D.

Hereditary Nonpolyposis Colorectal Cancer

Molecular Nature of Colon Tumors in Hereditary Nonpolyposis Colon Cancer, Familial Polyposis, and Sporadic Colon Cancer
Konishi M, Kikuchi-Yanoshita R, Tanaka K, et al (Tokyo Metropolitan Inst of Med Science; Tokyo Med and Dental Univ; Tokyo Metropolitan Komagome Hosp; et al)
Gastroenterology 111:307–317, 1996   4–25

Background.—Hereditary nonpolyposis colon cancer (HNPCC) is characterized by microsatellite instability. However, the mechanism of HNPCC carcinogenesis is not fully understood. The replication error (RER) and genetic changes between HNPCC and non-HNPCC tumors were compared to better define the nature of HNPCC tumors.

Methods.—Twenty-one cases of HNPCC, 389 of familial adenomatous polyposis, and 206 of sporadic tumors were assessed for RER and genetic changes. Polymerase chain reaction, single-strand conformation polymorphism, sequencing, and Southern hybridization were used.

Findings.—Ninety-five percent of tumors at all stages of HNPCC were RER-positive. Among familial adenomatous polyposis and sporadic tumors, RER positivity was 3% in adenoma and intramucosal carcinoma, 13% to 24% in invasive carcinoma, and 35% in carcinoma metastasis in liver. Fifty percent of RER-positive HNPCC tumors had germline and somatic mutations of *hMSH2* or *hMLH1* genes. By contrast, 6% of RER-positive non-HNPCCs had somatic mutation. Compared with non-HNPCC, HNPCC had significantly less frequent *APC*, *p53*, and K-*ras*-2 mutations and loss of heterozygosity of tumor-suppressor genes, but significantly more frequent transforming growth factor β type II receptor mutations (Table 4).

TABLE 4.—Summary of Frequency of Somatic Changes (%) in Replication Error[+] and Replication Error[−] Colorectal Carcinomas From Patients With Hereditary Nonpolyposis Colon Cancer (HNPCC) and Non-HNPCC Cancers

	No. of tumors analyzed*	Mutation or LOH									
			No. of tumors with somatic changes								
			Mutation				LOH/informative tumors				
RER type		*hMSH2* or *hMLH1*	*APC*	*p53*	*K-ras-2*	*TGF-βRII*	5q	8p	17p	18q	22q
HNPCC											
Severe RER[+]	15	8/15 (53)	3/15 (20)	2/15 (13)	1/15 (7)	11/15 (73)	1/10 (10)	1/10 (10)	1/10 (10)	1/6 (17)	1/10 (10)
[Severe RER[+]	9	8/9 (89)	2/9 (22)	2/9 (22)	0/9 (0)	7/9 (78)	0/5 (0)	0/5 (0)	0/6 (0)	0/4 (0)	0/5 (0)]†
Mild RER[+]	0										
RER[−]	1	0/1	1/1	0/1	0/1	0/1	0/1	—	0/1	—	—
FAP											
Severe RER[+]	2	0/1	1/2	0/2	1/2	0/1	0/2	—	0/2	0/2	0/2
Mild RER[+]	9	0/9 (0)	7/9 (78)	5/9 (56)	5/9 (56)	0/9 (0)	5/9 (56)	6/7 (86)	6/8 (75)	5/9 (56)	5/8 (63)
RER[−]	32	ND	11/25 (44)	6/13 (46)	11/22 (50)	0/20 (0)	13/23 (57)	6/12 (50)	9/15 (60)	8/14 (57)	4/19 (21)
Sporadic											
Severe RER[+]	5	1/5	0/4	2/5	0/5	2/5	1/3	2/2	1/3	0/1	1/2
Mild RER[+]	23	1/23 (4)	13/20 (65)	12/22 (55)	11/22 (50)	0/22 (0)	9/17 (53)	5/7 (71)	15/18 (83)	12/18 (67)	10/17 (59)
RER[−]	122	ND	21/56 (38)	37/55 (67)	24/79 (30)	0/76 (0)	49/89 (55)	42/64 (66)	65/82 (79)	50/86 (58)	33/83 (40)
P value,‡ severe RER[+] HNPCC											
vs. severe RER[+] non-HNPCC	0.1	0.7	0.4	0.5	0.1	0.6	0.05	0.6	0.7	0.5	
vs. total RER[+] non-HNPCC	0.0002	0.01	0.01	0.007	0.000001	0.03	0.0006	0.001	0.09	0.01	

*Carcinomas include invasive carcinoma and carcinoma metastasized to the liver.

†Data for carcinomas with identified germline mutation of *hMSH2* or *hMLH1* gene.

‡*P* values were determined by Fisher's exact test, with respect to total replication error *RER*)[+] hereditary nonpolyposis colon cancer (*HNPCC*) carcinomas and RER[+] non-HNPCC carcinomas.

Abbreviations: LOH, loss of heterozygosity; *FAP,* familial adenomatous polyposis; *ND,* not done.

(Courtesy of Konishi M, Kikuchi-Yanoshita R, Tanaka K, et al: Molecular nature of colon tumors in hereditary nonpolyposis colon cancer, familial polyposis, and sporadic colon cancer. *Gastroenterology* 111:307–317, 1996.)

Conclusions.—Replication error positivity is seen from an early stage of HNPCC carcinogenesis but in later stages of non-HNPCC. The development of most HNPCC tumors may occur through genetic changes different from those in the adenoma-carcinoma sequence, although a certain proportion develops through *APC* mutation.

▶ In their introduction, the authors provide a beautiful, concise summary of genetic alterations in colon cancer They point out that analysis of many tumors from patients with familial adenomatous polyposis (FAP) and sporadic colon cancer (SCC) have shown the following abnormalities: (1) Loss of heterozygosity (LOH) on chromosomes 5q, 8p, 17p, 18q, and 22q; (2) Mutation of the adenomatous polyposis coli (*APC*), *p53*, and K-*ras*-2 genes are major development mechanisms of colorectal cancers via the adenoma-carcinoma sequence; and (3) There is an accumulation of genetic changes in multiple tumor suppression genes:

- Inactivation of the *APC* gene is involved in the development of adenomas
- LOH of the *APC* gene is associated with future development of carcinoma
- Mutation and LOH of the *p53* gene is involved in the conversion of adenoma to carcinoma
- LOH on 18p, 18q, and 22q is involved in the progression from early to advanced carcinoma
- K-*ras* 2 mutations affects tumor growth

The development of most tumors in patients with SCC follows this sequence. However, HNPCC occurs in 3% to 6% of all colon cancer and, in addition, tumors from HNPCC patients appear to have different mechanisms then those from FAP and SCC. Therefore, the aim of the study was to clarify the nature of carcinogenesis in HNPCC. The major finding in this study is that colorectal HNPCC tumors have different molecular characteristics than FAP and SCC.

N.J. Greenberger, M.D.

Better Survival Rates in Patients With *MLH1*-Associated Hereditary Colorectal Cancer
Sankila R, Aaltonen LA, Järvinen HJ, et al (Univ of Helsinki; Helsinki Univ Hosp; Jyväskylä Central Hosp, Finland)
Gastroenterology 110:682–687, 1996 4–26

Background.—Hereditary nonpolyposis colorectal cancer is the most common inherited form of colorectal cancer. Studies have identified 4 predisposing genes to this disease. The prognosis of patients with hereditary nonpolyposis colorectal cancer may be better than that of patients with common sporadic colorectal cancer, but this hypothesis has not been confirmed. The survival rates of patients with hereditary nonpolyposis colorectal cancer and patients with common sporadic colorectal cancer were compared.

Methods.—Data from a nationwide cancer family registry were used. Colorectal cancer was diagnosed in 175 patients younger than 65 years from 39 families with hereditary nonpolyposis colorectal cancer; 120 of these patients were from families with germline mutations in the *MLH1* gene. Cumulative relative survival rates were calculated.

Results.—The overall 5-year cumulative relative survival rate was 65% for patients with hereditary nonpolyposis colorectal cancer, and 44% for patients with common sporadic colorectal cancer. In every stratum studied, the relative survival rate of patients with hereditary nonpolyposis colorectal cancer was better than the survival rate of patients with sporadic colorectal cancer.

Conclusions.—The natural history of colorectal cancer associated with the *MLH1* gene is different from that of sporadic colorectal cancer. In hereditary nonpolyposis colorectal cancer, it is possible that an impaired DNA repair mechanism increases mutation frequency, and that the same genetic defect responsible for tumor initiation and progression reduces cancer cell viability.

▶ This report from Finland, using the tools of molecular genetics to identify a precise high-risk population, is on the forefront of how we will prognosticate on therapeutic outcomes in the future. However, use of such powerful analytical tools requires a second ingredient: the capacity to identify and follow up not only with the patient, but with all living members of the family tree over a long period of time. This obviously requires a considerable investment in time and money. The rewards, however, would go beyond just the small segment of the population studied, but could extend to the population at large as more is learned in the defined population about the origins of their disease.

F.G. Moody, M.D.

Importance of Small Adenoma

Importance of Adenomas 5 mm or Less in Diameter That Are Detected by Sigmoidoscopy
Read TE, Read JD, Butterly LF (Lahey Hitchcock Med Ctr, Burlington, Mass)
N Engl J Med 336:8–12, 1997   4–27

Background.—Authorities disagree on the need for colonoscopy in patients with adenomas of 5 mm or less in diameter detected by sigmoidoscopy. The prevalence of proximal colonic neoplasms was determined prospectively in a large group of asymptomatic patients at average risk for colorectal cancer and with diminutive benign adenomatous polyps on screening flexible sigmoidoscopy.

Methods.—A total of 3,496 consecutive patients underwent sigmoidoscopy, 311 of whom were found to have neoplastic rectosigmoid polyps. One hundred eight were excluded because of a history of colonic neoplasia, symptoms, previous colonic assessment, or incomplete follow-up data. The remaining 203 patients underwent colonoscopy. Rectosigmoid ad-

TABLE 2.—Histologic Characteristics of Index Neoplastic Lesions Found at Flexible Sigmoidoscopy in 203 Asymptomatic Average-risk Patients

Characteristic	Rectosigmoid Adenoma ≤5 mm in Diameter (N = 137)	Rectosigmoid Adenoma 6–10 mm in Diameter (N = 52)	Rectosigmoid Adenoma ≥11 mm in Diameter (N = 14)
	no. of patients (%)		
Tubular adenoma	129 (94)	41 (79)	9 (64)
Tubulovillous adenoma	3 (2)	8 (15)	3 (21)
Villous adenoma	1 (1)	0	1 (7)
Adenoma with moderate-to-severe dysplasia	4 (3)	3 (6)	1 (7)

(Courtesy of Read TE, Read JD, Butterly LF: Importance of adenomas 5 mm or less in diameter that are detected by sigmoidoscopy. *N Engl J Med* 336:8–12, 1997. Reprinted by permission of *The New England Journal of Medicine*. Copyright 1997, Massachusetts Medical Society. All rights reserved.)

enomas 5 mm or less in diameter were designated diminutive, those 6–10 mm were designated small, and those 11 mm or greater were designated large.

Findings.—Neoplasms were detected in the proximal colon of 29% of the 137 patients with diminutive index polyps, 29% of the 52 patients with small index polyps, and 57% of the 14 patients with large index polyps. Advanced neoplasms were detected in 6%, 10%, and 29%, respectively. Two patients with diminutive index polyps had proximal carcinoma in situ. Another 2 in this group had proximal stage I carcinomas. Proximal stage III carcinoma was found in a patient with a large index polyp (Table 2).

Conclusions.—The prevalence of proximal colonic neoplasms, including advanced lesions, in asymptomatic average-risk patients with rectosigmoid adenomas of 5 mm or less in diameter is substantial. Colonoscopy is warranted in these patients.

▶ There is considerable controversy regarding the probability of discovering an advanced proximal neoplasm in patients found to have diminutive (less than 5 mm) or small (6–10 mm) polyps on flexible sigmoidoscopic examination. This carefully done study by Read and colleagues found that asymptomatic, average-risk patients with diminutive or small rectosigmoid adenomas on screening flexible sigmoidoscopic examination have a 29% prevalence of proximal neoplasms at colonoscopy. More disquieting was the finding that 4 patients with diminutive rectosigmoid adenomas had early stages of proximal lesions harboring frank carcinoma. The authors suggest that neoplastic changes in the distal colon may be a marker for neoplastic changes in the proximal colon, but appropriately caution that because they did not perform colonoscopy on a control group of patients who had no neoplasms at sigmoidoscopy, this association remains unproved.

N.J. Greenberger, M.D.

Prevalence of Colonic Polyps in Acromegaly

The Prevalence of Colonic Polyps in Acromegaly: A Colonoscopic and Pathological Study in 103 Patients

Delhougne B, Deneux C, Abs R, et al (Univ of Liège, Belgium; Univ of Paris; Univ of Antwerp, Belgium; et al)

J Clin Endocrinol Metab 80:3223–3226, 1995

4–28

Background.—Patients with acromegaly are thought to be at risk for adenomatous colonic polyps, which are considered to be preneoplastic lesions. However, this belief is based on studies of rather small series of patients without control groups. The prevalence of colonic polyps was determined in a prospective study of a large number of individuals with and without acromegaly.

Methods.—One hundred patients with acromegaly and 138 individuals without acromegaly were included. Colonoscopic and pathologic assessments were performed.

Findings.—The patients with acromegaly had a significantly higher prevalence rate of adenomatous polyps than did the control subjects— 22.3% vs. 8%, respectively. However, the difference in prevalence rates was significant only in male patients with acromegaly and control subjects. Patients with acromegaly who were younger than 55 years had a 20% prevalence rate of colonic polyps, which was significantly greater than the 3% prevalence rate in the control group. Adenomatous colonic polyps in patients with acromegaly were characterized by multiplicity and a location proximal to the splenic flexure. The duration of acromegaly was similar in patients with and without adenomatous polyps. The prevalence rate of hyperplastic colonic polyps was 24.3% in patients with acromegaly and 4.4% in the control group, also a significant difference (Table 1).

TABLE 1.—Colonic Polyps in Patients With Acromegaly vs. Control Subjects

	Acromegalic group	Control group	*P* Values
Adenomatous polyps	23/103 (22.3)	11/138 (8)	0.0024
Multiple adenomatous polyps	6/103 (5.8)	0/138 (0)	
Males with adenomatous polyps	14/49 (28.6)	3/55 (5.5)	0.0026
Females with adenomatous polyps	9/54 (16.7)	8/83 (9.6)	0.2899
<55 yr old with adenomatous polyps	14/70 (20.0)	2/66 (3.0)	0.0026
>55 yr old with adenomatous polyps	9/33 (27.3)	9/72 (12.5)	0.0635
Hyperplastic polyps	25/103 (24.3)	6/138 (4.4)	<0.001

Note: Percentages are given in parentheses.

(Courtesy of Delhougne B, Deneux C, Abs R, et al: The prevalence of colonic polyps in acromegaly: A colonoscopic and pathological study in 103 patients. *J Clin Endocrinol Metab* 80:3223–3226, 1995. Copyright The Endocrine Society.)

Conclusions.—Patients with acromegaly are at risk for colonic adenomatous polyp development. Colonoscopic screening is useful for detecting colonic cancer early.

▶ This study provides additional documentation that patients with acromegaly are at significant risk for the development of colonic adenomatous polyps. The new information provided is the greater risk of polyps found in men compared with women and the appreciable frequency of polyps (20% in this series) observed in patients younger than 55 years. Although the overall prevalence rate of adenomatous polyps was 22% (23 of 103 patients), no adenocarcinomas were discovered. The authors recommend that colonoscopy be part of the follow-up examination in patients with acromegaly. The genetic link between acromegaly and colonic polyps remains to be elucidated.

N.J. Greenberger, M.D.

Familial Juvenile Polyposis

Familial Juvenile Polyposis: Patterns of Recurrence and Implications for Surgical Management
Scott-Conner CEH, Hausmann M, Hall TJ, et al (Univ of Mississippi, Jackson; Baton Rouge Clinic, La)
J Am Coll Surg 181:407–413, 1995   4–29

Introduction.—Familial juvenile polyposis (FJP) is a rare condition that is inherited as an autosomal dominant trait. The risk to develop carcinoma is estimated to be 50% in this cohort. The standard recommendation for management of patients with FJP is subtotal colectomy with ileorectal anastomosis. A large kindred of patients with FJP was reviewed retrospectively to characterize distribution of disease and recurrence. From these findings and review of other published series, a strategy for management is described.

Methods.—Data collected in a registry since 1988 on 41 patients in a kindred with FJP were reviewed for patient history. Pathology samples were retrieved and reviewed. At the time of subtotal colectomy surgery, all patients were considered to be at risk for recurrence.

Results.—Of 34 living members of the kindred, 15 had undergone follow-up investigation at the time of review. Of the 15 patients, 11 had histologic findings of typical juvenile polyps (Fig 1). Of 8 patients who underwent surgical resection, all resected specimens had juvenile polyps, that numbered from 3 to more than 50. Juvenile polyps with foci of mild dysplasia were found in 6 colectomy specimens. One specimen contained a juvenile polyp with severe dysplasia. Three patients had coexisting adenomatous polyps, 1 patient had a villous adenoma, and 1 patient had polyps with coexisting juvenile and adenomatous elements. Seven of 8 patients who underwent resection were considered at risk of recurrence in the rectal remnant. Recurrent juvenile polyps were determined in 3 of the 7 patients at a mean of 36 months. Two patients underwent conversion to

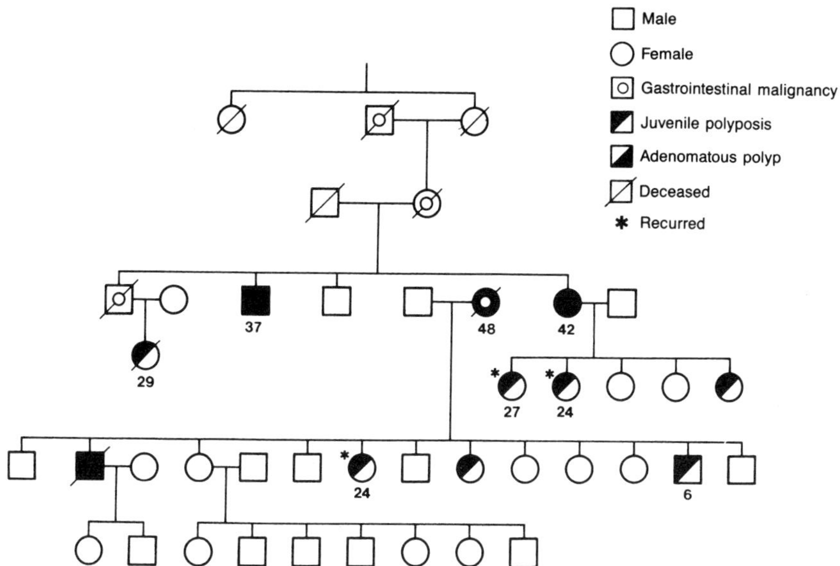

FIGURE 1.—Pedigree of kindred with familial juvenile polyposis. Ages are given for patients who underwent subtotal colectomy. (Courtesy of Scott-Conner CEH, Hausmann M, Hall TJ, et al: Familial juvenile polyposis: Patterns of recurrence and implications for surgical management. *J Am Coll Surg* 181:407–413, 1995. By permission of the *Journal of the American College of Surgeons.*)

total proctocolectomy with ileoanal anastomosis and J pouch. One of these patients had small juvenile polyps in the pouch at 40 months after conversion.

Conclusion.—Because of the propensity for recurrence of polyps, it is recommended that restorative proctocolectomy be the initial procedure in patients with FJP. Since juvenile polyps may recur in the ileal reservoir, it is recommended that these patients be followed closely.

▶ Familial juvenile polyposis is an autosomal dominant genetic disorder that carries with it a coin flip (50%) lifetime incidence of colon cancer. Clearly, families with this trait require careful screening and surveillance. Once polyposis occurs (usually in the right colon), subtotal colectomy is required, but even this procedure does not prevent recurrence in the rectum. It is important to note that, if polyps are found elsewhere in the gastrointestinal tract, the chance for malignancy remains equally high and usually occurs before 40 years of age.

F.G. Moody, M.D.

Surgical Considerations

Five-year Follow-up After Radical Surgery for Colorectal Cancer: Results of a Prospective Randomized Trial

Mäkelä JT, Laitinen SO, Kairaluoma MI (Oulu Univ, Finland)
Arch Surg 130:1062–1067, 1995   4–30

Background.—The value of intensive follow-up of patients who undergo curative resection for colorectal cancer has been unclear. The most appropriate follow-up program for these patients has not been determined. Old, conventional and new, intensified follow-up protocols were compared in a prospective, randomized trial.

Methods.—One hundred six patients had radical primary surgery for colorectal cancer and were randomized to participate in conventional or intensified follow-up programs for 5 years. Recurrence rates were recorded, and differences in detection methods and the effect of earlier detection on reoperability and survival were determined.

Results.—Recurrence of cancer was identified earlier in patients receiving intensified follow-up. The recurrence rate was 39% in patients given conventional follow-up and 42% in those given intensified follow-up. The most common method that showed recurrence in both groups was carcinoembryonic antigen determination. In patients given intensified follow-up, endoscopy and ultrasound were beneficial, but CT did not improve diagnostic methods. The mode of recurrence was similar for both groups. Radical resection was performed in 14% of patients in the conventional follow-up group and in 22% of patients in the intensified follow-up group. The five-year survival rate was 54% in patients given conventional follow-up and 59% in patients given intensified follow-up.

Conclusions.—Intensive follow-up of these patients did not lead to significant differences in resectability or 5-year survival rates. In patients receiving intensified follow-up, CT was not cost-efficient, ultrasonography was very effective in detecting metastases in the liver, and endoscopy was very effective in mucosal surveillance of the colon.

▶ The surgeons from the Department of Surgery in the Oulu University Hospital in Finland compared the relative merits of an intense rigorous follow-up to a conventional follow-up that required patients to receive rigid sigmoidoscopy on a yearly basis. The intense follow-up, which included colonoscopy at 3 months and yearly thereafter, CT scans on a yearly basis, and frequent flexsigmoidoscopic examinations (every 3 months) for patients with rectosigmoid cancers, led to naught. It turns out that yearly carcinoembryonic antigen analysis was the most sensitive tool for early detection, and early detection did not lead to prolonged survival. I guess a sensible approach is to perform a colonoscopy on all patients with colon cancer before the operation. Patients should receive another colonoscopy at 6 months or so, and then they should be followed up yearly with carcinoembryonic antigen analysis. It is not surprising that CT scans were of little value to the patients' welfare.

F.G. Moody, M.D.

Local Recurrence Rate in a Randomised Multicentre Trial of Preoperative Radiotherapy Compared With Operation Alone in Resectable Rectal Carcinoma
Swedish Rectal Cancer Trial (Univ of Uppsala, Sweden)
Eur J Surg 162:397–402, 1996   4–31

Background.—Previous studies have reported reduced local recurrence rates in patients who have resectable rectal carcinoma and receive preoperative irradiation. The effect of short-term, high-dose preoperative radiation therapy on local recurrence and postoperative mortality was evaluated in a prospective randomized trial.

Methods.—During a 3-year period, 1,168 patients who had resectable rectal carcinoma were randomly assigned to treatment with surgery alone or radiation therapy at 25 Gy in 5 fractions in 1 week and surgery within the next week. Operations that yielded tumor specimens with tumor-free margins were considered curative. The tumors were staged. Local recurrence rates after a minimum follow-up of 2 years were determined.

Results.—The overall local recurrence rates were 9% in the irradiated group and 24% in the surgery alone group. Significantly lower local recurrence rates were also seen in the irradiated group than in the surgery alone group among patients who had curative operations and among patients who had all stages of disease, regardless of the type of surgical procedure. Distant metastases developed within 2 years in 17% of the irradiated group and in 20% of the surgery alone group among those with curative operations.

Conclusion.—Short-term, high-dose preoperative radiation therapy reduces the local recurrence rate by approximately 65% in patients who have resectable rectal carcinoma. Longer follow-up is needed to determine the effect of preoperative radiation therapy on overall survival.

▶ The Swedish surgeons have a knack for conducting randomized trials that provide useful information. High-dose preoperative irradiation (25 Gy in 5 fractions in 1 week) reduces the local recurrence rate in patients who undergo resection of a rectal cancer. The results are impressive, and the radiation therapy as given appeared to incur no increased morbidity compared with operation alone. Further, surgery was delayed only for a 2-week period. It will be interesting to see whether this approach will prolong survival.

F.G. Moody, M.D.

Surgical Cure for Early Rectal Carcinomas (T1): Transanal Endoscopic Microsurgery *vs.* Anterior Resection

Winde G, Nottberg H, Keller R, et al (Westfälische Wilhelms-Univ of Münster, Germany)
Dis Colon Rectum 39:969–976, 1996   4–32

Introduction.—Anterior resection (AR), the gold standard for the treatment of rectal cancer, has yielded good results in regard to local recurrence and 5-year survival. Local resection using transanal endoscopic microsurgery (TEM) provides good overview within the rectal cavity and allows precise handling of neoplastic lesions. Morbidity, mortality, and survival rates of AR and TEM were compared prospectively to determine objective advantages of TEM in 52 patients with adenocarcinomas.

Methods.—Patients with early rectal carcinomas (T1) were randomly divided into 2 groups of 26 patients each and assigned to undergo either AR or TEM. Operative time, blood loss, length of hospitalization, mortality, early and late morbidity, postoperative analgesic opiate demand, and survival rates were compared for the 2 procedures.

Results.—Patients who underwent TEM had significantly lower operative time, intraoperative blood loss, length of hospital stay, and need for postoperative opiates than patients who underwent AR. Early morbidity rates for TEM and AR were 20.8% and 34.5%, respectively. Late complications occurred in 4.1% and 8% of patients in the TEM and AR groups, respectively. There was no intraoperative or early postoperative mortality in either group. Survival rates were similar for both groups.

Conclusions.—Transanal endoscopic microsurgery is associated with low morbidity, low local recurrence, and a shorter hospital stay. It should be preferred over AR for early rectal cancer because of superior overview during surgery and safer suturing after meticulous full wall thickness excision.

▶ Transanal endoscopic microsurgery is as effective as low AR for the treatment of early rectal cancer. Although the numbers in this controlled trial are small. the results are unequivocal. There is less morbidity and time spent in the hospital, with comparable survival in the microsurgery group. The key is precise preoperative staging. It is not clear how many patients were excluded because of unanticipated extension of the lesion.

F.G. Moody, M.D.

Laser Therapy for Villous Adenomas

Endoscopic Nd:YAG Laser Therapy for Villous Adenomas of the Colon and Rectum

Hyser MJ, Gau FC (St Francis Hosp, Evanston, Ill)
Am Surg 62:577–580, 1996   4–33

Background.—Villous adenomas are soft, sessile tumors with frondlike projections found mainly in the rectosigmoid colon. They also occur in the cecum and elsewhere in the colon. The outcomes of endoscopic laser treatment in a group of patients with villous adenomas were compared with the outcomes of other treatment strategies.

Methods.—Thirty-four patients with villous tumors of the colon and rectum underwent endoscopic Nd:YAG laser treatment between 1983 and 1995. The patients were 20 women and 14 men aged 31 to 93 years. Tumors were benign in 23 patients and contained carcinoma in situ in 11. Patients with invasive carcinomas were excluded. Six tumors were located in the cecum, 1 in the descending colon, 2 in the sigmoid colon, and 25 in the rectum. The mean number of total treatments per patient was 3.3. Only 1 patient required general anesthesia. Twenty-four received IV demerol. The tumors ranged from 2 to 12 cm in the largest dimension. One fourth of the tumors were 50% to 100% circumferential. In 4 patients, tumors were recurrent after transanal excision.

Findings.—Complications included mild stricture, occurring in 2 patients; self-limited bleeding in 2; and pinhole colovaginal fistula in 1. One treatment was incomplete. Also, there was 1 recurrence in the cecum that was carcinoma in situ at resection. No missed cancers occurred during the 1- to 120-month follow-up. The mean total cost for the entire treatment per patient was $3,627.

Conclusion.—Endoscopic Nd:YAG laser therapy is a safe and effective outpatient treatment for villous tumors of the colon and rectum. The complication rate is lower than in most reported series of patients undergoing surgery. Sphincter dysfunction, incontinence, or fecal fistula is avoided with endoscopic Nd:YAG laser therapy. Invasive carcinoma can be ruled out with close follow-up and repeated biopsy. Endoscopic Nd:YAG laser therapy is the procedure of choice for patients with villous adenomas of the colon and rectum.

▶ Hyser and Gau present results in their treatment of villous tumors of the colon and rectum by Nd:YAG laser that are almost too good to believe. In fact, several surgeons attending the presentation at the Midwest Surgical Association asked questions such as you probably have in mind. For example, doesn't treatment of circumferential lesions in this way lead to stricture and wouldn't neoplastic degeneration in a large lesion be overlooked? The results, however, speak for themselves; the stricture and recurrence rate were remarkably low.

F.G. Moody, M.D.

31 Diverticular Disease

The Hartmann Procedure: First Choice or Last Resort in Diverticular Disease?
Belmonte C, Klas JV, Perez JJ, et al (Univ of Minnesota, Minneapolis)
Arch Surg 131:612–617, 1996   4–34

Introduction.—The Hartmann procedure, used in the surgical management of diverticular disease, is associated with high morbidity and mortality and requires lengthy hospitalization for colostomy closure. Thus at the study institution, primary anastomosis is preferred in all cases when the patient is medically stable and the bowel ends are healthy. Results of this approach for 227 patients treated from 1988 to 1993 were reported.

Patients and Methods.—The patients had a mean age of 66 years; 143 were women and 84 were men. Surgery was elective in 86%, emergent in 8%, and urgent in 5%. Three types of operations were performed: primary resection with anastomosis, primary resection with anastomosis and diverting ileostomy, and primary resection with the Hartmann procedure. Choice of procedure was based on patient condition and experience of the operating team. Case records were reviewed retrospectively for morbidity, mortality, leak rates, and length of hospitalization, and patients were categorized for pathologic stage.

Results.—There were 23 patients in clinical/pathologic stage 0 (no inflammation), 40 in stage I (chronic inflammation), 53 in stage II (acute inflammation with or without microabscesses), 61 in stage III (pericolonic or mesenteric abscess), 39 in stage IV (pelvic abscess), and 11 in stage V (purulent or fecal peritonitis). Fifty patients, including 32 in stages II or III, had fistulas. Primary anastomosis was performed in 200 patients, 17 with and 183 without proximal diversion. Twenty-two of 27 patients who had the Hartmann procedure were in clinical/pathologic stages IV or V. Colostomy closure has been performed in 70% of this group. Morbidity, 23% overall, increased with worsening disease and reached 36% in the stage V group. An anastomotic leak occurred in 4 patients, all of whom were treated successfully. Three perioperative deaths all resulted from sepsis in stage IV patients. Both length of stay and morbidity were increased in cases of colostomy closure after the Hartmann procedure (13 days, 33%) vs. ileostomy closure (5 days, 7%).

Conclusion.—Removal of the affected bowel with minimal patient morbidity and mortality is the primary goal of surgery for diverticular disease.

Although the Hartmann procedure is popular, this approach is associated with high morbidity and mortality. Colostomy closure may be difficult, and one third of patients retain their stomas for life. But for almost all patients with disease stages 0 through III, resection and primary anastomosis should be possible.

▶ I appreciated the opportunity to upgrade my knowledge of the contemporary management of diverticular disease of the colon. The results suggest to me that the colorectal surgeons at the University of Minnesota have provided strong evidence that the Hartmann procedure should be used only in extreme cases when an anastomosis should be avoided at the time of resection or a permanent stoma is the best option for the patient's circumstances. CT-guided percutaneous drainage of pericolic abscesses has made a dramatic change in how we approach patients with advanced disease. The discussion of this paper presented to the 102nd Scientific Session of the Western Surgical Association (1995) is worth reading, because it reflects the current trend toward resection and reanastomosis even in complex cases. Dr. Goldberg's closing comments are highly recommended to those who treat this common disease. It is filled with high-quality "pearls."

F.G. Moody, M.D.

32 Miscellaneous

Bowel Dysfunction in Spinal Cord Injury

Bowel Dysfunction in Spinal-cord–injury Patients

Glickman S, Kamm MA (Charing Cross Hosp, London; St Mark's Hosp, London)

Lancet 347:1651–1653, 1996

4–35

Background.—Patients with traumatic spinal cord injury (SCI) face many problems in addition to motor paralysis, including sensory loss, spasticity, pain, and bladder and bowel dysfunction. Once the patients have adapted to impaired mobility, the major problem frequently is bowel dysfunction. The magnitude of bowel dysfunction in patients with SCI was investigated.

Methods.—The study included 115 consecutive patients with SCI. There were 89 men and 25 women, with a median age of 37.5 years. The median time since SCI was 62 months. Forty-eight percent of the injuries were cervical, 47% thoracic, and 5% lumbar. The patients provided information on their bowel function before and after SCI, and their perceptions of their disabilities and symptoms. They also were assessed on the Hospital Anxiety and Depression Scale.

TABLE 1.—Percentage of Patients ($n = 115$) With Preinjury and Postinjury Bowel Disorders and Symptoms

Diagnosed bowel problems	Preinjury	Postinjury	P Values
Any bowel problem	21	50	0.0001
Irritable bowel syndrome	2	2	1.0
Haemorrhoids	16	23	0.17
Prolapse	1	2	1.0
Polyps	4	1	0.38
Anal fissure	3	6	0.29
Diarrhoea	1	14	0.0001
Constipation	5	30	0.0001
Malabsorption	0	0	..
Inflammatory bowel disease	0	0	..
Cancer	0	0	..
Nausea	3	19	0.0001
Vomiting	4	7	0.34

TABLE 3.—Percentage of Patients ($n = 115$) Using Bowel Initiating Methods Before and After Injury

Methods of opening bowel	% of patients using method preinjury	% of patients using method postinjury	P Values
Using one or more method	20	95	0.0001
Straining >25%	9	20	0.01
Oral laxatives	5	29	0.0001
Supplemental fibre	2	17	0.0001
Digital stimulation	0	53	0.0001
Manual evacuation	1	68	0.0001
Suppositories	1	49	0.0001
Enemas	0	11	0.0002
Reflex	2	20	0.0001
Self-induced spasms	0	6	0.02
High-fibre diet	6	23	0.0001
Electrical implant	0	2	0.5
Other	4	6	0.5

(Courtesy of Glickman S, Kamm MA: Bowel dysfunction in spinal-cord–injury patients. *Lancet* 347:1651–1653, 1996. Copyright by The Lancet Ltd., 1996.)

Results.—Compared with their pre-injury state, the patients were much more likely to have nausea, diarrhea, constipation, and fecal incontinence after SCI (Table 1). Ninety-five percent of the patients used 1 or more techniques to initiate defecation, most frequently manual evacuation and digital stimulation (Table 3). Half were dependent on others for help in toileting, and half took longer than 30 minutes to complete their toileting procedure. Fifty-four percent of patients reported that bowel function was a distressing problem. Distress was linked to the time needed for bowel management and the frequency with which incontinence occurred. The time needed for bowel management also was significantly correlated with anxiety and depression scores. On a scale of 0 to 10, with 10 indicating the maximum perceived problem, the patients' mean rating for bowel management was 5.1, compared to 6.8 for loss of mobility.

Conclusions.—For patients with SCI, bowel dysfunction is a major source of physical and psychological problems. They may have constipation, diarrhea, and nausea. They often require help with toileting, which can be a time-consuming process. These patients' well-being may improve with improved management of bowel dysfunction.

▶ This study demonstrates that bowel function is a major physical and psychological problem in patients with SCI. Indeed, many patients rated their bowel management problems almost as bothersome as their loss of mobility using the Hospital Anxiety and Depression Scale questionnaire.[1] Most patients required medications and many required personal assistance to achieve defecation.

N.J. Greenberger, M.D.

Reference

1. Zigmond AS, Snaith RP: The Hospital Anxiety and Depression Scale. *Acta Psychiatr Scand* 67:361–370, 1983.

Laparoscopic Colorectal Surgery

Laparoscopic Colorectal Surgery: Ascending the Learning Curve

Reissman P, Cohen S, Weiss EG, et al (Cleveland Clinic Florida, Fort Lauderdale)
World J Surg 20:277–282, 1996   4–36

Objective.—The use of laparoscopic colorectal surgery is expanding rapidly, despite the lack of prospective, randomized trials demonstrating its benefits. A substantial learning curve is expected with laparoscopic colorectal surgery, given the unfamiliarity of the technique and the new instruments involved. The results of 100 laparoscopic and laparoscopy-assisted colorectal procedures were prospectively assessed.

Methods.—The first 100 laparoscopic colorectal surgical procedures performed in one institution by one surgical team from 1991 through 1994 were evaluated. Variables analyzed included the type and length of the procedure, intraoperative and postoperative complications, the need for conversion to open surgery, the duration of postoperative ileus, and hospitalization.

Patients and Findings.—The patients consisted of 60 males and 40 females; mean age, 49 years. Inflammatory bowel disease was the most frequent indication for surgery, (n = 34), followed by cancer (n = 15). The experience included 36 total abdominal colectomies (TACs), most involving creation of an ileoanal reservoir; 39 segmental resections of the colon and small bowel; 8 rectal resections; 7 diverting stomas; 7 reversals of Hartmann's procedure; and 3 miscellaneous procedures. Seven patients required conversion to open surgery. There were 26 complications in 22 patients, including 5 cases of enterostomy, 6 of hemorrhage, 4 of intra-abdominal abscess, 4 of prolonged ileus, 2 wound infections, and 1 case each of anastomotic leakage, aspiration, cardiac arrhythmia, upper gastrointestinal bleeding, and postoperative small-bowel obstruction. None of the patients died during the postoperative period.

Results.—The complication rate declined from 42% in the early part of the experience to 27% in the middle part and 12% in the late part. The decline in complication rate was associated with the declining number of TAC procedures performed. The overall complication rate in TAC procedures was 42%, compared with 9% in segmental resections and 12% in nonresectional procedures. Mean operating times were 4.0, 2.5, and 1.6 hours, respectively, and the mean duration of ileus was 3.5, 3.0, and 2.0 days. Patients undergoing TAC procedures stayed in the hospital a mean of 8.4 days, compared with 7.0 days for those undergoing segmental resections and 6.8 days for those undergoing nonresectional procedures.

Conclusions.—Laparoscopic colorectal surgery is established as a feasible technique. The complication rate declines as experience is gained. However, morbidity is also affected by the type of procedure performed, with TAC procedures having a higher complication rate than other types of procedures. Laparoscopic colorectal surgery is safe for use in selected cases of benign disease or for palliative purposes in patients with malignancies. It should be used for curative resections in cancer patients only as a part of prospective, randomized trials.

▶ Reissman and associates clearly establish 2 distinct components of the learning curve associated with the performance of laparoscopic colorectal surgery. Regarding morbidity over time, complication rates for the early, intermediate, and late part of the experience were 42%, 27%, and 12%, respectively. As expected, total colectomy was more technically demanding and was associated with a 42% complication rate. The latter should be performed in centers in which the surgeons have already mastered the less complicated, safer procedures.

F.G. Moody, M.D.

Visible Rectal Bleeding in a Primary Care Population

History of Visible Rectal Bleeding in a Primary Care Population: Initial Assessment and 10-Year Follow-up
Helfand M, Marton KI, Zimmer-Gembeck MJ, et al (Oregon Health Sciences Univ, Portland; St Marys Med Ctr, San Francisco; Dartmouth Med School, Hanover, NH)
JAMA 277:44–48, 1997   4–37

Background.—Visible rectal bleeding occurs fairly commonly in the general population. Whether this symptom, reported in a screening review of systems, necessitates assessment, and the accuracy of a defined protocol for the assessment of such bleeding was investigated in a prospective study.

Methods.—Two hundred ninety-seven patients with visible rectal bleeding were identified from 1 cohort using an 8-item review of systems. Sixty-eight percent of these patients completed a specified protocol, consisting of double-contrast barium enema (DCBE) examination, rigid sigmoidoscopy, and a follow-up assessment after 6–12 months. Ten years later, the diagnosis in 131 of 141 patients whose initial assessment suggested no cause or a benign anorectal cause of bleeding was verified.

Findings.—Serious disease was diagnosed in 24% of the initial group of 201. Twenty-six patients had polyps, 9 had inflammatory bowel disease, and 13 had colon cancer. The diagnosis was not predicted by the symptoms. Neither DCBE nor rigid sigmoidoscopy alone was sensitive enough to be used by itself. However, together they had a sensitivity and specificity of 0.96 and 0.76, respectively, for the diagnosis of polyps, cancer, or inflammatory bowel disease.

Conclusions.—Rectal bleeding reported during a review of systems was associated with a high likelihood of serious abnormalities. All adults should be asked about visible rectal bleeding, and those with this symptom should undergo visualization of the entire colon.

▶ This prospective study revealed that asking patients who visited a general medicine clinic a question regarding visible rectal bleeding identified patients at high risk of harboring serious colonic disease. Of 201 patients with visible rectal bleeding, 48 (24%) had serious disease; of 46 patients who were followed up, cancer was found in 13, polyps in 26, and inflammatory bowel disease in 8. Importantly, clinical findings were not good predictors of the diagnosis. However, age and duration of bleeding less than 2 months did have statistically significant associations with cancer. The authors recommend that in adults who report visible blood in their stool, colonscopy to visualize the entire colon should be the diagnostic procedure of choice.

N.J. Greenberger, M.D.

Closure of Colostomies in Trauma Patients

Early Closure of Colostomies in Trauma Patients: A Prospective Randomized Trial
Velmahos GC, Degiannis E, Wells M, et al (Univ of the Witwatersrand, Johannesburg, Republic of South Africa)
Surgery 118:815–820, 1995   4–38

Background.—Up to 60% of colon injuries can be repaired primarily, but many will still require a temporary colostomy. It is generally agreed that closure of temporary colostomies should be performed within 3 months of initial construction. Closure of a colostomy during the initial admission may be beneficial physiologically as well as psychologically. The safety of early closure of colostomies has not been reported in a prospective, randomized trial. The outcome of same-admission construction and closure of loop and end colostomies after severe trauma to the colon was evaluated.

Methods.—Early or late closure of colostomy was performed in 38 patients with severe injury to the colon. Early closure was performed within 15 postoperative days, and late closure was performed after 90 postoperative days. The morbidity and mortality rates were recorded and compared.

Results.—The morbidity was similar for both groups of patients. The overall complication rate was 26.3%. Early closure was technically much easier, required less operating time, and caused less bleeding than late closure. End closure required more operating time and caused more bleeding than loop closure. Early closure resulted in slightly shorter hospitalization. Late end closure resulted in prolonged hospitalization.

Conclusions.—End or loop closure of colostomies within 15 days of initial injury was safe in these patients. Early closure is easier and faster than late closure and has a similar complication rate. Closure of loop colostomies is easier to perform, both early and late, than closure of end colostomies.

▶ This controlled trial from Johannesburg establishes the relative safety of early closure of colostomies that have been constructed at the time of treatment of traumatic colonic injuries. The authors make an important point: a loop colostomy should be used whenever possible because its closure is much safer and less prone to complications than an end colostomy.

F.G. Moody, M.D.

Delayed Hypersensitivity Response in SICU Patients

The Delayed Hypersensitivity Response and Host Resistance in Surgical Patients: 20 Years Later
Christou NV, Meakins JL, Gordon J, et al (McGill Univ, Montreal)
Ann Surg 222:534–548, 1995   4–39

Background.—A previous study reported an association between a lack of a delayed-type hypersensitivity response to ubiquitous antigens and increased mortality among surgical patients. The nature of immune dysfunction in anergic patients and its effects on clinical outcome were investigated.

Methods.—A total of 4,292 patients either undergoing elective major surgery or admitted to the surgical ICU between 1973 and 1994 were skin tested with 5 ubiquitous antigens and were classified as either reactive (response to at least 2 antigens), relatively anergic (response to 1 antigen), or anergic (response to none of the antigens). The patients were monitored for infection. Over a 3-year period, 249 patients undergoing elective surgery underwent thorough investigations of comorbidity, and delayed-type hypersensitivity skin testing was performed. The role of nutritional manipulation on immune function was evaluated by prospectively randomizing 3 groups of anergic and reactive surgical and surgical ICU patients to receive either a regular amino acid solution or a modified amino acid solution formulated to enhance immune responsiveness. β-cell antibody response was evaluated in control, elective reactive, elective anergic, ICU anergic, and ICU reactive patients tested with tetanus toxoid and Pneumovax immunization. Cytokine expression was evaluated in skin biopsies from control skin and skin injected with specific or irrelevant antigen analyzed with polymerase chain reaction. Nonspecific host defense was evaluated by measuring circulating and exudate polymorphonuclear neutrophils in reactive and anergic elective surgical patients.

Results.—The mortality rate was 5.5% in the elective surgery group and 22.3% in the surgical ICU group. Overall, the mortality rate was 3.1% in reactive patients, 11% in relative anergy patients, and 25.1% in anergic patients. Among the 3,081 patients with no pre-existing infection who underwent elective surgery, the mortality rate was 17.6% in the anergic patients and 2.1% in the reactive patients. Among the patients who experienced an infectious challenge, the mortality rate was 58.2% in anergic patients and 12.3% in reactive patients. Anergic patients tended to be older and have decreased pulmonary function, lower body mass index, higher Na_3/K_3, anemia, lower lymphocyte counts, decreased serum albumin and prealbumin levels, and increased α-2-macroglobulin levels. Despite these findings, the mortality rate of the comorbidity sample was only 1.6%. The type of parenteral nutritional supplementation had no effect on immune function measurements. Anergic patients had a reduced antibody response to tetanus toxoid, but made comparable amounts of polysaccharide antibody to healthy control subjects. T cells were present in skin biopsy specimens of reactive patients, but not in skin biopsy specimens of anergic patients. Anergic patients had a significant lack of mRNA expression of interleukin-3 and interferon-γ in the skin. There were no differences in polymorphonuclear neutrophils measurements between anergic and reactive patients.

Conclusions.—The susceptibility of anergic patients to infection-related mortality appears to be related to an absence of T-cell function.

▶ The McGill surgeons provide the first and last word on delayed hypersensitivity responsiveness and surgical morbidity. A wealth of information is presented; the bottom line is anergy is a bad prognostic sign for patients in critical care units and is no longer a problem these days for patients undergoing elective surgery. The relationship between anergy and sepsis-related mortality in sick and injured patients deserves further study.

F.G. Moody, M.D.

Continence After Ripstein Rectopexy

Continence Is Improved After the Ripstein Rectopexy: Different Mechanisms in Rectal Prolapse and Rectal Intussusception?
Schultz I, Mellgren A, Dolk A, et al (Danderyd Hosp, Stockholm)
Dis Colon Rectum 39:300–306, 1996   4–40

Background.—Anal incontinence often accompanies rectal prolapse and rectal intussusception. These conditions can be treated by transabdominal or perineal surgery. Ripstein rectopexy is one such procedure that is often used to treat rectal prolapse and rectal intussusception. The reasons for the frequent improvement in anal incontinence seen postoperatively are unclear. Changes in anal canal pressure after Ripstein rectopexy in patients with rectal prolapse and postoperative changes in anal continence in patients with rectal intussusception were studied.

Methods.—Ripstein rectopexy was performed in 42 patients (mean age, 60 years; 41 women, 1 man) with rectal prolapse or rectal intussusception in a prospective study. Anorectal manometry was performed preoperatively and postoperatively. Anal continence was graded into 4 groups. Follow-up was 6 months.

Results.—Preoperatively, maximum resting pressure was higher in patients with rectal intussusception than in patients with rectal prolapse. Postoperatively, maximum resting pressure increased in patients with rec-

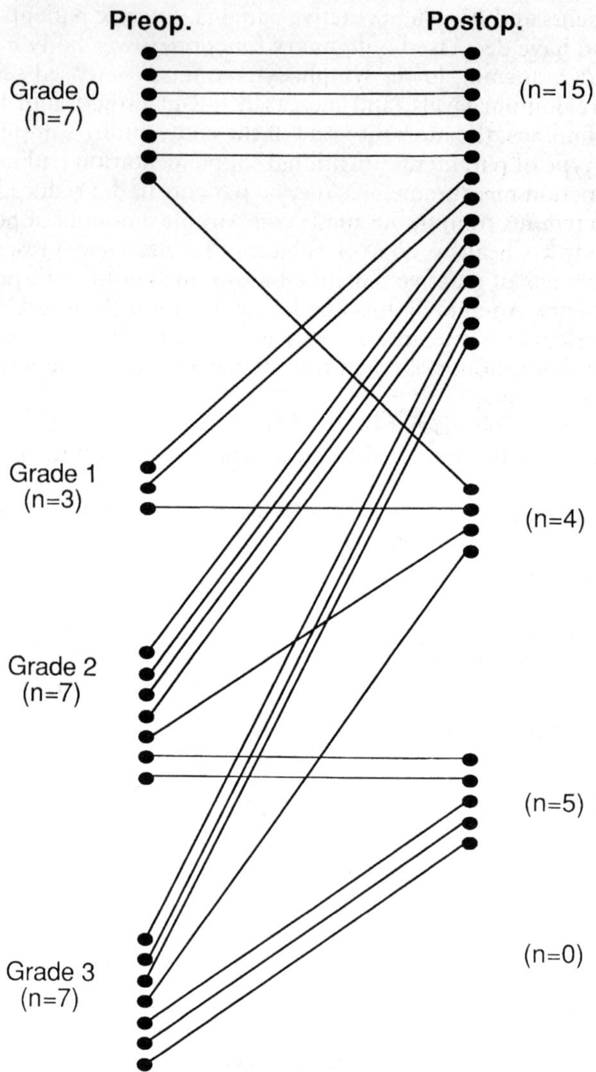

FIGURE 1.—Incontinence grading preoperatively (**Preop.**) and postoperatively (**Postop.**) of patients with rectal prolapse (n = 24). (Courtesy of Schultz I, Mellgren A, Dolk A, et al: Continence is improved after the Ripstein rectopexy: Different mechanisms in rectal prolapse and rectal intussusception? *Dis Colon Rectum* 39:300–306, 1996.)

tal prolapse after 6 months, but not after 7 days. There was no increase in maximum squeezing pressure. In patients with internal rectal procidentia, maximum resting pressure and maximum squeezing pressure did not increase. Continence improved in patients with rectal prolapse and rectal intussusception (Fig 1). Postoperatively, rectal emptying difficulties did not increase.

Conclusions.—In these patients, Ripstein rectopexy improved anal incontinence. The increase in maximum resting pressure in patients with rectal prolapse indicates that internal anal sphincter function was restored. A different mechanism of improvement in rectal intussusception is indicated by the lack of improvement in maximum resting pressure in patients with this condition.

▶ Anal incontinence represents an extremely unpleasant complication of rectal prolapse and intussusception. This group of Swedish surgeons, using anal manometry, have shown why the Ripstein rectopexy operation is successful in relieving this unpleasant symptom (Fig 1).

F.G. Moody, M.D.

PART FIVE

THE LIVER

Introduction

Familiar themes characterize this section. New insights into the epidemiology of hepatitis A indicate that patients may be infectious for at least 3 months. There are 5 articles on hepatitis B, 2 of which detail transmission from infected surgeons. Interesting, hepatitis B e antigen (HBeAG), which is a marker of infectivity, was absent in some of the surgeons. The difficult problem of preventing recurrent hepatitis B infection in liver transplantation patients using 2 modalities of therapy is discussed, i.e., hepatitis B immunoglobulin and lamivudine.

That 12 articles on hepatitis C are included in this section underscores the explosion of new information regarding this important infection. The natural history of chronic hepatitis and cirrhosis caused by the hepatitis C virus is detailed, indicating that 75% to 80% of patients have chronic hepatitis develop, 25% to 30% have cirrhosis develop, and as many as 5% develop hepatoma. The interval for development of cirrhosis is 20 years and for hepatoma, 30 years. A meta-analysis of interferon therapy of chronic hepatitis C indicates that the dose of interferon and duration of therapy both influence the likelihood of a favorable response. Although the majority of patients with chronic hepatitis C infection and cirrhosis who undergo liver transplantation have hepatitis C develop in the new liver, the overall 5- and 10-year survival rates in this group are not significantly different from those of individuals who undergo liver transplantation for other reasons. The 2 articles about hepatitis G indicate that infection is common, with approximately 1.7% of United States blood donors having positive test results. However, there is no convincing evidence that this agent causes chronic liver disease.

Five articles concern alcoholic cirrhosis and related problems. An interesting report on the treatment of alcoholic hepatitis with prednisone with a long-term follow-up of 1–2 years indicates that, although survival is enhanced during the first year, this beneficial effect is lost during the second year. Accordingly, patients with severe alcoholic hepatitis that fails to respond to corticosteroids after 6–12 months should then be considered for liver transplantation. The hepatic venous pressure gradient has been shown to have significant prognostic value and can be used to assess the response to treatment with β-blockers and in patients who have undergone a transjugular intrahepatic portosystemic shunt (TIPS) procedure. An extensive review of 100 patients with the hepatopulmonary syndrome provides insights into this interesting disorder. Furthermore, basal arterial PO_2 and PCO_2 values along with testing with 100% oxygen aid in identifying patients who are unlikely to benefit from liver transplantation. New insights into the natural history of primary biliary cirrhosis are gained from an extensive review of patients diagnosed when they were asymptomatic. Useful information on hemochromatosis, pyogenic hepatic abscess, and liver involvement with mastocytosis is also presented. Eight articles relate to liver neoplasms and 5 articles on additional surgical issues. An interesting article profiles an urban practice of hepatology. Not surprising, the most common problems were hepatitis C infection and primary biliary cirrhosis, and not alcoholic liver disease. That approximately 3.9 million Americans are believed to be infected with the hepatitis C virus explains the very large number of such patients who are being seen by hepatologists.

Norton J. Greenberger, M.D.

33 Hepatitis A

Prolonged Fecal Excretion of Hepatitis A Virus in Adult Patients With Hepatitis A as Determined by Polymerase Chain Reaction
Yotsuyanagi H, Koike K, Yasuda K, et al (Univ of Tokyo; St Marianna Univ, Kawasaki, Japan)
Hepatology 24:10–13, 1996   5–1

Introduction.—Fecal excretion of hepatitis A virus (HAV) reportedly stops soon after symptoms develop in the infected patient. Efforts to

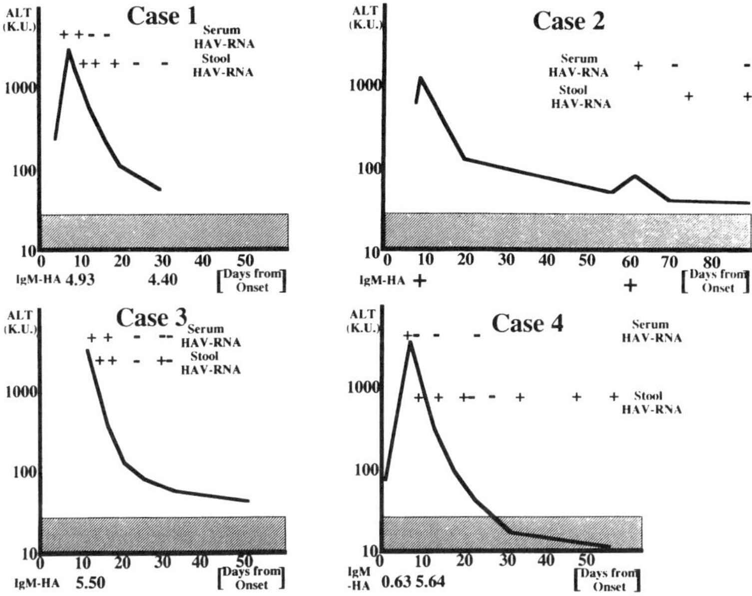

FIGURE 4.—Representative cases of patients with hepatitis A whose stools were hepatitis A virus (*HAV*) RNA–positive. In case 1, HAV RNA was detected in the patient's stool until day 18 after clinical onset, but not on day 24 or thereafter. In case 2, the patient's stool remained HAV RNA–positive until day 89, with consistently elevated alanine transaminase (*ALT*) levels. The patient in case 3 showed intermittent fecal shedding of the virus for about 30 days from clinical onset. The patient in case 4 also demonstrated intermittent fecal excretion of HAV RNA into his stool. In this patient, reappearance of shedding of HAV in stool occurred after serum ALT levels had become normal. *Shaded areas* indicate the normal range of ALT levels. *Abbreviation: KU,* Karmen units. (Courtesy of Yotsuyanagi H, Koike K, Yasuda K, et al: Prolonged fecal excretion of hepatitis A virus in adult patients with hepatitis A as determined by polymerase chain reaction. *Hepatology* 24:10–13, 1996.)

control hepatitis A depend on accurate knowledge of the duration of fecal shedding. Although there have been reports of HAV detected in feces using polymerase chain reaction (PCR), there are few data on the duration of fecal HAV infection in adult patients. This issue was studied using a reverse transcriptase PCR (RT-PCR) method.

Methods and Findings.—The study included 10 patients with acute HAV who tested positive for IgM anti-HAV. A 2-stage RT-PCR was used to detect HAV RNA in fecal samples. Five patients showed viral RNA in their stools after the onset of clinical symptoms. Samples obtained within 10 days of the onset of illness were always positive. The duration of positivity was sometimes as short as a few days, sometimes as long as 3 months (Fig 4). Four patients had detectable HAV RNA after serum alanine transaminase (ALT) levels had peaked, continuing in 1 case until after ALT levels had returned to normal.

Conclusions.—Patients with HAV infection can continue to shed virus in feces for months after the resolution of symptoms. During this time, they could be responsible for further transmission of the virus in the community. The patients' close contacts should receive hepatitis A prophylaxis—including HAV vaccination—even after lengthy delays in identification or diagnosis.

▶ Hepatitis A virus spreads mainly by the fecal-oral route. Both sporadic cases and epidemics of HAV infection have been reported. Because fecal shedding of the virus is so important in the pathogenesis of this disease, careful definition of such shedding is important for its control. Conventional teaching has been that patients continue to shed virus from the onset of jaundice or abnormal ALT levels until 2–4 weeks thereafter. The carefully done study by Yotsuyanagi and colleagues indicates that fecal shedding of HAV can continue for up to 3 months after the onset of illness, and even after the normalization of serum ALT levels. As the authors emphasize in their discussion, the practical implications of these findings are twofold: (1) careful attention to sanitation, hygiene, and thorough hand-washing is necessary even after patients with HAV enter the recovery phase; and (2) prophylaxis with HAV immunization is appropriate even when there is a delay in diagnosis.

N.J. Greenberger, M.D.

34 Hepatitis B

Transmission From Infected Surgeons

Transmission of Hepatitis B to Patients From Four Infected Surgeons Without Hepatitis B e Antigen

Heptonstall J, for the Incident Investigation Teams and Others (Public Health Lab Service Communicable Disease Surveillance Centre, London)

N Engl J Med 336:178–184, 1997   5–2

Introduction.—The transmission of hepatitis B virus (HBV) to patients from surgeons who carry hepatitis B e antigen (HBeAg) has been documented in numerous reports. Reported here are 4 unconnected instances of transmission of HBV to patients by 4 infected surgeons whose serum did not show HBeAg.

Case Reports.—All 4 patients were women and were seen for acute onset of jaundice (Table 1). None had received blood transfusions. Each patient had had surgery within the past 6 months. An investigation was begun, and members of each surgical team were tested for HBV carrier status. Three surgeons tested positive for hepatitis B surface antigen (HBsAg) and negative for antibody against hepatitis B core antigen (anti-HBc) IgM. One surgeon was known to be an HBeAg-negative carrier of HBV and continued to operate within existing guidelines. All other members of the 4 surgical teams were immune to HBV or uninfected. All patients recovered completely and no patients experienced fulminant hepatitis.

Methods.—Serum HBV DNA was amplified by a nested polymerase chain reaction from serum of the 4 infected surgeons and infected patients. Direct sequencing of the 2 regions of the HBV genome was executed. Patients who underwent surgeries by the infected surgeons were offered testing.

Results.—All 4 surgeons were carriers of HBV and none of them had detectable levels of HBeAg. It was not possible to distinguish the nucleotide sequences of HBV DNA from the surgeons and their corresponding infected patients. At least 2 other exposed patients who were offered screening probably acquired hepatitis B from their respective infected

TABLE 1.—Characteristics of the 4 Index Patients Whose Hepatitis B Virus (HBV) Infections Were Associated With Contact With HBV-Infected Surgeons

Characteristic	Patient 1	Patient 2	Patient 3	Patient 4
Sex	F	F	F	F
Age group (yr)	30–39	30–39	60–69	70–79
Date of onset of jaundice	June 1988	October 1993	August 1994	January 1995
HBV subtype	ayw	adw	ayw	ayw
Type of procedure	Elective cholecysectomy	Elective cesarean section	Elective hysterectomy and removal of ovarian cyst	Elective cholecystecto-my and nehprectomy
Interval between procedure and onset of jaundice (wk)	12	11	12	12
Blood transfusion	No	No	No	No
Sexual partner tested for HBV markers	Not tested	Anti-HBc-negative	Anti-HBc-negative	Not applicable
Other identified risk factors for HBV	None known	No	No	No
Identified source*	Surgeon 1	Surgeon 2	Surgeon 3	Surgeon 4
Role of infected surgeon in procedure	Main operator	Main operator	Assistant	Assistant

Abbreviation: Anti-HBe, antibodies against hepatitis B core antigen.

*All other members of the surgical teams were either immune to HBV or uninfected.

(Reprinted by permission of The New England Journal of Medicine, courtesy of Heptonstall J, for the Incident Investigation Teams and Others: Transmission of hepatitis B to patients from four infected surgeons without hepatitis B e antigen. *N Engl J Med* 336:178–184, copyright 1997, Massachusetts Medical Society. All rights reserved.)

surgeons. All surgeons made career changes that did not put patients a risk of exposure to the virus.

Conclusion.—Surgeons who are carriers of HBV with no detectable serum HBeAg can transmit the hepatitis B virus to their patients. Surgeons in the United Kingdom are allowed to perform procedures within guidelines if their serum contains HBsAg but not HBeAg.

▶ In the United Kingdom, health care workers in whom HBeAg is detected are not allowed to perform procedures involving a risk of exposure. However, carriers in whom HBeAg is not detectable may perform such procedures unless it can be shown that their participation is linked to the transmission of HBV infection. The data obtained in this study provide clear evidence that surgeons who are carriers of HBV who do not have HBeAg in their serum may, nonetheless, transmit the virus to patients. Furthermore, these findings illustrate the value of obtaining a detailed clinical history from patients with acute hepatitis B. As the authors emphasize in their discussion, a history of surgery in the 6 months before the onset of HBV infection without other evident risk factors should lead to a review of the HBV status of physician members of the surgical team.

N.J. Greenberger, M.D.

Transmission of Hepatitis B Virus to Multiple Patients From a Surgeon Without Evidence of Inadequate Infection Control
Harpaz R, von Seidlein L, Averhoff FM, et al (Ctrs for Disease Control and Prevention, Atlanta, Ga; Univ of California, Los Angeles; Los Angeles County Health Dept)
N Engl J Med 334:549–554, 1996   5–3

Purpose.—An outbreak of hepatitis B virus (HBV) associated with an infected thoracic-surgery resident is described. Possible mechanisms of transmission were investigated.

Methods.—Chart reviews, interviews, and serologic testing of thoracic-surgery patients were performed at the 2 hospitals where the infected resident had worked from July 1991 to July 1992. Hepatitis B surface antigen (HBsAg) subtypes and DNA sequences were obtained from the resident and from infected patients.

Findings.—Among the infected surgeon's 144 available patients, 13% had acute HBV infection. One of the 2 hospitals at which he had worked during this period was chosen for further study. At this hospital, none of the 124 patients of other thoracic surgeons had evidence of recent infection with HBV. No other common source of HBV infection was detected. The HbsAg subtype and partial HBV DNA sequences from the surgeon matched those from infected patients. Infection transmission was associated with cardiac transplantation but not with other surgical procedures. The infected surgeon was positive for hepatitis B e antigen and had high serum HBV DNA levels. The surgeon and hospital were in compliance with recommended infection-control procedures.

Conclusions.—Although this surgeon's technical skills were not a problem, his high levels of serum HBV DNA, combined with paper-cut–like lesions on his fingers obtained during suturing, could have contributed to disease transmission if glove failure occurred. This tragic outbreak could have been avoided had the surgeon been inoculated with HBV vaccine.

▶ The infected thoracic surgeon studied in this report transmitted HBV to at least 19 patients during surgery. Importantly, no patients undergoing procedures performed by other thoracic surgeons had evidence of recent infection. This outbreak occurred despite apparent compliance with recommended infection control practices, and specific events that led to transmission could not be identified. However, the authors point out some interesting observations in their discussion. They indicate that while participating in a 1-hour simulation of suture tying, the surgeon did acquire paper-cut–like lesions on his fingers, and both hepatitis B surface antigen and HBV and DNA were isolated from washings of his hands. It is conceivable that such lesions, combined with the failure of his gloves, may have allowed contamination of patients with HBV. Further, the authors point out that there is no conclusive evidence regarding the effectiveness of double gloves in protecting patients from blood-borne infections. This report underscores the importance that all physicians receive HBV vaccine.

N.J. Greenberger, M.D.

Long-term Follow-up After Interferon

Long-term Follow-up of HBeAg-Positive Patients Treated With Interferon Alfa for Chronic Hepatitis B
Niederau C, Heintges T, Lange S, et al (Heinrich Heine Univ, Düsseldorf, Germany; Ruhr Univ Bochum, Germany)
N Engl J Med 334:1422–1427, 1996   5–4

Introduction.—In patients with chronic hepatitis B, previously called chronic active hepatitis B, treatment with interferon-α (IFN-α) can increase the elimination rate of hepatitis B e antigen (HBeAg), which is often associated with the disappearance of hepatitis B virus (HBV) DNA. A few studies have suggested that IFN-α treatment can reduce inflammatory activity. However, improved clinical outcomes have yet to be demonstrated. The impact of IFN-α treatment on the clinical outcomes of patients with chronic hepatitis B was prospectively studied.

Methods.—The cohort study included 103 patients with chronic hepatitis B infection who were treated with IFN-α-2b. Treatment lasted for 4–6 months and was repeated for some patients in whom HBeAg was not eliminated. The patients were followed up for a mean of 50 months, and their clinical outcomes were compared with those of a group of untreated controls.

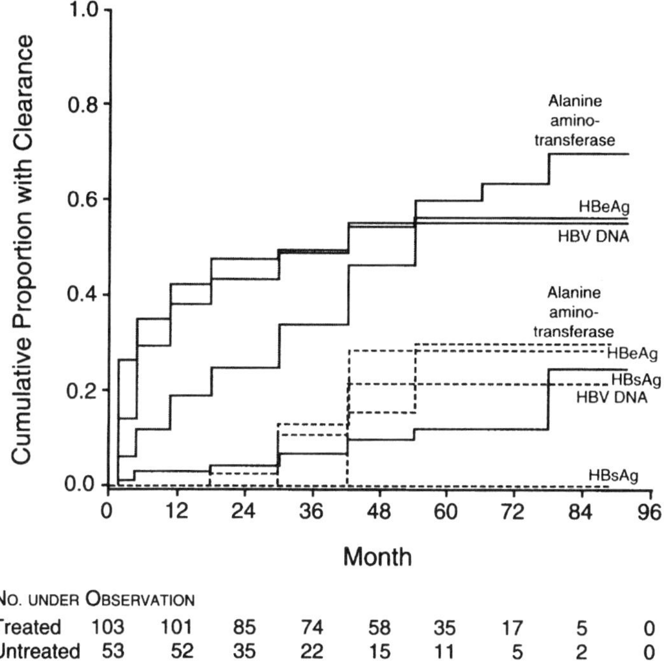

No. under Observation								
Treated	103	101	85	74	58	35	17	5	0
Untreated	53	52	35	22	15	11	5	2	0

FIGURE 1.—Cumulative clearance of HBeAg, HBV DNA, and HBsAG and normalization of alanine aminotransferase levels, calculated by the Kaplan-Meier method, in 103 patients with chronic hepatitis B treated with interferon alfa (*solid lines*) and 53 untreated patients (*dashed lines*). (Courtesy of Niederau C, Heintges T, Lange S, et al: Long-term follow-up of HBeAg-positive patients treated with interferon alfa for chronic hepatitis B. *N Engl J Med* 334:1422–1427. Copyright 1996, Massachusetts Medical Society. Reprinted by permission of *The New England Journal of Medicine*. All rights reserved.)

Findings.—With IFN-α treatment, HBeAg and HBV DNA became undetectable in 53 of the 103 patients. Only 10 patients became seronegative for hepatitis B surface antigen (HBsAg), however. The estimated 5-year cumulative clearance rate was 56% for HBeAg and 12% for HBsAg. In contrast, only 7 of 53 untreated controls became seronegative for HBeAg, and none became seronegative for HBsAg (Fig 1). In the treated group, 6 patients died of liver failure and 2 required liver transplantation; all of these patients remained positive for HBeAg. Of 8 treated patients who had complications of cirrhosis, 7 were persistently positive for HBeAg. Overall survival and survival free of clinical complications were significantly better in the IFN-α–treated patients (Fig 3). The best predictor of survival on regression analysis was clearance of HBeAg.

Conclusions.—For patients with chronic hepatitis B in whom HBeAg clears after IFN-α treatment, clinical outcomes are better than in untreated patients. Patients with elimination of HBeAg are at significantly reduced risk of death, liver transplantation, and severe clinical complications of cirrhosis. These data regarding the benefits of IFN-α treatment will be used in analyses of cost-effectiveness.

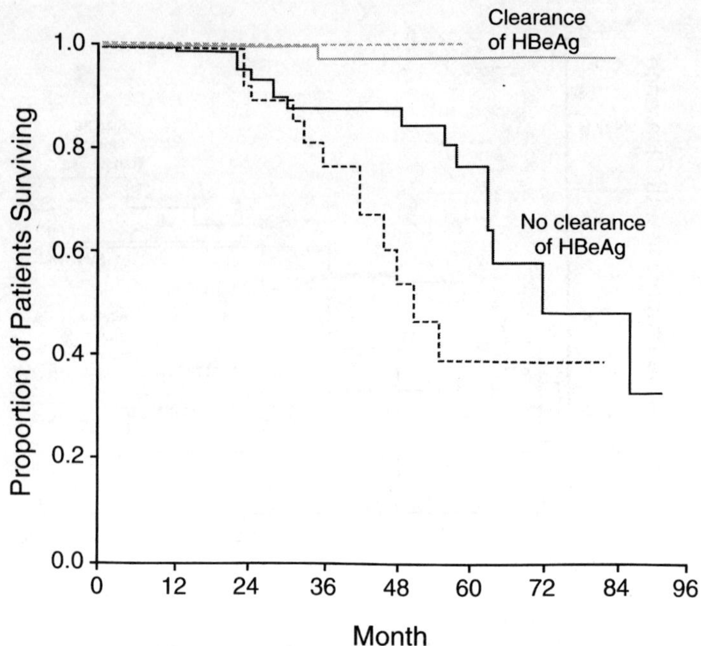

FIGURE 3.—Cumulative survival without complications among interferon-treated patients (*solid lines*) and untreated patients (*dashed lines*) who were HBeAg-negative at the end of follow-up, with the time until HBeAg seroconversion subtracted from the observation time, and among patients who had not yet lost HBeAg, with HBeAg seroconversion as a reason for censoring data. Survival was significantly longer among the patients in whom HBeAg was eliminated after interferon therapy than among those who did not have clearance ($P = 0.018$ by the proportional-hazards model). In the control group, survival was significantly longer among the patients who had spontaneous elimination of HBeAg than among those who did not ($P = 0.006$). (Courtesy of Niederau C, Heintges T, Lange S, et al: Long-term follow up of HBeAg-positive patients treated with interferon alfa for chronic hepatitis B. *N Engl J Med* 334:1422–1427. Copyright 1996, Massachusetts Medical Society. Reprinted by permission of *The New England Journal of Medicine*. All rights reserved.)

▶ That treatment of chronic hepatitis B with IFN-α results in improvement in serum aminotransferase levels and loss of HBV DNA is now well established. However, whether such improvement in liver tests translates into improved clinical outcomes has been an open question. The study by Niederau et al. provides convincing evidence that IFN-α treatment improves clinical outcomes. Overall survival and survival without clinical complications were significantly longer in patients who were seronegative for HBeAg after therapy with IFN-α than in those who remained seropositive. Whereas 53 of 103 patients treated with IFN-α lost HBeAg as well as HBV DNA, only 7 of 53 untreated patients spontaneously lost HBeAg and only 5 of the 7 lost their serum HBV DNA. Thus, in patients with chronic hepatitis B, clearance of HBeAg, which is much more likely to occur after treatment with IFN-α, is clearly associated with improved clinical outcomes.

N.J. Greenberger, M.D.

Moving?

I'd like to receive my *Year Book of Digestive Diseases* without interruption.
Please note the following change of address, effective:

Name: ____

New Address: ______________________________________

____

City: _________________________ State: ______ Zip: ______

Old Address: ______________________________________

____

City: _________________________ State: ______ Zip: ______

Reservation Card

Yes, I would like my own copy of *Year Book of Digestive Diseases*. Please begin my subscription with the current edition according to the terms described below.* I understand that I will have 30 days to examine each annual edition. If satisfied, I will pay just $77.95 plus sales tax, postage and handling (price subject to change without notice).

Name: ____

Address: ____

City: _________________________ State: ________ Zip: ______

Method of Payment
O Visa   O Mastercard   O AmEx   O Bill me   O Check (in US dollars, payable to Mosby, Inc.)

Card number: _________________________ Exp date: ___________

Signature: ____

LS-0909

*Your Year Book Service Guarantee:

When you subscribe to the *Year Book*, we'll send you an advance notice of future volumes about two months before they publish. This automatic notice system is designed to take up as little of your time as possible. If you do not want the *Year Book*, the advance notice makes it quick and easy for you to let us know your decision, and you will always have at least 20 days to decide. If we don't hear from you, we'll send you the new volume as soon as it's available. And, of course, the *Year Book* is yours to examine free of charge for 30 days (postage, handling and applicable sales tax are added to each shipment.).

BUSINESS REPLY MAIL
FIRST CLASS MAIL   PERMIT No. 762   CHICAGO, IL

POSTAGE WILL BE PAID BY ADDRESSEE

Chris Hughes
Mosby-Year Book, Inc.
161 N. Clark Street
Suite 1900
Chicago, IL 60601-9981

NO POSTAGE
NECESSARY
IF MAILED
IN THE
UNITED STATES

BUSINESS REPLY MAIL
FIRST CLASS MAIL   PERMIT No. 762   CHICAGO, IL

POSTAGE WILL BE PAID BY ADDRESSEE

Chris Hughes
Mosby-Year Book, Inc.
161 N. Clark Street
Suite 1900
Chicago, IL 60601-9981

NO POSTAGE
NECESSARY
IF MAILED
IN THE
UNITED STATES

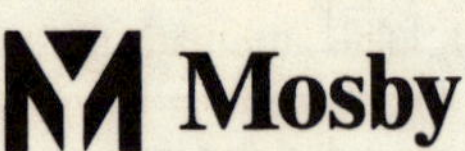

Mosby

Dedicated to publishing excellence

Prophylaxis in Liver Transplant Recipients Using Hepatitus B Immune Globulin

Prophylaxis in Liver Transplant Recipients Using a Fixed Dosing Schedule of Hepatitis B Immunoglobulin

Terrault NA, Zhou S, Combs C, et al (Veterans Affairs Med Ctr, San Francisco; Univ of California, San Francisco)
Hepatology 24:1327–1333, 1996

5–5

Background.—In liver transplant recipients who are positive for hepatitis B surface antigen (HBsAg), prophylactic hepatitis B immunoglobulin (HBIg) reduces the incidence of recurrent hepatitis B virus (HBV) infection and improves survival. The long-term effects of HBIg and an optimal schedule for its administration have yet to be defined; the efficacy of 1 protocol is described.

Methods.—Participating in the trial were 52 patients receiving liver transplants who were positive for HBsAg at the time of transplantation. Twenty-four patients received HBIg prophylaxis at a fixed dose of 10,000

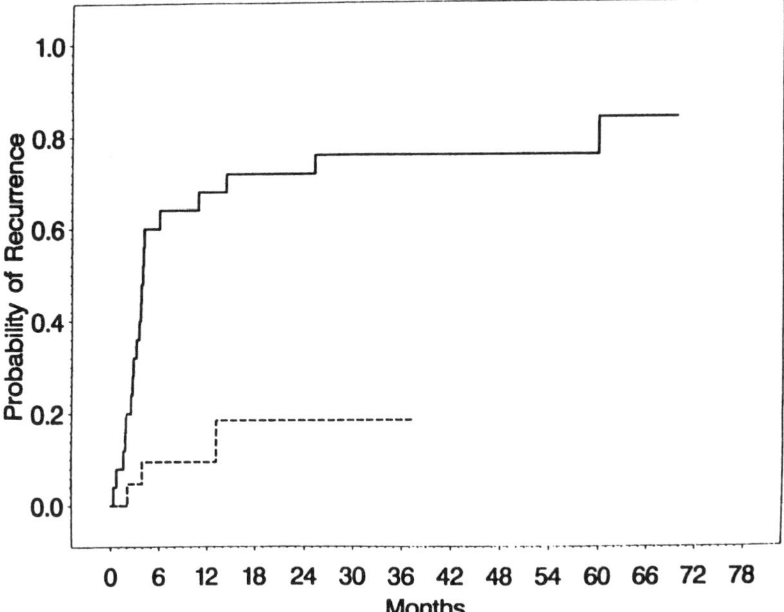

FIGURE 1.—Recurrence of hepatitis B virus (HBV) infection in each treatment subgroup. Recurrence of HBV (defined by the reappearance of hepatitis B surface antigen in the serum anytime after the eighth week posttransplantation) is shown according to the following treatment groups: hepatitis B immunoglobulin (HBIg) prophylaxis (*dashes*) (*n* = 24) and no prophylaxis (*solid line*) (*n* = 28). The x-axis shows the duration of follow-up in months, and the y-axis shows the probability of recurrence. The rate of reinfection was significantly less in the HBIg prophylaxis group than in the no-treatment group (*P* = 0.0002). Recurrence was not assessed in patients surviving for less than 8 weeks. (Courtesy of Terrault NA, Zhou S, Combs C, et al: Prophylaxis in liver transplant recipients using a fixed dosing schedule of hepatitis B immunoglobulin. *Hepatology* 24:1327–1333, 1996.)

IU monthly, and 28 were given no specific therapy. The mean duration of follow-up was 28.9 months.

Results.—2-year recurrence rate (reappearance of HBsAg) for treated patients was 19% and for control patients it was 76% (Fig 1). The titer of antibody to HBsAg varied significantly both over time and between patients in the treated group, which raises concern about its usefulness in guiding therapy. Nine patients remained negative for HBsAg after being treated with HBIg for at least 1 year; HBV DNA could be detected by polymerase chain reaction in the sera of 67%, the lymphocytes of 50%, and the liver of 57%.

Conclusions.—These data suggest that even in patients with indications of active viral replication before transplantation, a fixed monthly dose of HBIg can reduce the recurrence of hepatitis B surface antigenemia. Long-term administration of HBIg may be necessary, as evidenced by the presence of residual virus in the majority of treated patients. Larger, even longer-term studies may be needed to show a survival benefit.

▶ Recurrent HBV infection is common in patients undergoing liver transplantation for end-stage liver disease secondary to HBV infection. Such recurrence frequently results in reduced graft and patient survival. The study by Terrault et al. demonstrates that HBIG immunoprophylaxis using a fixed dose of 10,000 IU monthly prevents hepatitis B surface antigenemia both in patients with and in patients without indices of active viral replication. The reason why passive immunoprophylaxis is effective in preventing HBV reinfection is unknown.

Lamivudine and famciclovir are 2 other agents that may also be useful in preventing graft reinfection with HBV. Gutfreund et al. administered lamivudine at a dose of 100 mg/day orally to 5 HBsAg-positive patients before liver transplantation and for 18–22 months postoperatively. Posttransplant liver biopsies were negative for HBV DNA by polymerase chain reaction in 3 patients, and recurrent hepatitis B developed in 2 patients at 8–12 months. This preliminary study suggests that lamivudine as a single agent given before and after liver transplantation for prevention of graft reinfection with HBV can result in marked suppression of viral replication. However, there is also late failure apparently caused by the development of viral resistance.

Greilier et al.[2] treated 12 HBV DNA–positive patients with lamivudine, 100 mg/day for at least 4 weeks prior to liver transplantation. At 72 weeks after transplantation, 9 patients had lost HBsAg and remained negative for HBV DNA; 2 died and HBV DNA had reappeared in 1 patient. This study provides further support for the concept that lamivudine may prove useful in preventing recurrent hepatitis B after transplantation.

Rabinovitz et al.[3] treated 8 patients with recurrent HBV infection of their liver allograft with famciclovir at a dose of 300 mg 3 times daily adjusted for alterations in renal function. All were HBeAg and HBV DNA–positive. Three patients showed a 99% reduction in their HBV DNA levels, 1 had a 50% reduction, and 4 patients have not responded to famciclovir therapy. These provocative findings suggest that famciclovir may reduce HBV replication in a significant number of treated patients and that famciclovir therapy is safe.

N.J. Greenberger, M.D.

References

1. Gutfreund, KS, Fischer KP, Tippler G, et al: Late breakthrough of HBV uremia with lamivudine as a single agent for prevention of graft reinfection in liver transplantation for cirrhosis secondary to hepatitis B. *Hepatology* 24:285A, 1996.
2. Greilier C, Nutlmen D, Ahmed M, et al: Lamivudine prophylaxis against reinfection in liver transplantation for hepatitis B cirrhosis. *Lancet* 348:1212–1215, 1996.
3. Rabinovitz M, Dudson F, Rakela J: Famciclovir for recurrent hepatitis B infection after liver transplantation. *Hepatology* 24:282A, 1996.

Lamivudine in Post-Transplant Patients

Hepatitis-B–virus Resistance to Lamivudine Given for Recurrent Infection After Orthotopic Liver Transplantation

Bartholomew MM, Jansen RW, Jeffers LJ, et al (Univ of Miami, Fla; Glaxo Wellcome Inc, Research Triangle Park, NC; Univ of North Carolina, Chapel Hill)

Lancet 349:20–22, 1997   5–6

Introduction.—Recurrence of hepatitis B virus (HBV) is common in patients who undergo orthotopic liver transplantation because of chronic hepatitis B. The 3-year survival rate in patients with infected grafts is 54%. Lamivudine is a cytosine nucleoside analogue that has been shown to suppress HBV infection. The use of lamivudine was reported for 3 patients who underwent transplantation for end-stage chronic hepatitis B. The in vitro susceptibility of HBV to lamivudine was evaluated by infecting primary human hepatocytes with HBV serum collected before the start of treatment and after recurrence.

Methods.—Lamivudine was administered to 2 patients with recurrent HBV infection after transplantation. The third patient began receiving lamivudine 1 month before transplantation in an attempt to prevent HBV recurrence after transplantation. All 3 patients had good initial response to lamivudine. All patients experienced viral recurrence after 9–10 months of lamivudine. Serum samples obtained before treatment and after viral recurrence underwent DNA sequencing through a conserved polymerase domain (the tyrosine, methionine, aspartate, aspartate [YMDD] locus). Primary hepatocyte cultures were infected with HBV from serum collected before initiation of treatment and after recurrence.

Results.—All patients had 1 or 2 unique DNA changes that were detected in both pretreatment and posttreatment serum samples. All patients had a common mutation within the YMDD locus of the HBV polymerase gene during lamivudine treatment. One HBV polymerase mutation site was common to all 3 patients; the methionine codon of the YMDD locus. Mutations at this locus were detected in serum after recurrent infection but not in pretreatment serum. The HBV DNA concentrations in cultures infected with pretreatment serum were reduced to less than 6% of control cultures with lamivudine concentrations as low as 0.03 µmol/L. In cultures treated with serum obtained after recurrence, the HBV DNA concentrations did not drop below 20% of control values, even with lamivudine concentrations as high as 30 µmol/L.

Conclusion.—The initial response to lamivudine was good in the 3 patients evaluated. Findings give molecular and phenotypic characterization of HBV variants. Long-term follow-up is needed to determine the frequency of resistance to lamivudine monotherapy. It may be that HBV infection after transplantation may be best treated by combination drug therapy.

▶ Because orthotopic liver transplantation for patients with chronic HBV infection is often complicated by recurrence of HBV infection, there is considerable interest in strategies for reducing the risk of HBV recurrence. Although immunoprophylaxis with hepatitis B immunoglobulin is effective, it is costly and is associated with side effects. Lamivudine, a cytosine nucleoside analogue, inhibits hepadna virus replication in vitro and and has shown good results in small trials in the treatment of HBV infections in humans. In this report, the initial response to lamivudine in 3 patients suppressed HBV, but HBV recurred in all 3 patients 9–10 months after initiation of treatment. The molecular and phenotypic characterization of HBV variant isolated from the 3 patients indicates a common mechanism of lamivudine resistance for HIV and HBV that involves similar joint mutations in homologous domains of the viral polymerases.

N.J. Greenberger, M.D.

35 Hepatitis C

Epidemiologic Considerations in Transmission Studies

Transmission of Hepatitis C Virus by a Cardiac Surgeon

Esteban JI, Gómez J, Martell M, et al (Universitat Autònoma, Barcelona; Universitat de Valencia, Spain)
N Engl J Med 334:555–560, 1996   5–7

Introduction.—During a prospective analysis of the efficiency of immunoassays for hepatitis C virus (HCV) antibodies in reducing posttransfusion HCV, 2 patients were identified who had become infected with HCV shortly after open-heart surgery. Testing of blood donors did not reveal the source of infection. The infections were linked to a cardiac surgeon with chronic HCV. Epidemiologic and molecular evidence is provided that this surgeon may have transmitted HCV to 5 patients between 1988 and 1993.

Methods.—Among the 222 patients of the chronically infected surgeon who participated in this study, 6 contracted postoperative HCV (Table 1). All 6 patients had valve-replacement surgery. Nucleotide sequences from the hypervariable region at the junction of the coding regions for the E1 and E2 envelope proteins were sequenced from the surgeon, the 6 infected patients, and 10 controls infected with the same HCV genotype.

Findings.—Genotyping revealed that the surgeon and 5 of his 6 infected patients were infected with HCV genotype 3. The sixth patient had genotype 1 HCV and was believed to have contracted HCV from another source. An additional 13 patients had transfusion-associated genotype-1 HCV (Table 3). The average net genetic distance between the sequences from the 5 patients with HCV genotype 3 and those from the surgeon was 2.1%. The distance between the sequences from the patients and from controls infected with HCV genotype 3 was 7.6%. A phylogenetic tree analysis suggested a common epidemiologic origin of the viruses from the surgeon and his 5 infected patients.

Conclusions.—The results of this study suggest that a cardiac surgeon with chronic hepatitis may have transmitted HCV genotype 3 to 5 of his 222 patients during open-heart surgery. The exact mechanism of transmission was not uncovered. Glove perforation may have occurred during wire closure of the sternum, which is associated with percutaneous injuries.

TABLE 1.—Characteristics of the 6 Patients with Acute Hepatitis C Unrelated to Transfusions

Patient No.	Age (yr)	Sex	Type of Surgery	Date of Surgery (mo/yr)	Date of Sample Used for Sequencing (mo/yr)	Incubation Period (wk)	Interval to Seroconversion (wk)	Nature of Infection	Interferon Alfa-2b dose	Treatment outcome	HCV Genotype
1	73	M	Valve replacement	11/88	1/89	8	14	Chronic	3 million units twice a week for 6 months	Response followed by relapse	3
2	23	M	Valve replacement	2/89	4/89	6	18	Chronic	3 million units twice a week for 12 months	Sustained response	3
3	57	F	Valve replacement	3/89	6/89	12	16	Chronic	Untreated	—	1*
4	59	F	Valve replacement	5/89	7/89	8	8	Acute	3 million units twice a week for 12 weeks	Sustained response	3
5	66	F	Valve replacement	11/92	12/93†	6	12	Chronic	3 million units twice a week for 12 months	Sustained response	3
6	38	M	Valve replacement	7/93‡	9/93	6	8	Chronic	3 million units twice a week for 12 months	Sustained response	3

*The patient was considered to have infection from another undetermined source and was excluded from further analysis.

†By mistake, the sample used for sequencing was obtained 1 year after infection, just before interferon treatment; it was not an acute-phase sample.

‡The day after the initial procedure, the patient underwent emergency surgery to reposition a blocked aortic-valve prosthesis.

TABLE 3.—Incidence of Acute Hepatitis C (Transfusion-associated and Non–transfusion-Associated Cases) among 222 Patients of the HCV-Infected Surgeon

Date and Surgeon's Role During Procedure	Total No. of Patients	No. Followed Prospectively (%)	No. with Postoperative Hepatitis C	
			Related To Transfusion	Unrelated To Transfusion
1988				
Surgeon	31	12 (39)	2	1
Assistant	32	15 (47)	2	0
1989				
Surgeon	39	29 (74)	3	2
Assistant	81	58 (72)	6	1*
1990				
Surgeon	32	10 (31)	0	0
Assistant	59	18 (31)	0	0
1992				
Surgeon	58	7 (12)	0	1
Assistant	47	11 (23)	0	0
1993				
Surgeon	63	16 (25)	0	1
Assistant	68	21 (31)	0	0
1994				
Surgeon	64	10 (16)	0	0
Assistant	69	15 (22)	0	0
Total				
Surgeon	287	84 (29)	5	5†
Assistant	356	138 (39)	8	1*

Note: No patients were prospectively evaluated between May 1990 and June 1992.

*This patient (Patient 3 in Table 1) had hepatitis C virus genotype 1 and was considered to have another source of infection.

†$P = 0.03$.

(Courtesy of Esteban JI, Gomez J, Martell M, et al: Transmission of Hepatitis C Virus by a Cardiac Surgeon. *N Engl J Med* 334:555–560. Copyright 1996, Massachusetts Medical Society. All rights reserved.)

▶ The findings obtained in this study provide evidence that a cardiac surgeon with chronic HCV infection transmitted HCV to 5 of his patients during open-heart surgery. It is interesting to note that the surgeon reported an overall incidence of about 20 percutaneous injuries per 100 procedures, with most of these occurring in the course of tying wires during closure of the sternum. Other surgical colleagues of the index surgeon, however, also acknowledged frequent percutaneous injuries while closing the sternum with wires. The authors in their discussion also point out another interesting fact concerning transmission of various viral infections after needle-stick injuries. They cite evidence indicating that the average risk of HCV infection after needle-stick injury involving HCV-infected blood has ranged between 2% and 3%, as compared with the risk of infection with HBV, which is 10 times higher at 30%, and HIV, which is 10 times lower at 0.3%.

N.J. Greenberger, M.D.

Routes of Infection, Viremia, and Liver Disease in Blood Donors Found to Have Hepatitis C Virus Infection

Conry-Cantilena C, VanRaden M, Gibble J, et al (NIH, Bethesda, Md; Greater Chesapeake and Potomac Region American Red Cross, Baltimore, Md; Hosp Gen Vall d'Hebron, Barcelona; et al)

N Engl J Med 334:1691–1696, 1996

5–8

Objective.—There may be 3.5 million people in the United States who are carriers of the hepatitis C virus (HCV). For many of these carriers, the route of exposure, risk of transmission, and severity of associated liver disease are unclear. Blood donors were studied to assess the main routes of HCV transmission, the infectivity of individuals who are confirmed as anti-HCV–positive, and the link between anti-HCV positivity and liver disease.

Methods.—Four hundred eighty-one blood donors who were positive for HCV antibodies on a first-generation enzyme immunoassay were studied. A confirmatory second-generation recombinant immunoblot assay (RIBA) was performed in each donor. Each individual also underwent a risk factor assessment, physical examination, alanine aminotransferase and HCV serologic tests, and a polymerase chain reaction assay for HCV

TABLE 3.—Potential Risk Factors for Exposure to HCV in the Study Participants

Risk Factor	Results of Second-Generation RIBA			Multivariate Analysis*	
	positive (n = 248)	indeterminate (n = 102)	negative (n = 131)	odds ratio (95% CI)	P value
	number (percent)				
Transfusion	66 (27)	9 (9)	11 (8)	9.6 (4.4–20.7)	<0.001
Intranasal cocaine use	169 (68)	25 (25)†	14 (11)	8.0 (3.9–16.5)	<0.001
Intravenous drug use	103 (42)	5 (5)	2 (2)	12.5 (2.7–57.1)	0.001
Sexual promiscuity‡	132 (53)	27 (26)	31 (24)	3.0 (1.5–5.9)	0.002
Ear piercing among men§	42 (30)	7 (14)¶	0	‖	<0.05‖
Tattooing	52 (21)	9 (9)	5 (4)	—	—
Imprisonment	61 (25)	6 (6)	2 (2)	—	—
Needle stick**	10 (4)	1 (1)	2 (2)	—	—
Acupuncture	11 (4)	2 (2)	1 (1)	—	—

*The positive group was compared with the negative group in a logistic-regression model. P < 0.001 for all univariate comparisons between these groups, except in the case of needle stick and acupuncture (P > 0.05). *Dashes* indicate that the risk factor shown did not meet the criteria for inclusion in the model. CI denotes confidence interval.

†P = 0.003 for the univariate comparison with the negative group.

‡Defined as a history of sexually transmitted disease, sex with a prostitute, 5 or more sexual partners per year, or a combination of these.

§Among women, no significant differences were found between study groups. The percentages shown are based on a total of 139 men in the positive group, 50 in the group with indeterminate results, and 83 in the negative group.

¶P < 0.001 for the univariate comparison with the negative group.

‖Because no men who were negative for HCV by RIBA had pierced ears, the estimated relative odds is infinite. The P value shown was derived by approximation.

**Data refer to needle-stick injuries in health care workers.

Abbreviations: HCV, hepatitis C virus; *RIBA,* recombinant immunoblot assay.

(Courtesy of Conry-Cantilena C, VanRaden M, Gibble J, et al: Routes of infection, viremia, and liver disease in blood donors found to have hepatitis C virus infection. *N Engl J Med* 334:1691–1696. Copyright 1996, Massachusetts Medical Society. Reprinted by permission of *The New England Journal of Medicine.* All rights reserved.)

RNA. Sexual contacts and family members were tested to assess infectivity. In addition, some RIBA-positive donors underwent liver biopsy.

Results.—Two hundred forty-eight of 481 patients were RIBA-positive for HCV. The results of RIBA were indeterminate in 102 patients and negative in 131. The significant risk factors for HCV infection on logistic regression analysis were a history of blood transfusion, intranasal cocaine use, IV drug use, sexual promiscuity, and ear piercing among men (Table 3). Although 9 of 85 sexual partners tested were also anti-HCV–positive, 8 of them were IV drug users or had received transfusions. Eighty-six percent of HCV-positive donors were found to have HCV RNA, and 69% had laboratory evidence of chronic liver disease. Of 77 HCV-positive patients undergoing liver biopsy, 66 had mild-to-moderate chronic hepatitis and 5 had severe chronic hepatitis or cirrhosis; only 6 were free of signs of hepatitis.

Conclusions.—Risk factors for HCV infection among blood donors include a history of blood transfusion, intranasal cocaine use, IV drug use, sexual promiscuity, and ear piercing in men. A second-generation RIBA is helpful in confirming the presence on absence of HCV infection. Sexual transmission of HCV, if it occurs, is not very efficient. Many HCV-positive patients have biochemical and histologic evidence of chronic liver disease, although few have severe histologic lesions.

▶ It is currently estimated that as many as 3–4 million Americans are infected with HCV. Earlier epidemiologic studies had identified blood transfusions (especially before 1990), IV drug use, high-risk sexual behavior, tattooing, needle-stick exposure, acupuncture, and shared razors/toothbrushes as important risk factors. However, after going through this checklist with HCV-positive patients, approximately 30% to 40% have no clearly identifiable risk factor. The study by Conry-Cantilena et al. provides new insight into identifying 2 additional important risk factors; i.e., intranasal cocaine use and ear piercing among men. After this article appeared, I was able to determine that some of my patients with heretofore unexplained chronic hepatitis C had used intranasal cocaine, whereas others had previously undergone ear piercing. The other factor that patients are often initially reluctant to discuss concerns high-risk sexual behavior. In subsequent interviews, with detailed questioning, this often comes to light. In the context of hepatitis C, the definition for sexual promiscuity has varied; the one used by Conry-Cantilena et al. defines sexual promiscuity as any combination of the following: (1) a history of a sexually transmitted disease; (2) sex with a prostitute; (3) 5 or more sexual partners per year. I anticipate that current epidemiologic studies will indicate that only a small percentage of chronic hepatitis C patients will have no identifiable risk factor.

N.J. Greenberger, M.D.

The Risk of Transfusion-transmitted Viral Infections

Schreiber GB, for the Retrovirus Epidemiology Donor Study (Westat Inc, Rockville, Md; Univ of California, San Francisco; Univ of California, Los Angeles; et al)
N Engl J Med 334:1685–1690, 1996

5–9

Introduction.—There is ongoing concern about the safety of the blood supply. Efforts to monitor the safety of transfused blood and to assess the benefits of new screening tests require accurate information about the risks of transmitting infectious diseases by blood transfusion. Blood donated by seronegative donors during the infectious "window" period, before sero-conversion has occurred, poses the main threat to the safety of the blood supply. The risks of transmitting HIV and other viral infections in blood donated during the window period were assessed.

Methods.—The analysis included 586,507 individuals who gave blood on repeated occasions between 1991 and 1993, for a total of 2,318,356 allogeneic blood donations. The incidence of seroconversion was assessed for individuals whose donated blood passed all screening tests. These rates were then adjusted to reflect the estimated window period for each virus under consideration, i.e., HIV, human T-cell lymphotropic virus (HLTV), hepatitis C virus (HCV), and hepatitis B virus (HBV). Further reductions in risk that might accrue from the use of new and more sensitive screening tests were estimated as well.

Results.—The adjusted incidence rates of seroconversion were 3.37/100,000 person-year for HIV, 1.12/100,000 for HTLV, 4.32/100,000 for HCV, and 9.80/100,000 for HBV (Table 1). The estimated risks of giving blood during an undetected infection were 1 in 493,000 for HIV, 1 in

TABLE 1.—Crude and Adjusted Incidence Rates of Seroconversion Associated With Each of 4 Major Blood-borne Viruses

Virus*	Crude Rate			Adjusted Rate		
	no. of seroconversions	no. of person-yr	incidence rate per 100,000 person-yr	no. of seroconversions	no. of person-yr	incidence rate per 100,000 person-yr (95% CI)†
HIV	33	822,494	4.01	27	801,571	3.37 (2.22–4.76)
HTLV	9	822,417	1.09	9	801,572	1.12 (0.51–1.98)
HCV‡	16	330,924	4.84	14	324,356	4.32 (2.35–6.87)
HBV						
HBsAg	33	822,426	4.01	33	801,553	4.12 (2.83–5.64)
Total HBV§	—	—	9.54	—	—	9.80 (6.74–13.42)

*Markers for each virus were assayed.

†Among donors whose previous donations were unusable; CI denotes confidence interval.

‡Data are limited to donations screened by the second-generation enzyme immunoassay, the use of which began in March and April 1992.

§Data were adjusted for transient antigenemia by multiplying the incidence rate of hepatitis B surface antigen *(HBsAg)* seroconversion and the 95% confidence interval by 2.38, on the assumption that 42% of hepatitis B virus infections are detected by the assay for HBsAg.

Abbreviations: HTLV, human T-cell lymphotropic virus; *HCV,* hepatitis C virus; *HBV,* hepatitis B virus.

202,000 for HTLV, 1 in 641,000 for HCV, and 1 in 63,000 for HBV. The overall risk of donating during an infectious window period was 1 in 34,000—HBV and and HCV made up 88% of this risk. With new viral antigen or nucleic acid screening tests, it was estimated that the risk could be reduced by 27% to 72%.

Conclusions.—The risk that virus-infected blood will be undetected during the infectious window period for HIV, HTLV, HCV, and HBV is very small, and it should become smaller still with the introduction of new screening tests. The surveillance program used in this study, which includes data from 5 blood centers across the United States, will be useful in providing essential data on blood safety issues.

▶ This study attests to the remarkable progress that has been made in reducing the risk of transfusion-transmitted viral infections in the United States. This should reassure both patients and physicians that transfusion of donated blood is quite safe. Furthermore, with the use of new and more sensitive viral-antigen or nucleic acid and screening tests, the risks should be minuscule.

It will be recalled that as recently as 1984, the risk of having hepatitis, primarily hepatitis C, develop after coronary artery bypass surgery was approximately 8%. In 1997, the risk of transmitting hepatitis C by transfusion of screened blood is only 1 in 103,000 (95% confidence interval of 28,000–288,000).

N.J. Greenberger, M.D.

Hepatitis C Virus Genotypes in the United States: Epidemiology, Pathogenicity, and Response to Interferon Therapy
Zein NN, and the Collaborative Study Group (Mayo Clinic, Rochester, Minn; Univ of Miami, Fla; Univ of Vermont, Burlington)
Ann Intern Med 125:634–639, 1996   5–10

Background.—Hepatitis C virus infection is the major cause of post-transfusion non-A, non-B hepatitis. About 50% of these patients have chronic liver disease and about 20% have cirrhosis. A worldwide comparison of hepatitis C virus genomic sequences has revealed that there is significant heterogeneity of nucleotide sequences within various regions of the viral genome. On the basis of these genomic differences, hepatitis C virus has been classified into multiple genotypes. These genotypes may be associated with variant antigenic and biological properties, and with variable response rates to interferon therapy. The geographic distribution, clinical characteristics, and response rate to interferon therapy of various genotypes of hepatitis C virus were determined.

Methods.—Serum samples were obtained from 179 patients with hepatitis C virus and chronic liver disease. Ribonucleic acid was extracted by chaotropic lysis and isopropanol precipitation. Polymerase chain reaction was performed on the NS5 region, and automated direct sequencing and genotyping of desalted amplification products were performed.

Results.—Of the 179 patients, 104 had subtype 1a, 38 had subtype 1b, 4 had subtype 2a, 23 had subtype 2b, 8 had subtype 3a, and 2 had subtype 4a. There was no correlation between genotype and mode of acquisition (such as blood transfusion, injection drug use, or employment at a health care facility) or baseline histologic findings. Severe hepatitis occurred in 68% of patients with genotype 1a, 80% of those with genotype 1b, and 37% of those with genotype 2a or 2b. A complete biochemical response occurred after 6 months of interferon therapy in 28% of patients with subtype 1a and 26% of patients with subtype 1b; 71% of those with subtype 2a or 2b had a complete response to interferon therapy. A sustained biochemical response was seen in 13% of patients with genotype 1a, 7% of those with genotype 1b, and 18% of patients with genotype 2a or 2b.

Conclusions.—Hepatitis C virus genotypes 1a and 1b are the primary genotypes in the United States in patients with chronic hepatitis C. There is no correlation between genotype and mode of virus acquisition or histologic findings. More severe liver disease and lower response rates to interferon therapy were seen in patients with genotypes 1a or 1b than in patients with genotype 2a or 2b. These findings may help select patients for interferon therapy and predict outcome.

▶ It is estimated that as many as 3.5 million Americans have hepatitis C. Recent data indicate that 75% to 80% of hepatitis C patients subsequently have chronic hepatitis, 20% to 25% have cirrhosis, and less than 5% have hepatoma. The most vexing unanswered question is why the disease progresses from chronic hepatitis to cirrhosis in approximately one third of patients with chronic hepatitis. The average time interval to development of cirrhosis is 20 years.

The study by Zein, et al. provides important information on hepatitis C virus (HCV) genotypes in the United States. Hepatitis C virus genotypes 1a and 1b are the most common HCV genotypes and seem to be associated with more severe liver disease and a lower response rate to interferon therapy.

The following factors are associated with an unfavorable response to interferon therapy: age >40, presence of cirrhosis, HCV genotypes, high serum HCV-RNA levels, coinfection with hepatitis B, coinfection with HIV, high hepatic iron content, and longer duration of disease. No doubt other prognostic factors will be identified in the future.

N.J. Greenberger, M.D.

Outbreak of Acute Hepatitis C Following the Use of Anti–Hepatitis C Virus–Screened Intravenous Immunoglobulin Therapy

Healey CJ, Sabharwal NK, Daub J, et al (John Radcliffe Hosp, Oxford, England; Univ of Oxford, England; Univ of Edinburgh, Scotland; et al)
Gastroenterology 110:1120–1126, 1996   5–11

Introduction.—A batch of the IV immunoglobulin (Ig) therapy Gammagard was withdrawn in February 1994 after being linked to cases of acute hepatitis C infection. In the United Kingdom, 36 patients had received injections from this batch at 19 local centers. Also identified were 12 patients who underwent Gammagard therapy at these centers during the same period but whose injections did not come from the suspected batch. These 48 patients were the subject of an epidemiologic study.

Methods.—Several patients had abnormal liver test results after receiving Gammagard from a particular batch. The same batch was associated with cases of acute hepatitis C in Spain. Physicians of patients who received IV Ig therapy from this batch and physicians of patients treated with another batch of Gammagard were sent a questionnaire to complete and asked to provide laboratory results for the 2 groups of patients. The genotype and subtype of representative samples from several centers were determined to establish whether the hepatitis C virus (HCV) infections were caused by the same virus.

Results.—Forty-six of the 48 patients had questionnaires returned. None had a history of illicit IV drug use, tattoos, or sexual contact with individuals with hepatitis. One patient whose injections were from the suspected batch had a history of lichen planus, but none of the others had evidence of an HCV-related disorder. Twenty-eight of 34 exposed patients (82%) became positive for HCV RNA. Two of the 6 who tested negative for HCV RNA had abnormal liver function and subsequently converted to anti–HCV antibody–positive. The mean time from exposure to the first positive HCV polymerase chain reaction test result was 37.5 days. Jaundice developed in 27% of the exposed patients, and 79% had abnormal liver transferase levels. Twenty-one virus isolates, including an isolate from the implicated batch, demonstrated evidence of transmission from a single source in that they were genotype 1a and virtually identical by sequence analysis of the NS5 region.

Discussion.—Use of this batch of Gammagard, made from blood screened for anti-HCV antibody, was associated with the transmission of acute hepatitis C. Analysis of viral isolates implicated a single donor. Both the anti-HCV screening and the production method failed. Because of the possibility of seronegative but HCV RNA–positive donations, the risk of HCV infection will continue (Table 2). It is important to carefully document batch numbers and provide regular biochemical monitoring for all IV Ig recipients.

▶ Recent reports[1] documented an outbreak of hepatitis C in patients undergoing IV immunoglobulin therapy. A total of 110 suspected cases of HCV

TABLE 2.—Summary of Previous Outbreaks of Hepatitis C Virus Infection in Patients Undergoing Intravenous Immunoglobulin Therapy

Country	Year	Study	Product	Outbreak	HCV PCR	Cirrhosis
United Kingdom	1983	Lane, Lever et al.	British Blood Products Laboratory, Elstree	12/12 IV Ig-treated patients contracted non-A, non-B hepatitis	5/5 positive	3 cases by 1986
United States	1988	Ochs et al.	Hyland Therapeutics Division, California	7/16 IV Ig-treated patients contracted non-A, non-B hepatitis	10/15 positive	2 cases by 1986
Sweden	1988	Bjorkander et al.	Gammonativ, Kabivitrium	16/77 treated patients contracted non-A, non-B hepatitis	8/10 positive	3 cases in initial report
Scotland	1989	Williams et al.	Scottish National Blood Transfusion Service	4/34 treated patients contracted non-A, non-B hepatitis	3/4 positive	Not known
Sweden	1986	Weiland et al.	Gammonative, Kabivitrium	4 patients with non-A, non-B hepatitis	Not known	2 cases in initial report
Sweden	1986	Hammarstrom and Smith	Not reported	1 patient with non-A, non-B hepatitis	1/1 positive	1 in initial report
Norway/ Sweden	1994	Bjoro et al.	Gammonativ, Kabivitrium	17 HCV-positive by PCR from 54 patients treated 1982-1986	17/54 positive	5 cases by 1994
United Kingdom	1994	Healey (present study)	Gammagard; Baxter-Hyland	28 HCV-positive by PCR from 36 patients exposed to one batch of IV	28/34 positive	Not known
United States	1994	MMWR	Gammagard; Baxter-Hyland	110 suspected cases of HCV infection treated with Gammagard	Not known	Not known

Abbreviations: Ig, immunoglobulin; *HCV,* hepatitis C virus; *PCR,* polymerase chain reaction.
(Courtesy of Healey CJ, Sabharwal NK, Daub J, et al: Outbreak of acute hepatitis C following the use of anti–hepatitis C virus–screened intravenous immunoglobulin therapy. *Gastroenterology* 110:1120–1126, 1996.)

infection occurred in patients treated with Gammagard.[2] The report by Healey et al. discusses 34 patients in the United Kingdom monitored since exposure to a contaminated batch of Gammagard. Hepatitis C virus infection developed in 30, with anti-HCV antibody developed in 28 who were also positive for HCV RNA; 2 were found to have abnormal liver tests with negative HCV antibody tests. Virus isolates were genotype 1a and virtually identical by sequence analysis, findings consistent with transmission from a single source. Jaundice developed in 9 of 34 patients, and 27 of 34 had abnormal aminotransferase levels. It is too early to tell whether the course of hepatitis C infection in these patients will be accelerated as has been documented in other immunodeficient patients infected with HCV.

N.J. Greenberger, M.D.

References

1. Bjoro MD, Froland SS, Yun Z: Hepatitis C infection in patients with primary hypogammaglobulinemia after treatment with contaminated immune globulin. *N Engl J Med* 331:1607–1611, 1994.
2. Meeks EL, Beach MJ: Outbreak of hepatitis C associated with intravenous immunoglobulin administration—United States, October 1993–June 1994. *MMNR Morb Mortal Wkly Rep* 43:505–509, 1994.

Chronic Hepatitis and Cirrhosis

The Long-term Pathological Evolution of Chronic Hepatitis C

Yano M, Kumada H, Kage M, et al (Nagasaki Chuo Natl Hosp Inst, Ohmura-shi, Japan; Toranomon Hosp, Tokyo; Kurume Univ, Japan; et al)
Hepatology 23:1334–1340, 1996   5–12

Background.—At least 60% of patients with acute hepatitis C virus (HCV) infection experience chronic hepatitis, and approximately half this group have insidious progression to cirrhosis. Little is known about the rate of progression and histopathologic pathways to cirrhosis. The pathologic progression of chronic hepatitis C was studied.

Methods.—Seventy patients with HCV infection were followed up continuously for more than 5 and up to 26 years. The mean follow-up was 9 years. During this time, a mean of 4 biopsy specimens were obtained per patient. Each specimen was scored for portal/periportal necroinflammation, lobular necroinflammation, the sum of these scores (final grade), and fibrosis (Table 1). The scores then were correlated with disease progression and transition to cirrhosis.

Results.—Cirrhosis developed in half the patients during follow-up. Cirrhosis developed in all patients who had high-grade necroinflammation on their initial biopsies and were followed up for 10 years and in 96% of patients who had intermediate-grade necroinflammation and were followed up for 17 years. In contrast, cirrhosis developed in just 30% of patients with low-grade necroinflammation after 13 years' follow-up. Within 10 years, all patients with septal fibrosis with incomplete nodularity had cirrhosis (Fig 4).

TABLE 1.—Histologic Evaluation of Liver Biopsy Specimens

Grading

Portal Inflammation		Lobular Inflammation		Final Grade
None or minimal	0	None	0	0
Portal inflammation	1	Inflammation but no necrosis	1	2
Mild limiting plate (lymphocytic piecemeal) necrosis	2	Spotty necrosis or acidophilic bodies	2	4 5
Moderate limiting plate (lymphocytic piecemeal) necrosis	3	Severe focal cell damage	3	6 7
Severe limiting plate (lymphocytic piecemeal) necrosis	4	Bridging necrosis	4	8

Staging

Stage	Degree of Fibrosis	Hepatic Architecture
1	None or too mild to affect size of portal tracts	Portal tracts not appreciably enlarged; no septa
2	Mostly periportal	Enlarged portal tracts, periportal fibrosis, or portal-to-portal septa but *without* architectural distortion
3	Septal	Prominent septal fibrosis *with* architectural distortion; no cirrhosis
4	Cirrhotic	Probable or definite cirrhosis

Findings
1. Lymphoid aggregated (yes, no).
2. Lymphoid follicles with germinal center (yes, no).
3. Nonsuppurative cholangitis with duct damage (yes, no).
4. Macrovesicular fatty changes (no, mild, moderate, severe).
5. Sinusoidal inflammation (no, mild, moderate, severe).
6. Septal fibrosis (yes, no).
7. Septal fibrosis incomplete nodularity (yes, no).
8. Cirrhosis (yes, no).

(Courtesy of Yano M, Kumada H, Kage M, et al: The long-term pathological evolution of chronic hepatitis C. *Hepatology* 23:1334–1340, 1996.)

Conclusions.—The grade and stage of liver biopsy lesions in patients with chronic hepatitis C reflect the long-term outcomes of the disease. Patients whose initial biopsies show high-grade necroinflammation, septal fibrosis, and regions of nodularity are likely to have advanced cirrhosis during the next 10 years or so. Other pathologic findings—such as lymphoid aggregates, steatosis, or cholangitis—are not prognostically significant.

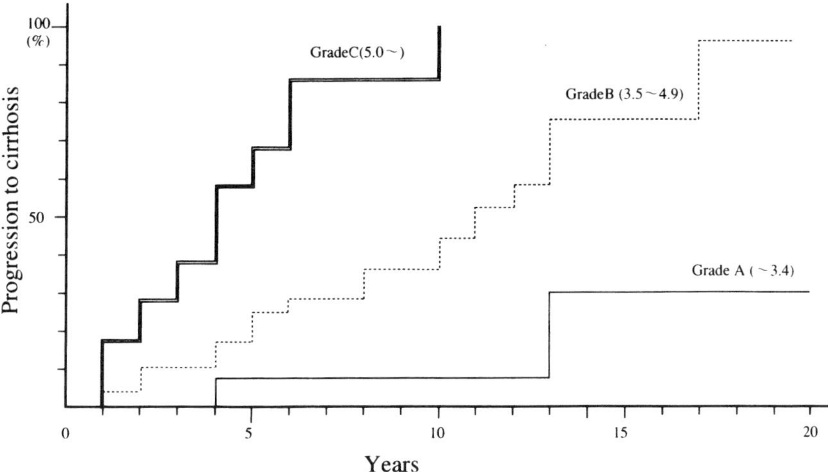

FIGURE 4.—Graphic depiction of patients who had progression to cirrhosis, with the cumulative rate of progression over time shown according to the final grade of necroinflammation on initial biopsy. Cirrhosis developed in 9 of 11 patients with initial grade C lesions who were followed up for more than 10 years. Of 40 patients with initial grade B lesions, 23 were followed up for 17 years and 22 had progression to cirrhosis. Of 19 patients with initial grade A lesions, 13 were followed up for more than 13 years, and 4 had progession to cirrhosis. (Courtesy of Yano M, Kumada H, Kage M, et al: The long-term pathological evolution of chronic hepatitis C. *Hepatology* 23:1334–1340, 1996.)

▶ It is now recognized that for every 100 patients in whom acute hepatitis C develops, approximately 75% will have chronic hepatitis, 25% to 30% will have cirrhosis of the liver, and fewer than 5% will have a hepatoma. The reason that only 50% to 65% of patients with chronic hepatitis have *non-progressive disease* and 35% to 50% have insidious progression to cirrhosis over 20–25 years is largely unknown. The study by Yano and colleagues provides important new information that addresses this vexing question. These investigators studied a mean of 4 liver biopsies obtained from 70 HCV-positive patients during a mean interval of 8.8 years (range 1–26 years). The biopsy specimens were assessed to determine the histologic features that could be predictive of prognosis. The key observations were that a high grade of necroinflammatory changes, septal fibrosis, and regions of nodularity on the initial biopsy specimens identified patients who were at high risk for the development of advanced cirrhosis in the ensuing decade. Conversely, cirrhosis developed in only 30% of patients with low-grade necroinflammatory changes on the initial biopsy specimens after a 13-year interval. That cirrhosis developed in half the patients in the study may reflect a selection bias, because lower rates of progression have been described in other cohorts.

N.J. Greenberger, M.D.

Morbidity and Mortality in Compensated Cirrhosis Type C: A Retrospective Follow-up Study of 384 Patients

Fattovich G, Giustina G, Degos F, et al (Univ of Verona, Italy; Università di Padova, Italy; Hopital Beaujon, Paris; et al)
Gastroenterology 112:463–472, 1997   5–13

Background.—The long-term prognosis of chronic liver disease associated with hepatitis C infection has not been well documented. The morbidity and survival of patients with compensated cirrhosis type C were assessed.

Methods.—Three hundred eighty-four patients with cirrhosis who were seen at 7 European tertiary referral centers were included. All had biopsy-proved cirrhosis; abnormal serum aminotransferase levels; no cirrhosis-related complications; and no evidence of hepatitis A or B viruses or metabolic, toxic, or autoimmune liver disease. The mean follow-up was 5 years.

Findings.—Ninety-eight percent of the 361 patients tested had positive antibodies against hepatitis C virus. The risks of hepatocellular carcinoma and of decompensation were 7% and 18%, respectively, at 5 years. Thirteen percent of the patients died, 70% from liver disease. Five-year survival probability was 91%, and 10-year survival probability was 79%. Fifty-three percent of the patients were treated with interferon-α. The 5-year estimated survival probability for treated patients was 96%, and for untreated patients, it was 95%, after adjustment for clinical and serologic differences at baseline.

Conclusions.—The life expectancy of patients with compensated cirrhosis type C appears to be relatively long. This is consistent with morbidity data that indicate an indolent disease course.

▶ This important study provides a wealth of information about the clinical course of compensated cirrhosis associated with hepatitis C. More than 250 patients with biopsy-proved cirrhosis but without any clinical evidence of decompensation were observed for a mean of 5 years after referral to tertiary hospitals. I would like to reiterate briefly the most important findings in the study.

• The cumulative probability of decompensated cirrhosis developing after diagnosis was 12% at 3 years, 18% at 5 years, and 29% at 10 years, giving a yearly incidence of 3.9%. Decompensation was defined by the development of ascites, variceal bleeding, encephalopathy, or jaundice.

• The probability of survival after diagnosis of decompensated cirrhosis was 91% at 5 years and 79% at 10 years, yielding a yearly incidence of mortality of 1.9% during the first 5 years.

• The cumulative probability of hepatocellular carcinoma developing was 7% at 5 years and 14% at 10 years, yielding a yearly incidence of 1.4% per year.

The data obtained indicate that a high proportion of patients with compensated cirrhosis do well for at least 10 years, as clinically overt liver disease occurred in 29% of patients at the end of the observation. The important conclusion, however, seems clear, and that is that progression of chronic hepatitis C occurs gradually and inexorably over time. As Dienstag points out in an accompanying editorial,[1] although chronic hepatitis C has a negligible clinical impact during the first 2 decades in the majority of patients, end-stage liver disease does occur in at least 20% of patients observed for a sufficiently long period. Dienstag also emphasizes that the data provided by Fattovich et al. support the notion that we should be treating earlier in the disease before progression is too advanced for therapy to be effective. A vexing problem is identifying which patients who have early disease are likely to benefit from treatment. It is clear that other studies are needed to resolve this important question.

N.J. Greenberger, M.D.

Reference

1. Diensthe JL: The natural history of hepatitis C and what we should do about it. *Gastroenterology* 112:651–655, 1997.

Meta-analysis of Interferon in Randomized Trials

Meta-analysis of Interferon Randomized Trials in the Treatment of Viral Hepatitis C: Effects of Dose and Duration
Poynard T, Leroy V, Cohard M, et al (Hôpital Michallon, Grenoble, France)
Hepatology 24:778–789, 1996
                                                                5–14

Background.—Since the first meta-analysis of randomized clinical trials of interferon therapy for acute or chronic hepatitis C published in 1991, 88 new studies have appeared. The original meta-analysis was expanded to include these latest references. Specifically, the benefits of higher doses or longer treatment duration were compared with the value of a standard interferon regimen in patients with chronic hepatitis.

Methods and Findings.—Seventeen studies of treated vs. control patients and 16 studies comparing different interferon regimens were analyzed. A standard regimen of 3 MU 3 times per week for 6 months was associated with an increase of the complete alanine transaminase (ALT) response rate by 45% and an increase of the sustained (ALT) response rate by 21%. The natural course was less than 2% of spontaneous responses. A significant dose effect was noted on the sustained response rate at 12 months, the mean increase being 17%. However, this effect was not observed at 6 months. A significant duration effect was noted on the sustained response rate at a dose of 3 MU (mean, 16%) and 6 MU (mean, 20%), 3 times a week. In the treatment of acute hepatitis, 3 months of interferon therapy was significantly more effective than control, as evidenced by differences in complete ALT response rates, sustained response rates during the 12 months after treatment, and hepatitis C virus RNA clearance.

Conclusions.—The best efficacy-to-risk ratio is attained with 3 MU 3 times a week for at least 12 months in patients with chronic hepatitis C not previously treated with interferon. Patients with acute hepatitis should be given inteferon-alfa at a dosage of at least 3 MU 3 times a week for 3 months.

▶ This meta-analysis provides important up-to-date guidelines on interferon treatment of viral hepatitis C and indicates that both *dose* and *duration* of treatment influence outcome. The following findings bear reemphasis:

• Prior standard therapy with interferon in a dosage of 3 million units thrice weekly for 6 months resulted in an initial 45% response rate (normalization of ALT) and a sustained response rate of 21%.

• Therapy with 6 million units thrice weekly for 6 months resulted in a modest increase in sustained response rate (mean = 17%)

• There was a significant *duration* effect with sustained response rates significantly greater after 12 months of therapy with both the 3.0 and 6.0 million units thrice weekly dosage regimens.

• From a cost-effective and efficacy risk point of view the regimen of choice at this time appears to be 3.0 million units thrice weekly for 12 months.

• Importantly, patients with acute viral hepatitis type C respond quite favorably to treatment with 3.0 million units of interferon given thrice weekly for 3 months.

The important end point of interferon therapy remains clearance of the hepatitis C virus (HCV) as evidenced by loss of serum HCV-RNA demonstrated by a sensitive technique such as polymerase chain reaction.

N.J. Greenberger, M.D.

Hepatitis C Fulminant Failure

Hepatitis C Virus–Associated Fulminant Hepatic Failure
Farci P, Alter HJ, Shimoda A, et al (NIH, Bethesda, Md; Rancho Los Amigos Med Ctr, Downey, Calif; Georgetown Med Ctr, Washington, DC)
N Engl J Med 335:631–634, 1996   5–15

Introduction.—In patients with fulminant hepatic failure, only a single serum sample is typically obtained and that is usually late in the course of the disease. Reported is a patient with hepatitis C virus (HCV)-associated fulminant hepatitis in whom serial serum samples were able to be collected. The availability of this serum provided the opportunity to demonstrate a temporal association between HCV infection and the development of fulminant hepatitis.

Case Report.—Man, 68, received 39 units of red-cell concentrate, 15 units of platelets, 21 units of fresh-frozen plasma, and 2 units of plasma cryoprecipitate during coronary artery bypass grafting and aortic valve replacement. The surgery occurred in March of 1990, about 2 months before the introduction of anti-HCV screening for blood donors. Four weeks after discharge, the patient was readmitted for increasing malaise and nausea. His serum alanine aminotransferase concentration was 4,493 U/L, compared with 27 U/L at discharge. Icterus, progressive encephalopathy, and coagulopathy developed. The patient died in an hepatic coma on the 11th hospital day. The peak serum bilirubin concentration was 15 mg/dL and the longest prothrombin time was 70 seconds.

Methods.—All serum samples were tested for the presence of hepatitis B virus DNA, hepatitis G virus RNA, and anti-HCV. At biopsy, liver tissue was stained for HCV antigen encoded by the fourth nonstructural gene and the percentage of antigen-positive cells was calculated.

Results.—Serum HCV viremia was not detected before or 1 week after multiple transfusions. It was detected when the patient was readmitted to the hospital 5 weeks after the transfusions and remained for 11 days until his death (Fig 1). The anti-HCV antibodies were not detected in serum before surgery but were detected by a second-generation enzyme immu-

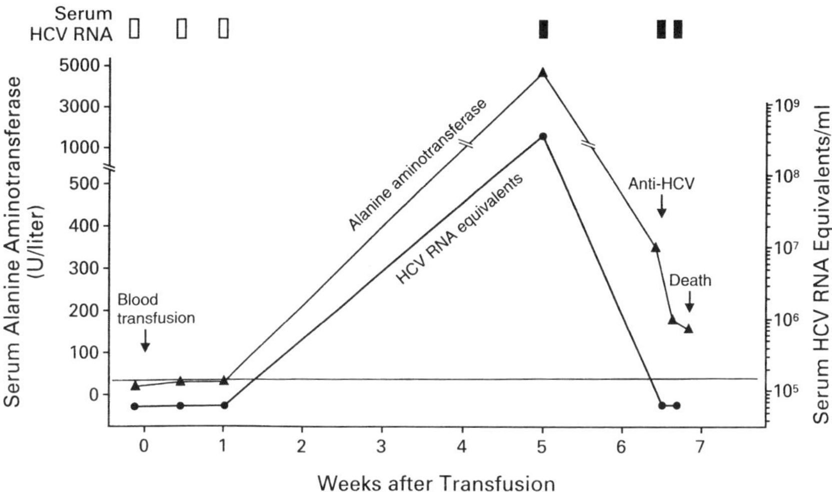

FIGURE 1.—Biomechanical, serologic, and molecular profiles of fulminant hepatitis C in a patient who acquired hepatitis C virus *(HCV)* Infection after blood transfusion for heart surgery. *Open bars* indicate negative assays for serum HCV RNA by polymerase chain reaction; *solid bars* indicate positive assays. A logarithmic scale is used to show the titer of serum HCV RNA. The *horizontal line* indicates the limit of sensitivity of the assay. Anti-HCV was detected by a second-generation enzyme 1 day before the patient's death. (Reprinted by permission of *The New England Journal of Medicine,* courtesy of Farci P, Alter HJ, Shimoda A, et al: Hepatitis C virus–associated hepatic failure. *New Engl J Med* 335:631–634. Copyright 1996, Massachusetts Medical Society. All rights reserved.)

noassay 1 day before the patient died. The level of HCV viremia increased in parallel with serum alanine aminotransferase concentrations, then quickly decreased below the level of sensitivity, despite the fact that serum HCV was continuously detected by polymerase chain reaction (PCR) until the patient died (Fig 1). Sequencing confirmed that the viral strain at 5 weeks and just before the patient's death was the same and showed genetic heterogeneity within each of the 2 isolates.

Conclusion.—Fulminant hepatic failure can be caused by HCV. The presence of serum HCV RNA by PCR is the earliest and most valuable marker for the diagnosis of fulminant hepatitis C.

▶ This study clearly shows that hepatitis C infection can result in fulminant hepatic failure. In this patient, the detection of serum HCV RNA was the earliest marker for the diagnosis of fulminant hepatitis C, being first demonstrated 5 weeks after transfusion (see Fig 1). By contrast, HCV antibody (HCV Ab) was first detected only 1 day before the patient's death. This suggests that in fulminant hepatitis with a rapid course, there may not be sufficient time for the development of HCV antibodies. Because HCV RNA is the earliest marker for diagnosis of hepatitis C and usually becomes positive within 1 to 2 weeks, a negative test for HCV RNA in a patient with fulminant hepatitis makes it very unlikely that the patient has HCV infection.

N.J. Greenberger, M.D.

Outcome After Liver Transplantation

Long-term Outcome of Hepatitis C Virus Infection After Liver Transplantation

Böker KHW, Dalley G, Bahr MJ, et al (Inst of Pathology, Hannover, Germany)
Hepatology 25:203–210, 1997   5–16

Background.—Hepatitis C virus (HCV)-related liver disease is a major indication for liver transplantation; however, within a few weeks of transplantation, reinfection of the grafted liver occurs in the majority of patients. The initial course of posttransplantation hepatitis C is usually mild, but the long-term prognosis is not clear. The clinical, biochemical, and histologic course after liver transplantation in 71 patients with HCV infection was monitored for as long 12 years.

Findings.—Patients were RNA-positive for HCV infection after liver transplantation because of either reinfection or de novo infection. The cumulative survival rate 2 years after transplantation was 67%, after 5 years it was 62%, and after 10 years it was 62%. These values did not differ significantly from those of HCV-negative patients who received transplants for other nonmalignant diseases (Fig 1). The presence of hepatocellular carcinoma at transplantation was the main factor determining long-term survival. Whereas deaths in the first year after transplantation were caused by rejection or infectious or cardiovascular problems, deaths after 12 months occurred exclusively because of recurrence of hepatocellular carcinoma. The majority of patients showed biochemical and histo-

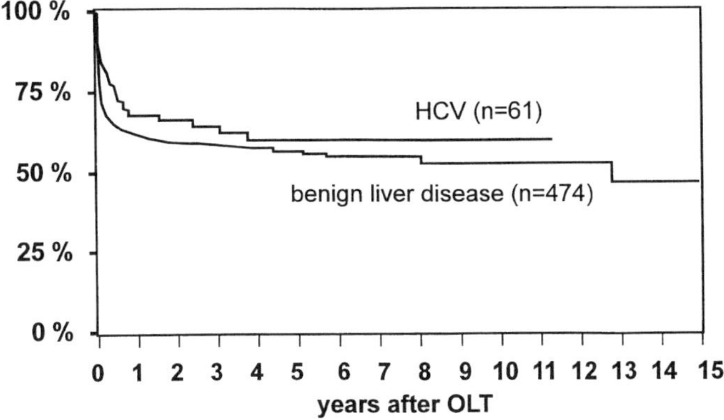

FIGURE 1.—Cumulative survival of patients who underwent orthotopic liver transplantation (*OLT*) for hepatitis C–related disease vs. patients who received transplants for other nonmalignant indications. Patients with concomitant hepatocellular carcinoma are not excluded from the hepatitis C group. Patients with hepatitis B–related diseases are included in the nonmalignant indication group. *Dotted line*, hepatitis C virus (*HCV*) infection (*n* = 61); *straight line*, nonmalignant indications except HCV (*n* = 474). The difference between the groups is not statistically significant; *P* = 0.25 (log rank test). (Courtesy of Böker KHW, Dalley G, Bahr MJ, et al: Long-term outcome of hepatitis C virus infection after liver transplantation. *Hepatology* 25:203–210, 1997.)

logic evidence of hepatitis, but only 22% complained of symptoms (hepatitis was the cause of these symptoms in 82%). Positivity for HCV RNA disappeared in a prolonged, ongoing fashion in 2 patients. Neither age, sex, severity of pretransplant liver disease, cold ischemic time of the graft, duration of the procedure, transfusion, number of rejection episodes, nor long-term immunosuppressive regimen was related to the severity of posttransplantation hepatitis. Inflammatory activity was decreased only by initial short-term therapy with interleukin-2 receptor antibodies. Histologic examination revealed inflammation in 88% of the biopsy specimens and fibrosis in 24%.

Conclusions.—These data indicate that in the majority of patients with HCV infection after liver transplantation, chronic hepatitis does develop. Approximately 16% of the patients experience a carrier state without significant laboratory abnormalities. Another 60% of the patients show biochemical abnormalities but do not experience clinical signs of the disease. In approximately 25% of the patients, symptomatic disease develops. The disease course is similar to that of nontransplanted HCV-infected patients; clinical signs are generally mild but signs of graft fibrosis appear within the first decade in 10% or more of the patients.

▶ This study provides important information on the clinical, biochemical, and histologic course of 71 patients with HCV infection after liver transplantation who were monitored for up to 12 years. Cumulative survival at 2, 5, and 10 years was not significantly different from that in patients transplanted for other nonmalignant diseases without HCV infection. While it appears that chronic hepatitis develops in the majority of patients with HCV infection after liver transplantation, the carrier state without significant laboratory abnormalities occurs in approximately 16% biochemical abnormalities without symptoms occur in approximately 60%, and symptomatic disease occurs in a quarter of the patients. These findings show posttransplantation hepatitis C to be a rather mild disease in most cases and also shows that there is no excess mortality because of the disease in the first decade after transplantation.

N.J. Greenberger, M.D.

Long-term Outcome of Hepatitis C Infection After Liver Transplantation

Gane EJ, Portmann BC, Naoumov NV, et al (King's College School of Medicine and Dentistry, London; Innogenetics, Ghent, Belgium)
N Engl J Med 334:815–820, 1996   5–17

Background.—Liver transplantation is commonly performed because of cirrhosis related to hepatitis C virus (HCV) infection. However, persistent viremia occurs in more than 95% of patients, and HCV infection in the graft can recur within 4 weeks after transplantation. The natural history of HCV infection in liver transplant recipients was studied, including the contribution of HLA mismatches and viral genotypes to the severity of recurrent HCV disease.

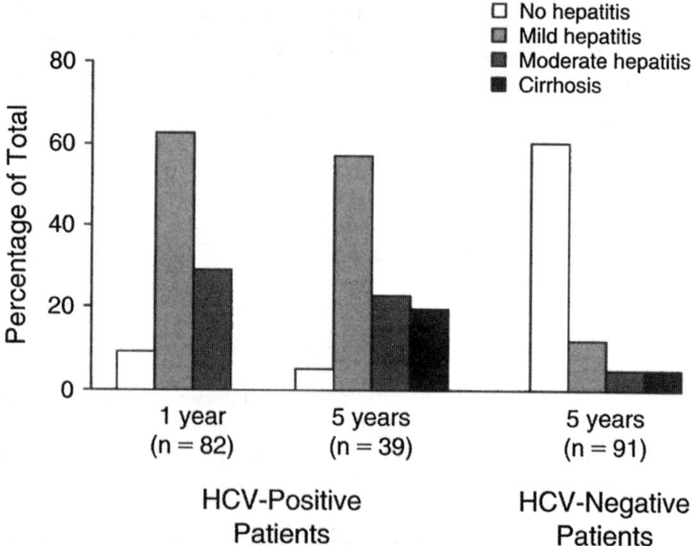

FIGURE 1.—Biopsy findings 1 and 5 years after liver transplantation in recipients with hepatitis C virus (HCV) infection after transplantation and in those without HCV infection. The number of patients in each group is given in parentheses. *P* < 0.001 for the comparison of each variable between the HCV-positive and HCV-negative groups at 5 years. (Courtesy of Gane EJ, Portmann BC, Naoumov NV, et al: Long-term outcome of hepatitis C infection after liver transplantation. *N Engl J Med* 334:815–820. Copyright 1996, Massachusetts Medical Society. Reprinted by permission of *The New England Journal of Medicine*. All rights reserved.)

Methods.—A total of 149 liver transplant recipients with HCV infection were studied. The natural outcome of HCV infection was assessed during a median follow-up of 36 months. A group of non–HCV-infected liver transplant recipients were analyzed for comparison. Pathologic review was conducted on 528 liver biopsy specimens obtained from the HCV-infected patients, including scheduled 1-year and 5-year specimens.

Results.—The HCV-infected patients had a cumulative survival of 79% at 1 year, 74% at 3 years, and 70% at 5 years. These were similar to the survival rates recorded for the non–HCV-infected recipients. Among HCV-infected recipients who survived longer than 6 months, the most recent liver biopsy specimens showed no signs of chronic hepatitis in 12%, mild chronic hepatitis in 54%, moderate chronic hepatitis in 27%, and cirrhosis in 8% (Fig 1). Patients infected with HCV genotype 1b had more severe graft injury, whereas the immunosuppressive regimen used and the extent of donor-recipient HLA mismatching had no significant impact on the severity of recurrent disease.

Conclusions.—In patients receiving liver transplants for HCV-related cirrhosis, persistent HCV infection can cause severe graft damage, particularly in those with HCV genotype 1b. However, 5-year graft and overall survival are comparable for liver transplant recipients with and without HCV infection. Liver biopsies to assess the extent of HCV-related damage to the liver graft could help to select patients who could benefit from antiviral therapy.

▶ Persistence of hepatitis C viremia after liver transplantation is almost universal, and recurrence of HCV infection in the graft is also common. Gane et al. have investigated the natural history of HCV infection in liver transplant recipients to determine the impact of such infection on the *morphologic characteristics* of the graft and the *long-term outcome*. They found that HCV infection frequently recurs after liver transplantation for HCV-induced cirrhosis. Although earlier reports suggested that HCV is a benign disorder after liver transplantation, Gane et al. found that moderate chronic hepatitis developed in 27% of the patients after a median of 35 months *and* that the disease progressed to cirrhosis in 8% after a median of 51 months. There appeared to be an accelerated rate of graft damage in those patients infected with HCV genotype 1b. Whether such patients would benefit from antiviral therapy remains an open question. Despite the above problem, the cumulative survival rates at 1, 3, and 5 years after transplantation were comparable between 149 patients with and 623 patients without HCV infection.

N.J. Greenberger, M.D.

Clinical Behavior and Antiviral C Cell-Mediated Immune Response

Different Clinical Behaviors of Acute Hepatitis C Virus Infection Are Associated With Different Vigor of the Anti-viral Cell-mediated Immune Response

Missale G, Bertoni R, Lamonaca V, et al (Università di Parama, Italy; Azienda Ospedaliera di Reggio Emilia, Italy; Università di Milano, Italy; et al)
J Clin Invest 98:706–714, 1996   5–18

Background.—Immune-mediated mechanisms, specifically the antiviral T-cell response, are believed to play a critical role in the pathogenesis of hepatitis C. Peculiar features of the T-cell response that are associated with recovery vs. viral persistence were examined by studying the HLA class II–restricted proliferative T-cell response to hepatitis C virus (HCV) proteins sequentially from the early clinical stages of disease.

Methods.—Participants included 21 patients with acute HCV infection; follow-up lasted an average of 44 weeks. The peripheral blood T-cell proliferative response to core, E1, E2, NS3, NS4, and NS5 recombinant antigens and synthetic peptides was analyzed and alanine aminotransferase (ALT) levels were measured.

Results.—Normalization of ALT values occurred in 12 of 21 patients (group 1) largely within 3–7 weeks. Values for ALT remained primarily above the normal range in 9 patients (group 2) with persistent viremia. All

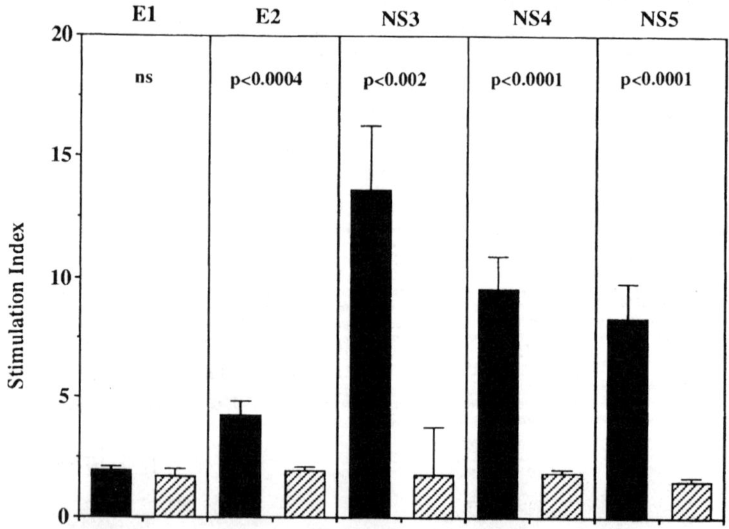

FIGURE 4.—Comparison of the strength of T-cell responses to hepatitis C virus proteins in patients with different outcomes of infection (*solid bars,* patients who normalized ALT; *crosshatched bars,* patients with persistently elevated ALT). (Courtesy of Missale G, Bertoni R, Lamonaca V, et al: Different clinical behaviors of acute hepatitis C virus infection are associated with different vigor of the anti-viral cell mediated immune response. Reproduced from *J Clin Invest* 98:706–714, by copyright permission of The American Society for Clinical Investigation.)

but 2 patients in group 1 experienced clearance of HCV RNA from serum. Patients in group 1 showed significantly more vigorous and more frequently detectable T-cell proliferative responses to all HCV antigens except E1 (Fig 4). Sequential evaluation of these responses showed that the difference between groups was detectable very early in the acute stage of infection and continued throughout.

Conclusions.—These data suggest that HCV disease resolution and infection control may be critically determined by the vigor of the T-cell response during the early stages of infection. A vigorous antiviral T-cell response appears to be associated with the ability of the host to show normal ALT levels and to recover, either transiently or permanently, from hepatitis C.

▶ This study suggests that the relative strength of the T-cell response to HCV proteins in the acute phase of hepatitis C may represent a critical determinant of disease resolution and control of infection. Additional factors contribute to the *progression* of chronic hepatitis C. Kobayashi and other investigators[1] have shown that more severe progression of chronic hepatitis C is seen in patients showing genotype 1b as compared with genotype 2. For an excellent brief review of hepatitis C genotypes, see the review article by Zein and Persing.[2]

N.J. Greenberger, M.D.

References

1. Kobayashi M, Tanaka E, Sodeyama T, et al: The natural course of chronic hepatitis C: A comparison between patients with genotypes 1 and 2 hepatitis C virus. *Hepatology* 23:695–699, 1996.
2. Zein NW, Persing DH: Hepatitis C genotypes: Current trends and future implications. *Mayo Clin Proc* 71:458–467, 1996.

36 Hepatitis G

Molecular Cloning and Disease Association of Hepatitis G Virus: A Transfusion-transmissible Agent
Linnen J, Wages J Jr, Zhang-Keck Z-Y, et al (Genelabs Technologies, Redwood City, Calif; Ctrs for Disease Control and Prevention, Atlanta, Ga; NIH, Bethesda, Md; et al)
Science 271:505–508, 1996   5–19

Background—Despite the availability of sensitive and specific assays to detect the known hepatitis viruses, no cause can be identified for some cases of posttransfusion and community-acquired hepatitis. Thus, there may be unknown causative viruses. The cloning and disease associations of a new transfusion-transmitted hepatitis virus, designated hepatitis G virus (HGV), are reported.

Findings.—The new RNA virus was isolated from the plasma of a patient with chronic hepatitis. The entire 9,392-nucleotide genome, encoding a 2,873 amino-acid polyprotein, was identified by extension from an immunoreactive complementary DNA clone. Comparative studies suggested that HGV was closely related to GB virus C (GBV-C) and more distantly related to hepatitis C virus, GBV-A, and GBV-B. Patient studies showed an association between HGV and acute and chronic hepatitis; HGV RNA was found in 15% of patients with acute non–A through E hepatitis and 18% of patients with acute hepatitis C. In addition, HGV RNA was detected in about 1.5% of potential blood donors with or without an elevated alanine aminotransferase level. Evidence of HGV transmission by blood transfusion was observed in patients with post-transfusion hepatitis (Table 1).

Conclusion.—This virus is distributed globally, can be detected in the United States blood donor population, and can be transmitted by transfusion. Studies of the pathogenesis, epidemiology, and natural history of HGV infection are needed.

▶ The hepatitis alphabet soup continues. Hepatitis G virus is the latest addition to well-characterized hepatitis viruses A, B, C, D, and E. The blood-borne nature of HGV has been clearly shown by Linnen et al. who demonstrated the development of HGV RNA in the serum of patients *after*, but not before, transfusion. They have also provided evidence indicating that HGV infection can persist for years.

TABLE 1.—Frequency of Hepatitis G Virus Viremia in People Who Have Hepatic Disease, Are at Risk for Exposure to Parenterally Transmitted Infectious Agents, or Are Volunteer Blood Donors

Condition	Origin	Patients (n)	Total HGV+	HGV only	HGV+ and HBV+	HGV+ and HCV+	HGV+, HBV+, and HCV+
		Liver disease					
Post-transfusion	US	12	2	2	0	0	0
non-A-E hepatitis	AUS	1	1	0	0	0	0
Chronic non-A-C	SA	48	6	6	0	0	0
hepatitis	EU	110	9	9	0	0	0
Suspected non-A-E hepatitis	EU	12	1	1	0	0	0
Chronic HBV	EU	72	7	0	7	0	0
Chronic HCV	EU	96	18	0	0	18	0
Hepatocellular carcinoma	EU	30	2	0	1	1	0
Alcoholic hepatitis	EU	49	6	6	0	0	0
Autoimmune hepatitis	EU	53	5	5	0	0	0
Primary biliary cirrhoses	EU	58	1	0	0	1	0
		Parenteral exposure risk					
Hemophilia	EU	49	9	0	0	8	1
Multiply transfused anemia	EU	100	18	11	1	6	0
Intravenous drug use	EU	60	20	6	1	11	2
		Volunteer blood donors					
Accepted donations	US	769	13	13	0	0	0
Rejected donations (ALT > 45 IU/ml; fresh)	US	214	5	4	0	0	1
Rejected donations (ALT > 45 IU/ml; frozen)	US	495	6	4	0	1	1

Abbreviations: *HGV*, hepatitis G virus; *HBV*, hepatitis B virus; *HCV*, hepatitis C virus; *Non–A–E*, non–A through E; *non–A–C*, non–A through C; *ALT*, alanine aminotransferase; *US*, United States; *AUS*, Australia; *SA*, South America; *EU*, Europe.

(Reprinted with permission, courtesy of Linnen J, Wages J Jr, Zhang-Keck Z-Y, et al: Molecular cloning and disease association of hepatitis G virus: A transfusion-transmissible agent. *Science* 271:505–508. Copyright 1996, American Association for the Advancement of Science.)

Another interesting finding is that HGV antibodies have been demonstrated in 1.7% of 779 volunteer blood donors with normal alanine aminotransferase (ALT) levels. The fact that the prevalence of HGV was nearly the same (1.5%) in 709 excluded donors with normal ALT levels raises the question of whether HGV causes liver disease in healthy blood donors.

Antibodies to HGV have also been demonstrated in patients with chronic liver disease, but the frequent finding of the concurrent presence of other hepatitis viruses (notably HCV and HBV) further clouds the issue of whether HGV per se causes chronic liver disease. For a thoughtful and authoritative brief review for this landmark paper, see the commentary by Pessoa and Wright.[1]

N.J. Greenberger, M.D.

Reference

1. Pessoa MG, Wright TC: Hepatitis G: A virus in search of a disease. *Hepatology* 24:461–463, 1996.

Infection With Hepatitis GB Virus C in Patients on Maintenance Hemodialysis
Masuko K, Mitsui T, Iwano K, et al (Masuko Inst for Medical Research, Aichi-Ken, Japan; Murayama Hosp, Tochigi-Ken, Japan; Yamanashi Med Univ, Japan; et al)
N Engl J Med 334:1485–1490, 1996   5–20

Background.—The hepatitis GB virus C (HGBV-C) is a recently discovered non-A, non-E hepatitis virus that resembles but is not a genotype of hepatitis C virus (HCV). There is little information on the mode of transmission and clinical manifestations of HGBV-C. A reverse-transcription–polymerase-chain-reaction (RT-PCR) assay was used to test a series of maintenance hemodialysis patients for HGBV-C infection.

Methods.—Five hundred nineteen patients were tested. The RT-PCR assay used nested primers deduced from the nonstructural region of HGBV-C to identify HGBV-C RNA in serum. Eight patients with HGBV-C

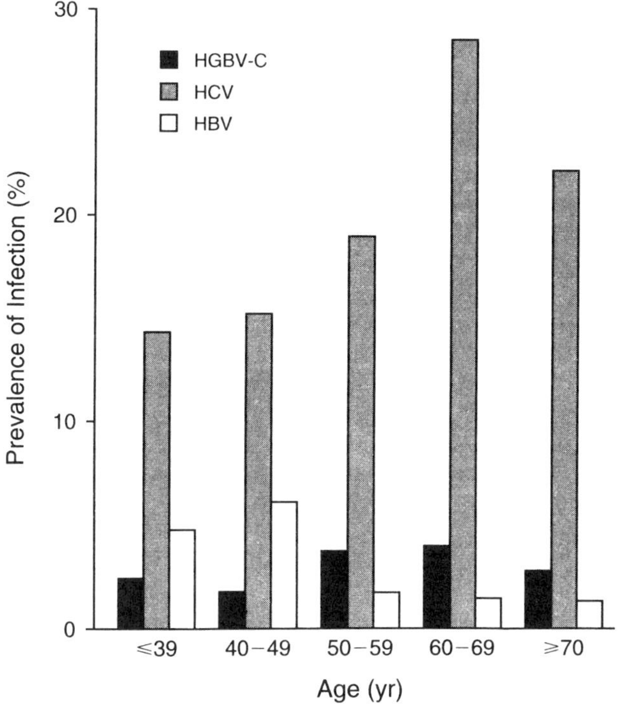

FIGURE 1.—Age-specific prevalence of hepatitis GB virus C (HGBV-C), hepatitis C virus (HCV), and hepatitis B virus (*HBV*) among 519 patients on maintenance hemodialysis. The detection of HCV RNA on reverse-transcription–polymerase-chain-reaction assay was considered to indicate infection with HCV, and a positive test for hepatitis B surface antigen was considered to indicate infection with HBV. (Courtesy of Masuko K, Mitsui T, Iwano K, et al: Infection with hepatitis GB virus C in patients on maintenance hemodialysis. *N Engl J Med* 334:1485–1490. Copyright 1996, Massachusetts Medical Society. Reprinted by permission of *The New England Journal of Medicine.* All rights reserved.)

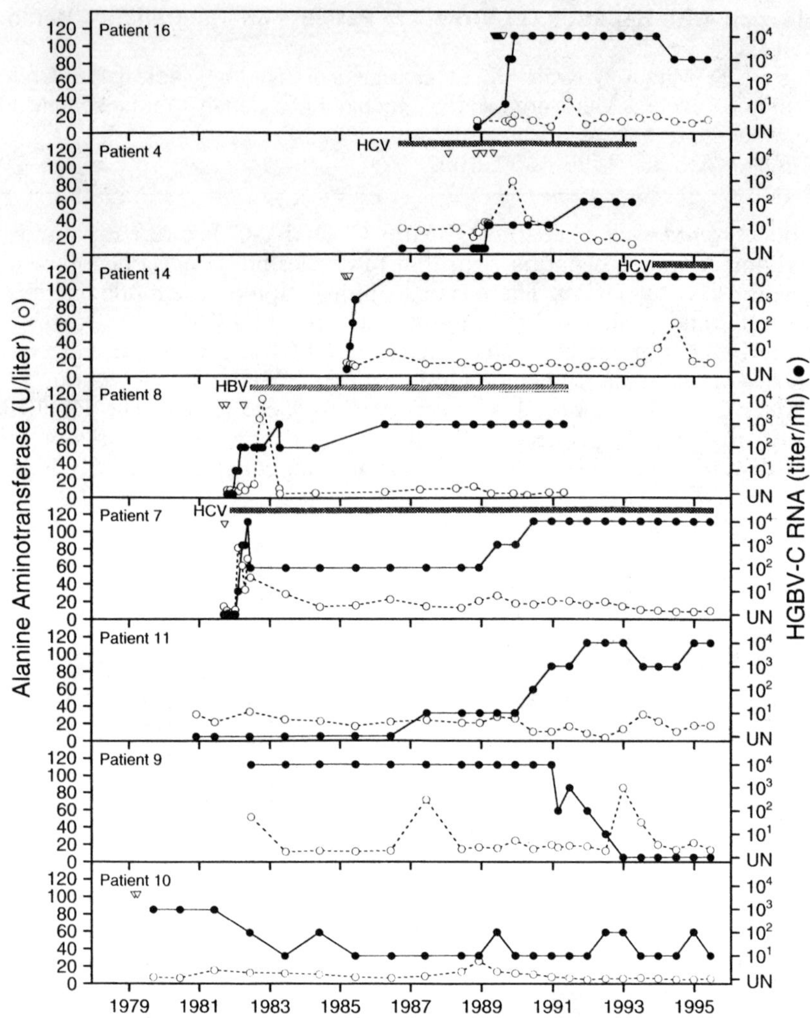

FIGURE 2.—Serum alanine aminotransferase levels and titers of HGBV-C RNA in 8 patients on maintenance hemodialysis. The patients had been followed since the start of dialysis. Each *inverted triangle* represents a transfusion. Patients 4, 7, 8, and 14 were also infected with hepatitis C virus (HCV) or hepatitis B virus (*HBV*). *Abbreviation: UN*, undetectable. (Courtesy of Masuko K, Mitsui T, Iwano K, et al: Infection with hepatitis GB virus C in patients on maintenance hemodialysis. *N Engl J Med* 334:1485–1490. Copyright 1996, Massachusetts Medical Society. Reprinted by permission of *The New England Journal of Medicine*. All right reserved.)

infection were followed up for 7–16 years to gain insight into the transmission, persistence, and evolution of HGBV-C.

Results.—Three percent of the hemodialysis patients were found to have HGBV-C RNA, compared with 1% of healthy blood donors. The age-specific prevalence of HGBV-C was similar to that of HCV, with a peak in the seventh decade of life (Fig 1). Of the 16 patients with HGBV-C RNA, 7 also had HCV infection, although none had active liver disease. The follow-up study suggested that HGBV-C was transmitted by blood transfusion; IV drug use may also have played a role. Serum alanine aminotransferase levels were not elevated in the patients with HGBV-C infection, suggesting that it did not cause liver inflammation (Fig 2).

Conclusions.—The rate of HGBV-C infection among hemodialysis patients may be higher than previously thought. Blood transfusion appears to be an important source of transmission, although other routes are possible as well. Hepatitis GB virus C causes persistent infections but it does not appear to cause inflammation of the liver.

▶ The hepatitis G virus (HGV) and the HGBV-C are now considered to be closely related isolates of the same virus, in large part because the amino acid sequences of the 2 agents are more than 95% homologous. Several issues of the HGV/HGBV-C virus are both intriguing and incompletely understood:

* Preliminary studies indicate that HGV/HGBV-C has been found in 1% to 2% of volunteer blood donors in the United States.[1]

* HGV/HGBV-C is transmitted by transfusions.

* The interval between transfusions and the appearance of HGV/HGBV-C in serum appears to range between 13 and 17 weeks.

* HGV/HGBV-C accounts for only a small minority of cases of hepatitis without a defined cause.

* Although a small number of patients with chronic liver disease of uncertain etiology do have evidence of HGV/HGBV-C infection, the vast majority of patients with prospectively observed HGV infection have no evidence of associated liver inflammation or liver disease.

As Alter[1] emphasizes, the incompletely resolved aspects of HGV/HGBV-C infection are whether it causes acute liver injury, and whether it alone leads to serious chronic liver disease.

N.J. Greenberger, M.D.

Reference

1. Alter HJ: The cloning and clinical implications of HGV and HGBV-C. *N Engl J Med* 334:1336–1337, 1996.

37 Liver Transplantation

UCLA Liver Transplantation: Analysis of Immunological Factors Affecting Outcome
Dawson S III, Imagawa DK, Johnson C, et al (Univ of California Los Angeles School of Medicine; UCI School of Medicine, Orange, Calif; Univ of California Los Angeles Tissue Typing Lab)
Artif Organs 20:1063–1072, 1996   5–21

Background.—The immunologic factors influencing graft and patient survival after orthotopic liver transplantation (OLT) are not understood well. One series was analyzed retrospectively to increase understanding of such factors.

Methods and Findings.—Between 1988 and 1993, 938 first and 1,146 total OLTs were performed at 1 center. At 1 year, 89% of black patients and 80% of whites were still alive. One-year survival rates did not differ between whites and Hispanics. Asians had a 1-year survival rate of 50%, even after the exclusion of hepatitis B. Asian patients positive for hepatitis B surface antigen had a survival rate of only 21%. Patients with panel reactive antibody (PRA) of less than 10% did not have a graft or patient survival advantage compared with patients with PRAs of more than 10%. A positive antidonor flow cytometry crossmatch was correlated with a reduced graft survival at 1 year ... compared with flow-negative recipients. One-year graft survival for patients with no HLA-DR mismatches was 74%; for 1 DR mismatch, 57%; and for 2 DR mismatches, 59%.

Conclusions.—Asian OLT recipients who received transplants for hepatitis B had poor outcomes because of aggressive recurrent disease. Although patients with PRA exceeding 10% are more likely to have a positive crossmatch, most OLT patients are not sensitized. The 1-year survival rate is significantly reduced in patients with a positive antidonor flow cytometry crossmatch. Patients with no DR mismatches have better graft and patient survival rates than those with 1 or 2 DR mismatches.

▶ This review of the total OLT experience at UCLA during a 5-year period (1988–1993) reveals some interesting observations. The ethnicity observations regarding 1-year survival were as follows: blacks, 89%; whites, 80%; and Asians, 50%. The Hispanics had similar experiences to whites. The high rate of attrition in Asian patients was attributed to recurrence of hepatitis B in the transplanted liver. The 1-year survival was remarkably low in Asian patients who were positive for hepatitis B surface antigen (21%). The article contains a wealth of immunologic information that would be of interest to those who understand and deal with panel reactive antibodies and HLA-DR matching.

F.G. Moody, M.D.

Graft Function and Outcome of Older (≥60 Years) Donor Livers
Washburn WK, Johnson LB, Lewis WD, et al (New England Deaconess Hosp, Boston; Harvard Med School, Boston)
Transplantation 61:1062–1066, 1996   5–22

Introduction.—Liberalization of donor selection criteria would be an easy and readily available method of increasing the supply of donor organs. Although many donor livers are refused without inspection if the donor is older than 50 years, the program at the study institution considers livers from donors 60 years or older. Graft function and outcome were compared in 2 groups of patients: 29 (group A) received livers from donors 60 years or older and 194 (group B) from donors younger than 60 years.

Patients and Methods.—Groups A and B were matched for recipient diagnosis and severity of disease. Liver donors for the 2 groups had similar liver, renal, and hematologic studies before donation. All older donors and all but 2 of the younger donors were ABO identical or compatible with the recipients. Donors and recipients were evaluated for variables related to outcome.

Results.—The mean donor age was 63.7 years for group A and 30.7 years for group B. Most older donors died of intracerebral bleeding (76%), whereas the most common cause of death among younger donors was a closed head injury (42%). During the first 10 postoperative days, the 2 groups of liver recipients did not differ significantly in levels of alanine aminotransferase and aspartate aminotransferase and in prothrombin time. On postoperative days 6–10, group A grafts were significantly more cholestatic than group B grafts. One-year patient survival rates were 58.6% for group A vs. 79.2% for group B; 1-year graft survival rates were 44.8% and 74.5%, respectively. Four of the 12 deaths in the first year in group A were completely unrelated to allograft function. Exclusion of these deaths yielded patient and graft survival rates of 68% and 52%, still significantly lower than the rates of group B. Donor sex appeared to be unrelated to outcome.

Discussion.—Although livers transplanted from older donors can function well initially, patient and graft survival rates are significantly better when the donor is younger than 60 years. In the 2 groups of recipients, donors were similar in laboratory values and in pretransplant liver biopsies and differed significantly only in age and cause of death. Because risk factors related to poor outcome with older donors are not yet understood, these grafts should be used after careful selection and retransplanted promptly if function is poor.

► Livers from older donors appear to reflect their age when they are engrafted into needy recipients. This is a shame because older people have a higher likelihood of dying and are probably pretty generous with donating their body parts, and terminal strokes are a fairly common way to leave this world. It appears that older livers are more susceptible to prolonged ischemia times. Furthermore, they seem to be more cholestatic for reasons that we do not entirely understand. I have been impressed with how sturdy the liver appears to be in patients who are 60 years or even much older when it remains in their body. It would be important to expand the donor pool by learning more about why older livers do not appear to "like" being put into younger patients.

F.G. Moody, M.D.

---

10 Years of Pediatric Liver Transplantation
Andrews W, Sommerauer J, Roden J, et al (Univ of Texas Southwestern Med Ctr, Dallas; Children's Med Ctr of Dallas)
J Pediatr Surg 31:619–624, 1996   5–23

Introduction.—Although approximately 20% of patients awaiting liver transplantation are children, few studies have examined long-term outcomes in the pediatric population. Ten-year patient and graft survival rates were reviewed retrospectively, and factors affecting survival were analyzed.

Patients and Methods.—From October 1984 to October 1994, 202 children underwent 225 liver transplantations. Biliary atresia, present in 45% of cases, was the most common reason for transplantation. Children ranged in age from 6 weeks to 19 years (mean, 5.14 years); there were 104 girls and 98 boys. In the early years of the program, immunosuppression was cyclosporine- and steroid-based. Azathioprine and antilymphocyte preparations were added to the protocol after 1990. Screening for Epstein-Barr virus by polymerase chain reaction was performed posttransplantation and at regular intervals for 2 years.

Results.—Overall patient survival rates were 76% at 1 year, 70% at 5 years, and 61% at 10 years; corresponding overall graft survival rates were 71%, 63%, and 59%. Neither age at the time of transplantation nor race had a significant impact on survival. Children with metabolic disease, however, had a substantially higher overall survival rate (90% at 5 years) than those with acute hepatic failure (43% at 5 years). Nine-year survival rates for patients with biliary atresia, hepatitis, and the other diagnoses ranged from 62% to 69%. Although 7-year graft survival was lower for ABO-incompatible than for ABO-identical groups, the difference was not significant. Forty-eight of the 60 deaths occurred during the first year, and most (42%) were the result of sepsis. After the first year, lymphoproliferative disease and preoperative or postoperative complications each accounted for 3 deaths. Mean operating time, mean amount of blood loss, and the average period of hospitalization all decreased during the study period, despite an increase in pretransplant illness severity, as reflected in patient priority status. A decrease in early deaths from sepsis increased the patient survival rate to 88% for 1993–1994.

Conclusion.—Pediatric liver transplantation has undergone enormous advances during the last decade. New protocols based on an analysis of the etiology of deaths have reduced the number of deaths related to the patient's pretransplant condition, to surgical complications, and to the complications of immunosuppression. Deaths from unpredictable causes, including lymphoproliferative disease and pulmonary complications, remain a problem.

▶ Few advanced techniques in surgery can match liver transplantation in children in the life years achieved. The transplant team from the University of Texas at Dallas reports a 10-year experience, which reveals the remarkable advances made in the field. As expected, biliary atresia tops the list of indications (45%), but the remaining diseases that required transplantation are equally disabling or lethal. An overall survival during the past 2 years of 87% is a remarkable achievement.

F.G. Moody, M.D.

38 Alcoholic Cirrhosis and Related Problems

Prediction of Risk of Liver Disease

Prediction of Risk of Liver Disease by Alcohol Intake, Sex, and Age: A Prospective Population Study

Becker U, Deis A, Sørensen TIA, et al (Univ of Copenhagen; Hvidovre Hosp, Denmark; Copenhagen Health Services)
Hepatology 23:1025–1029, 1996
5–24

Background.—The risk of alcohol-induced liver damage developing is known to increase with the amount of alcohol consumed, but the dose-effect relation has not been determined. A large population-based cohort was followed for 12 years to assess the association between self-reported current alcohol intake and the risk of future liver disease.

Patients and Methods.—The study population was drawn from The Copenhagen City Heart Study. Complete information was available for 13,285 individuals between 30 and 79 years of age who completed the

TABLE 1.—Alcohol Intake by Sex, Number of Incident Cases of Alcohol-induced Liver Disease, and Cirrhosis

			Alcohol-Induced Liver Disease		Alcohol-Induced Cirrhosis	
Alcohol Intake	Men *(n)*	Women *(n)*	Men *(n)*	Women *(n)*	Men *(n)*	Women *(n)*
Beverages per week (g alcohol per week)						
<1 (<12)	625	2,472	15	17	10	5
1–6 (12–72)	1,183	3,079	18	23	6	7
7–13 (84–156)	1,825	1,019	32	20	7	9
14–27 (168–324)	1,234	543	29	11	11	4
28–41 (336–492)	585	72	31	4	20	3
42–69 (504–828)	388	29	34	1	25	0
= 70 (= 840)	211	20	25	1	17	0
Total	6,051	7,234	184	77	96	28

(Courtesy of Becker U, Deis A, Sørensen TIA, et al: Prediction of risk of liver disease by alcohol intake, sex, and age: A prospective population study. *Hepatology* 23:1025 1029, 1996.)

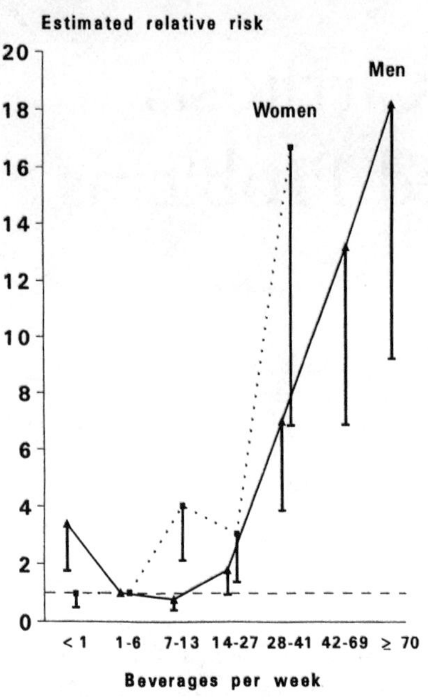

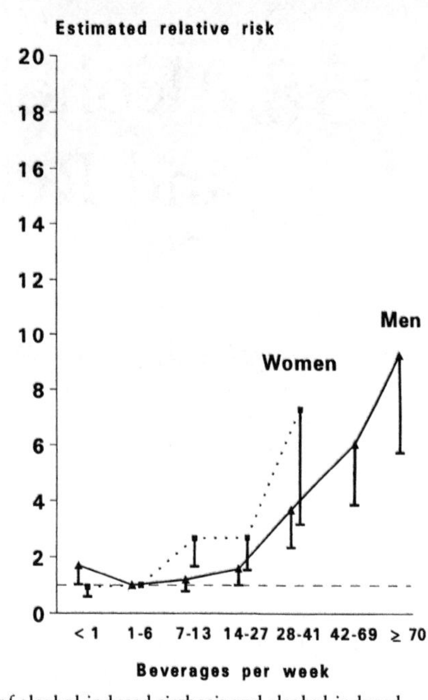

FIGURE 1.—Relative risk estimates for development of alcohol-induced cirrhosis and alcohol-induced liver disease as a function of the individual alcohol intake classified as <1 beverage (<12 g); 1–6 beverages (12–72 g); 7–13 beverages (84–156 g); 14–27 beverages (168–324 g); 28–41 beverages (336–492 g); 42–69 beverages (504–828 g); >70 beverages (>840 g). The group with an alcohol intake of 1–6 beverages (12–72 g) per week is the reference group (relative risk = 1). The *vertical lines* are estimated lower 95% confidence limits. (Courtesy of Becker U, Deis A, Sørensen TIA, et al: Prediction of risk of liver disease by alcohol intake, sex, and age: A prospective population study. *Hepatology* 23:1025–1029, 1996.)

alcohol intake questionnaire. Participants were asked to respond to multiple-choice questions concerning the frequency and type (beer, wine, or spirits) of alcohol consumption. After 12 years, register-based information was obtained on death or hospital discharge with a liver-related diagnosis suggestive of alcohol-induced liver disease. The risk function between alcohol intake and liver diseases was analyzed by multiplicative Poisson regression models.

Results.—There were 261 cases of alcohol-induced liver disease (184 men and 77 women), resulting in 98 deaths during the observation period. Alcohol-induced cirrhosis occurred in 96 men and 28 women, yielding incidence rates of 0.2% per year in men and 0.03% per year in women (Table 1). Risk for the development of cirrhosis and liver disease was lowest among those whose alcohol intake ranged from 1 to 6 beverages per week. Above this level, a steep dose-dependent increase in relative risk was observed (Fig 1). With an intake of 7–beverages per week for women and 14–27 beverages per week for men, the relative risk was higher than 1. For any given level of alcohol intake, the relative risk of developing alcohol-related liver disease and alcohol-induced cirrhosis was significantly higher for women than for men.

Conclusion.—Both men and women demonstrated a dose-dependent increase in the relative risk of developing alcohol-induced liver disease. Previous studies have indicated that women are more vulnerable to alcohol, and in this cohort the risk increased more steeply for women than for men with increasing alcohol intake.

▶ This carefully done study provides additional support for the concept that the likelihood of alcoholic liver disease developing is directly related to dose and duration of alcohol use. I think it is important for physicians to quantify a patient's alcohol intake in a manner similar to quantifying cigarette consumption. A simple and easy to use reference system is as follows: 1 oz of whiskey, gin, or vodka contains up to 10 or 11 g of alcohol, one 12-oz can of beer has 10 or 11 g of alcohol, and 4 oz of wine has 10 or 11 g. Thus if a patient drinks 6 bottles of beer per day, they are ingesting approximately 60–66 g of alcohol per day. One dose of alcohol in each of the above quantities is equivalent to one unit. More potent ales and beers may have as much as 12 g per bottle, so this number could rise to 72 g per day. Evidence exists to support the concept that more than 30 g of alcohol per day is capable of causing liver injury in women and more than 60 g of alcohol per day is capable of causing liver injury in men. Most authorities have suggested that alcohol consumption in quantities greater than 3 units per day or 21 units per week constitutes excessive consumption of alcohol.

That factors other than alcohol consumption are important in the development of alcoholic liver disease is clearly evident. One such factor is hepatitis C, which potentiates the likelihood of alcoholic liver disease developing. It would have been interesting if the study by Becker et al. had carried out additional studies to determine the proportion of their patients with alcohol-induced liver disease who actually were hepatitis C positive. Similar prospective studies should surely take this factor as well as other factors into consideration.

N.J. Greenberger, M.D.

Treatment of Alcoholic Hepatitis With Prednisone: Long-term Follow-up

Survival and Prognostic Factors in Patients With Severe Alcoholic Hepatitis Treated With Prednisolone
Mathurin P, Duchatelle V, Ramond MJ, et al (Hôpital Beaujon, Clichy, France; Hôpital Antoine Béclère, Clamart, France; CNRS URA, Paris)
Gastroenterology 110:1847–1853, 1996   5–25

Introduction.—Severe alcoholic hepatitis carries a high mortality rate. Although corticosteroid treatment can reduce short-term mortality, the independent prognostic factors are unknown. Prognostic factors and long-term survival were evaluated in patients with severe alcoholic hepatitis treated with corticosteroids.

TABLE 1.—Clinical and Biochemical Features

Characteristics	Randomized prednisolone group	Randomized placebo group	Prednisolone-open group
No. of patients	32	29	61
Age (*yr*)	48.3 ± 2.1	48.2 ± 1.6	49.5 ± 1.2
Sex (M/F)	10/22	9/20	28/33
Ascites (no. of patients)	24	25	43
Hepatic encephalopathy (no. of patients)	9	10	16
Serum bilirubin (*μmol/L*)	239.0 ± 34	222.6 ± 21	262.7 ± 19.6
Prothrombin time (% of normal)	42.1 ± 1.9	40.2 ± 3.1	40.9 ± 1.3
Serum albumin (*g/L*)	28.7 ± 1.1	26.3 ± 1.6	30.9 ± 0.8
Serum creatinine (*μmol/L*)	70.2 ± 4.9	88.3 ± 12.7	108.6 ± 15
White blood cells (*/mm^3*)	13,003 ± 1962	14,100 ± 1706	12,902 ± 946
Polymorphonuclear count (*/mm^3*)	10,441 ± 1885	12,659 ± 1558	10,721 ± 989
Discriminant function	42 ± 3	41 ± 3	46 ± 2

(Courtesy of Mathurin P, Duchatelle V, Ramond MJ, et al: Survival and prognostic factors in patients with severe alcoholic hepatitis treated with prednisolone. *Gastroenterology* 110:1847–1853, 1996.)

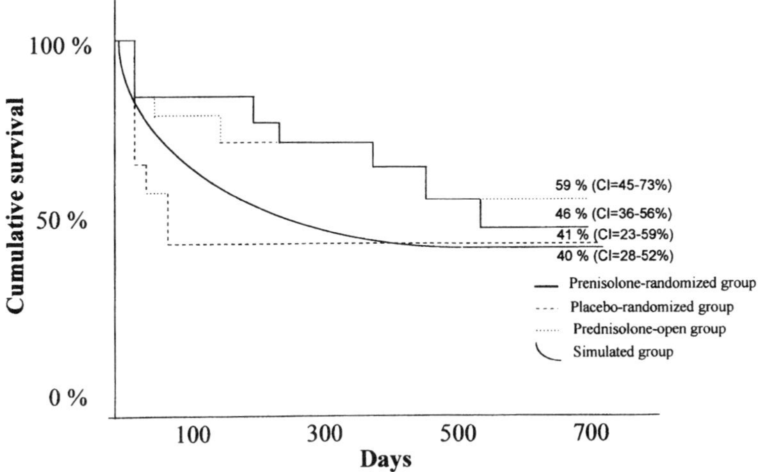

FIGURE 1.—Survival at 2 years in 32 prednisolone-randomized patients, 29 placebo-randomized patients, 61 prednisolone-open patients, and 61 simulated patients. (Courtesy of Mathurin P, Duchatelle V, Ramond MJ, et al: Survival and prognostic factors in patients with severe alcoholic hepatitis treated with prednisolone. *Gastroenterology* 110:1847–1853, 1996.)

Methods.—A total of 61 patients from a previous randomized trial were studied: 32 were treated with prednisolone (group 1) and 29 were untreated (group 2). Another 61 patients were treated openly with prednisolone after the end of the randomized trial (group 3) (Table 1). Also, a group of 61untreated controls were simulated using the Beclere model. Survival and independent prognostic factors were assessed.

Results.—One-year survival was 69% in group 1 and 71% in group 3, compared with 41% in group 2 and 50% in the simulated group 4. By 2 years, however, there were no significant differences in survival (Fig 1). One-year survival was 76% for prednisolone-treated patients with a marked liver polymorphonuclear infiltrate, compared with 53% of the other patients. Steroid-treated patients with polymorphonuclear counts of greater than 5,500/mm^3 also had better 1-year survival than other patients (77% vs. 40%). Both of these factors were independently correlated with 1-year survival in the prednisolone-treated patients (Table 1).

Conclusions.—In patients with severe alcoholic hepatitis, prednisolone therapy can improve survival rate for at least 1 year. There is no significant treatment effect after 1 year, suggesting that patients whose condition does not improve after 6–12 months of prednisolone therapy should be evaluated for liver transplantation. Among steroid-treated patients, liver polymorphonuclear infiltrate and polymorphonuclear count are independent prognostic factors.

▶ Several previous studies have shown that corticosteroid therapy significantly decreased *short-term* mortality in patients with severe alcoholic hepatitis. This effect was demonstrated in patients with hepatic encephalopathy and/or a clearly abnormal discriminant function value; the latter is based on the formula 4.6 × (patients' prothrombin time minus control prothrombin time) plus the serum bilirubin. A value greater than 32 is considered markedly abnormal.

Long-term survival of severe alcoholic hepatitis has not been studied extensively. The report by Mathurin et al. provides important new information on (1) long-term survival in severe alcoholic hepatitis; (2) factors associated with a favorable outcome; and (3) duration of effect of corticosteroid therapy after receipt of 40 mg of prednisolone for 1 month. From the graph in Figure 1, note that prednisolone clearly reduced mortality at the 1-year mark but that this effect disappears at 2 years. This finding prompted the authors to recommend that evaluation for liver transplantation should be undertaken between 6 and 12 months in patients with severe alcoholic hepatitis who did not improve after corticosteroid therapy.

Another interesting finding in this report is that patients with marked peripheral blood neutrophils and/or extensive polymorphonuclear infiltration in liver biopsy specimens were more likely to benefit from corticosteroid therapy.

N.J. Greenberger, M.D.

Prognostic Value of Hepatic Venous Pressure Gradient

Prognostic Value of Hepatic Venous Pressure Gradient Measurements in Alcoholic Cirrhosis: A 10-Year Prospective Study
Vorobioff J, Groszmann RJ, Picabea E, et al (Sanatorio Parque and Fundación Villavicencio, Rosario, Argentina; West Haven Veterans Affairs Med Ctr, Conn; Yale Univ, New Haven, Conn)
Gastroenterology 111:701–709, 1996   5–26

Objective.—Thirty patients with alcoholic cirrhosis and portal hypertension were studied to determine the prognostic value of sequential measurement of portal pressure. This parameter was measured in only 1 previous study of nonbleeding portal hypertensive cirrhotic patients.

Patients and Methods.—The patients were 23 men and 7 women with a mean age of 53 years. The diagnosis of cirrhosis was established by findings of liver biopsy and/or laparofibroscopy. At the time of the study, all patients had abstained from alcohol for at least 4 weeks. None had a history of variceal bleeding or hemorrhage, but all had esophageal varices. The severity of liver disease was graded according to Pugh's criteria. Portal pressure was determined by the hepatic venous pressure gradient (HVPG), which was obtained by subtracting the free hepatic venous pressure from the wedged hepatic venous pressure. The patients were urged to abstain from alcohol and were monitored for a mean period of 42 months. End points of the study were the first episode of upper gastrointestinal bleeding related to portal hypertension and/or death.

Results.—Seventeen patients died during the observation period. At the first follow-up (median, 10 months), the HVPG increased in 7 nonsurvivors, was unchanged in 4, and decreased in 6. Among survivors, the HVPG decreased in 10, was unchanged in 1, and increased in 2 (Fig 1). Upper

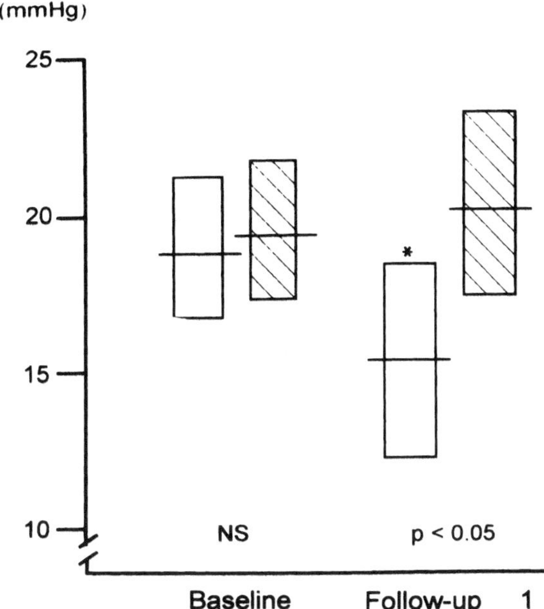

FIGURE 1.—Hepatic venous pressure gradient (*HVPG*) in survivors (*open bars*; n = 13) and non-survivors (*bars with diagonal lines*; n = 17). When compared with the baseline value and that in nonsurvivors, a significant reduction in HVPG (95% confidence intervals) was observed in survivors at follow-up 1 (median, 10 months). *P < 0.01 vs. baseline. (Courtesy of Vorobioff J, Groszmann RJ, Picabea E, et al: Prognostic value of hepatic venous pressure gradient measurements in alcoholic cirrhosis: A 10-year prospective study. *Gastroenterology* 111:701–709, 1996.)

gastrointestinal bleeding occurred in 10 patients during follow-up. When compared with bleeders, nonbleeders showed a significant reduction in HVPG at the initial follow-up (Fig 2). Sixteen of 21 patients who abstained from alcohol during the first follow-up period had a decrease in HVPG. In contrast, the HVPG increased in 8 of 9 nonabstainers. Decreases in HVPG were also associated with lower Pugh scores at follow-up and absence of ascites.

Conclusion.—Sequential measurements of portal pressure in nonbleeding patients with alcoholic cirrhosis offer prognostic information on the development of portal hypertensive–related bleeding and survival. On multivariate analysis, portal pressure at initial follow-up had the best prognostic and independent value for both bleeding and survival. Abstinence and early pharmacologic treatment may improve outcome.

▶ Measurement of the HVPG response to pharmacotherapy also provides useful prognostic information on the long-term risk of variceal bleeding. Feu et al.[1] prospectively investigated 69 cirrhotic patients receiving continuous propranolol therapy after an episode of variceal hemorrhage. The HVPG was measured before and after 3 months of drug therapy. A decrease in HVPG of 20% or greater accurately predicted the likelihood of rebleeding. The cumu-

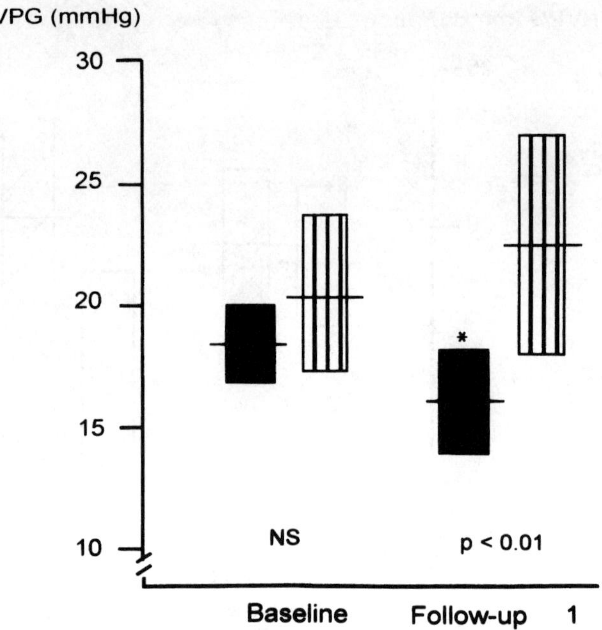

FIGURE 2.—Hepatic venous pressure gradient (*HVPG*) in nonbleeders (*solid bars*; n = 20) and bleeders (*bars with vertical lines*; n = 10). When compared with the baseline value and that in bleeders, a significant reduction in HVPG (*95% confidence intervals*) was observed in nonbleeders at follow-up 1 (median, 10 months). *P < 0.05 vs. baseline. (Courtesy of Vorobioff J, Groszmann RJ, Picabea E, et al: Prognostic value of hepatic venous pressure gradient measurements in alcoholic cirrhosis: A 10-year prospective study. *Gastroenterology* 111:701–709, 1996.)

lative probability of bleeding at 1, 2, and 3 years was 4%, 9%, and 9%, respectively, in patients with a decrease in HVPG of 20% or greater. Conversely, the risk of rebleeding was 28%, 39%, and 66% at the same time intervals in patients with a decrease in HVPG of 20% or greater.

N.J. Greenberger, M.D.

Reference

1. Feu F, Garcia-Pagan JC, Bosch J: Relation between partial pressure response to pharmacotherapy and risk of recurrent variceal hemorrhage in patients with cirrhosis. *Lancet* 346:1056–1059, 1995.

Portal Hypertension, Sclerotherapy, Transjugular Intrahepatic Portosystemic Shunts, Prophylactic Antibiotics with Bleeding

Nadolol Plus Isosorbide Mononitrate Compared With Sclerotherapy for the Prevention of Variceal Rebleeding

Villanueva C, Blanzó J, Novella MT, et al (Hosp de la Santa Creu i Sant Pau, Barcelona)
N Engl J Med 334:1624–1629, 1996
5–27

Introduction.—Patients who have had 1 episode of bleeding from esophageal varices need treatment to prevent further episodes of bleeding. Sclerotherapy is more effective in the prevention of rebleeding than β-blocker therapy; however, there is no difference in survival, and the rebleeding rate after sclerotherapy is still as high as 50%. The combination of isosorbide mononitrate and propranolol reduces portal pressure to a greater extent than propranolol alone. Sclerotherapy was compared with the combination of isosorbide mononitrate and nadolol for the prevention of rebleeding in patients with esophageal varices.

Methods.—Eighty-six cirrhotic patients with endoscopically diagnosed bleeding esophageal varices were studied. They were randomly assigned to receive either repeated endoscopic sclerotherapy or treatment with nadolol and isosorbide-5-mononitrate. Nadolol was given in an initial dose of 80

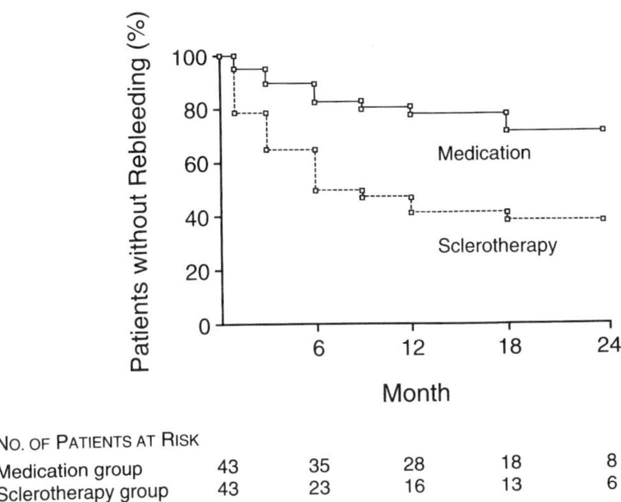

FIGURE 1.—Actuarial probability of remaining free of rebleeding in the medication and sclerotherapy groups. The probability of remaining free of rebleeding was significantly higher among the patients treated with nadolol plus isosorbide mononitrate than among those treated with sclerotherapy ($P = 0.001$). The difference was also significant when the 7 patients in the medication group who did not receive nadolol because of contraindications (in 3 patients) or complications (in 4) were not included in the analysis ($P = 0.003$). (Two of these 7 patients had rebleeding.) (Courtesy of Villanueva C, Blanzó J, Novella MT, et al: Nadolol plus isosorbide mononitrate compared with sclerotherapy for the prevention of variceal rebleeding. *N Engl J Med* 334:1624–1629. Copyright 1996, Massachusetts Medical Society. Reprinted by permission of *The New England Journal of Medicine*. All rights reserved.)

mg once daily, adjusted according to the resting heart rate. Oral isosorbide was then added, at a dose of up to 40 mg twice daily. Nadolol was chosen over propranolol because it permits once-daily dosing and is not metabolized by the liver. The 2 groups were compared for the primary outcomes of rebleeding, death, and complications. Baseline and 3-month hepatic venous pressure gradient measurements were performed in 31 patients in the isosorbide-nadolol group.

Results.—The 2 groups were comparable at baseline, and both were followed up for a median of 18 months. Rebleeding occurred in 23 patients in the sclerotherapy group vs. 11 in the isosorbide-nadolol group (Fig 1). Patients receiving isosorbide-nadolol had a greater actuarial probability of remaining free of all rebleeding episodes related to portal hypertension and variceal bleeding (Table 3). There were 9 deaths in the sclerotherapy group and 4 in the isosorbide-nadolol group, a nonsignificant difference. Sixteen patients had complications of sclerotherapy, whereas 7

TABLE 3.—Rebleeding in the Study Groups*

Variable	Medication Group (N = 43)	Sclerotherapy Group (N = 43)
Rebleeding (no. of patients)†	11	23
Site of rebleeding (no. of patients)		
Esophageal varices‡	9	22
Esophageal ulcer§	0	5
Portal hypertensive gastropathy¶	0	4
Gastric varices	1	2
Undetermined‖	2	3
Other**	1	1
No. of rebleeding episodes	16	48
No. of rebleeding episodes per patient††	0.3 ± 0.6	1.1 ± 1.2
Rebleeding index‡‡	15.5 ± 7.6	12.1 ± 9.7
Transfusions (units)††		
Mean	2.6	4.9
Median	2	4
Range	0–9	0–12
Treatment failure (no. of patients)§§	3	16
Hospital days¶¶	23 ± 13	31 ± 14
No. of hospital admissions not due to rebleeding	10	14

*Plus-minus values are means ± SD. The mean dose of nadolol was 110 ± 70 mg per day, and the mean dose of isosorbide mononitrate was 70 ± 18 mg per day. The mean number of sclerotherapy sessions performed was 5 ± 1.6.

†$P = 0.001$, by the log-rank test, for the comparison between the groups. In the medication group, 1 additional patient had rebleeding from a peptic ulcer. If this patient is included, the P value is 0.002.

‡$P = 0.002$, by the log-rank test, for the comparison between the groups. In the medication group, 9 patients had 12 rebleeding episodes from esophageal varices. In the sclerotherapy group, 22 patients had 33 rebleeding episodes from esophageal varices.

§$P = 0.02$, by the log-rank test, for the comparison between the groups.

¶$P = 0.03$, by the log-rank test, for the comparison between the groups.

‖Three patients had more than 1 potential bleeding site at endoscopy, and 2 patients (both in the sclerotherapy group) did not undergo endoscopy.

**One patient in the medication group had reflux esophagitis, and 1 patient in the sclerotherapy group had rectal varices.

††$P = 0.001$ for the comparison between the groups.

‡‡The rebleeding index was calculated by dividing the months of follow-up by the number of rebleeding episodes plus 1. This index reflects the time free of rebleeding during follow-up. $P = 0.025$ for the comparison between the groups.

§§$P < 0.001$, by the log-rank test, for the comparison between the groups.

¶¶$P = 0.02$ for the comparison between the groups.

(Courtesy of Villanueva C, Blanzó J, Novella MT, et al: Nadolol plus isosorbide mononitrate compared with sclerotherapy for the prevention of variceale bleeding. *N Engl J Med* 334:1624–1629. Copyright 1996, Massachusetts Medical Society. Reprinted by permission of *The New England Journal of Medicine*. All rights reserved.)

had complications of isosorbide-nadolol therapy. Thirteen of 31 patients in the isosorbide-nadolol group had more than a 20% decline in the hepatic venous pressure gradient, and just 1 of these patients had rebleeding. In contrast, 8 of 18 patients with smaller decreases in the pressure gradient had episodes of rebleeding.

Conclusions.—For patients with esophageal varices, the combination of isosorbide mononitrate and nadolol is more effective than sclerotherapy in preventing episodes of rebleeding. The complication rate is lower with isosorbide-nadolol, and survival may tend to be better as well. The isosorbide-nadolol combination improves many factors related to rebleeding.

▶ Patients who have bled from esophageal varices are at high risk for further bleeding and death. Although several effective modes of therapy are available to reduce the risk of rebleeding (endoscopic sclerotherapy, endoscopic band ligation, β-blockers, transjugular intrahepatic portosystemic shunts), the search continues for therapy that will not only further decrease the risk of rebleeding, but also enhance survival.

The study by Villanueva et al. indicates that after an acute episode of variceal bleeding has been controlled, therapy with nadolol plus isosorbide mononitrate has substantial advantages over injection sclerotherapy. Rebleeding was significantly less common with combined medication therapy. Importantly, there was also a trend toward improved survival, although the difference between the groups did not reach statistical significance ($P = 0.07$).

A relevant recent study by Feh et al.[1] suggests that measurement of the hepatic venous pressure gradient response to pharmacotherapy will provide useful prognostic information on the long-term risk of variceal rebleeding. In 69 cirrhotic patients receiving propranolol therapy after an episode of variceal bleeding, the hepatitic venous pressure gradient (HVPG) was measured before and after 3 months of β-blocker therapy. In 25 patients in whom the HVPG had fallen 20% or more, only 2 rebled. By contrast, rebleeding occurred in 23 of 44 patients in whom the HVPG fell less than 20%; in 8 patients in whom the HVPG fell to 12 mm Hg or less, none rebled. These data help explain the variable outcomes in cirrhotic patients being maintained on β-blockers to prevent variceal rebleeding. These findings are applicable to the study by Villanueva et al. in that the HVPG fell an average of 16% in the nadolol-isosorbide group but actually increased by 6% in the sclerotherapy group. This could explain the difference in the rebleeding rate.

N.J. Greenberger, M.D.

Reference

1. Feh F, Garcia-Pagan JC, Bush J, et al: Relation between portal pressure response to pharmacotherapy and risk of recurrent variceal hemorrhage in patients with cirrhosis. *Lancet* 346:1056–1059, 1995.

Transjugular Intrahepatic Portosystemic Shunts for Patients With Active Variceal Hemorrhage Unresponsive to Sclerotherapy

Sanyal AJ, Freedman AM, Luketic VA, et al (Virginia Commonwealth Univ, Richmond; Carolinas Med Ctr, Charlotte, NC)
Gastroenterology 111:138–146, 1996

5–28

Background.—The generally acknowledged initial treatment of choice for active hemorrhage from esophageal varices is endoscopic sclerotherapy. However, patients at greatest risk of nonresponse to emergent sclerotherapy are also those least likely to tolerate more invasive therapy. Such patients may be treated with surgical portal decompression or portosystemic venous disconnection at the gastroesophageal junction, but those with tense ascites, renal failure, severe encephalopathy, active sepsis, or aspiration pneumonia may have a mortality rate of 70% to 90%. The efficacy and safety of transjugular intrahepatic portosystemic shunt (TIPS), performed semiurgently after initial stabilization of patients with active bleeding despite emergent sclerotherapy, was prospectively evaluated.

Methods.—Participating were 30 patients with actively bleeding esophageal or contiguous gastric varices despite sclerotherapy who were considered at high risk of dying if treated with emergent portocaval shunt. These patients were stabilized via balloon tamponade and vasopressin/nitroglycerin. Within 12 hours, patients underwent TIPS, in which portal decompression was achieved by creating a parenchymal tract between the hepatic vein and the intrahepatic portion of the portal vein; patency is maintained via an expandable metal stent and angiographic techniques.

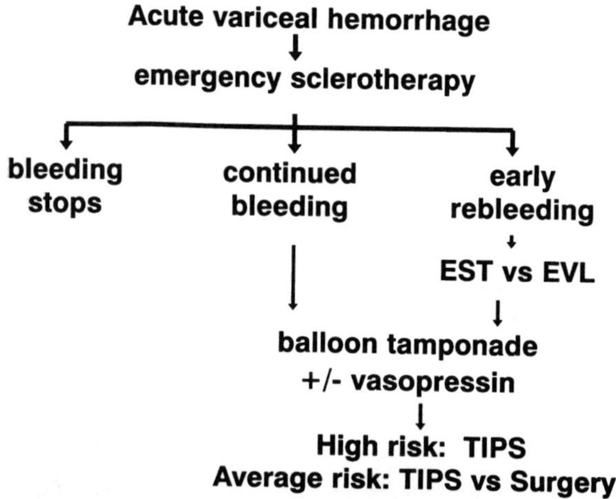

FIGURE 4.—An algorithm for the management of active variceal hemorrhage. *Abbreviations: EST,* endoscopic sclerotherapy; *EVL,* endoscopic variceal ligation; *TIPS,* transjugular intrahepatic portosystemic shunt. (Courtesy of Sanyal AJ, Freedman AM, Luketic VA, et al: Transjugular intrahepatic portosystemic shunts for patients with active variceal hemorrhage unresponsive to sclerotherapy. *Gastroenterology* 111:138–146, 1996.)

Within 24 hours after TIPS, balloon tamponade and vasopressin/nitroglycerin were discontinued.

Results.—Hemostasis was accomplished in 29 of the 30 patients in whom TIPS could be successfully placed. The survival rate was 63% after 30 days and 60% after 6 weeks; patients without aspiration had a 6-week survival rate of 90%. Of the original cohort, 46% were alive after a median follow-up of 920 days. Encephalopathy developed in 8 patients, early rebleeding in 2, and late rebleeding in 4. Within 6 months, 6 of 11 patients had stent stenosis requiring dilation.

Conclusion.—These data show that TIPS is a highly effective salvage technique for high-risk patients with active variceal hemorrhage after endoscopic sclerotherapy. An algorithm for the management of active variceal hemorrhage is given (Fig 4).

▶ Endoscopic sclerotherapy (EST) achieves initial hemostasis in 80% to 90% of cases and decreases the risk of early rebleeding. However, EST may fail in elderly patients with advanced liver failure, ascites, and encephalopathy and in patients with large, actively spurting varices. The authors have carried out an important study to determine the efficacy and safety of TIPS in patients with varices bleeding actively despite emergent EST. The results are impressive. TIPS was successfully placed in 29 of 30 patients and achieved hemostasis in all. Importantly, the 6-week survival rate was 60% and after a median follow-up of 920 days, 46% of the original 30 patients were alive. Thus, in this select group of patients hemorrhaging actively and at very high risk of dying, TIPS was highly successful as a salvage technique. The authors also provide a useful algorithm for managing acute variceal hemorrhage (see Fig 4).

N.J. Greenberger, M.D.

Systemic Antibiotic Prophylaxis After Gastrointestinal Hemorrhage in Cirrhotic Patients With a High Risk of Infection

Pauwels A, Mostefa-Kara N, Debenes B, et al (Hôpital Saint Antoine, Paris)
Hepatology 24:802–806, 1996
5–29

Background.—Bacterial infection is common in patients with gastrointestinal hemorrhage, and is most commonly caused by enteric bacteria. Intestinal decontamination may be effective prophylactic treatment. Disadvantages of intestinal decontamination include difficulty in administering oral antibiotics to patients with active bleeding, infections caused by bacteria other than Gram-negative bacilli in up to 50% of cases, and a risk of infection that varies from patient to patient. Patients with a Child-Pugh's class C or rebleeding have a high risk of infection. That patients who have a Child-Pugh's class C or rebleeding have a high rate of infection was confirmed, and the effectiveness of antibiotic prophylaxis for bleeding in patients with cirrhosis and gastrointestinal hemorrhage was evaluated.

TABLE 3.—Incidence and Types of Bacterial Infections in the 3 Groups of Patients

	Group 1 (n = 55)		Group 2 (n = 34)		Group 3 (n = 30)
Patients with infections	10(18.2)‡	*	18(52.9)‡	*	4(13.3)‡
Proved infections	8		16		2
Bacteremia	3		13		2
SBP	4		7		1
Respiratory	1		3		0
Urinary	2		2		0
Meningitis	0		1		0
Possible infections	2		2		2
Patients with sepsis syndrome or septic shock	2(3.6)	*	12(35.3)	†	2(6.6)

*$P < 0.001$.
†$P < 0.01$.
‡Values in parentheses are percentages.
Abbreviation: SBP, spontaneous bacterial peritonitis.
(Courtesy of Pauwels A, Mostefa-Kara N, Debenes B, et al: Systemic antibiotic prophylaxis after gastrointestinal hemorrhage in cirrhotic patients with a high risk of infection. *Hepatology* 24:802–806, 1996.)

Methods.—There were 119 patients with cirrhosis and gastrointestinal hemorrhage who were divided into 3 groups. Group 1 consisted of 55 patients with a low risk of infection: a Child-Pugh's class A or B and no rebleeding. Group 2 consisted of 34 patients with a high risk of infection who served as controls. Group 3 consisted of 30 patients who received ciprofloxacin and a combination of amoxicillin and clavulanic acid for 3 days after hemorrhage.

Results.—Patients in group 2 had a significantly higher risk of bacterial infections and more serious infections than patients in group 1 (Table 3). Sepsis or septic shock occurred in 66.7% of patients with infection in group 2, but in only 20% of patients with infection in group 1. Patients in group 3 had a much lower risk of bacterial infection than patients in group 2. In the first 4 weeks, 8 patients from group 2 and 4 patients from group 3 died (Table 4). Three patients in group 2 and 1 patient in group 3 died

TABLE 4.—Mortality at 4 Weeks, Length of Stay in ICU, and Antibiotic Costs in the 3 Groups of Patients

	Group 1 (n = 55)		Group 2 (n = 34)		Group 3 (n = 30)
Mortality at 4 wk	5(9.1)*		8(23.5)		4(13.3)
Hemorrhage	4		1		2
Septic shock	1		3		1
Liver failure	0		4		1
Length of stay in ICU (d)	3.4 ± 0.3	‡	7.4 ± 1.1		6.5
Antibiotic costs (US$)	38 ± 16	‡	208 ± 63	†	167

Note: Other comparisons between groups 1 and 2, and between groups 2 and 3 were not statistically significant.
*Values in parentheses are percentages.
†$P < 0.05$.
‡$P < 0.001$.
(Courtesy of Pauwels A, Mostefa-Kara N, Debenes B, et al: Systemic antibiotic prophylaxis after gastrointestinal hemorrhage in cirrhotic patients with a high risk of infection. *Hepatology* 24:802–806, 1996.)

of septic shock. Diarrhea was the only adverse effect seen in patients given antibiotic prophylaxis. Antibiotic therapy cost $208 per patient in group 2 and $167 per patient in group 3.

Conclusions.—Patients with cirrhosis and a Child-Pugh's class C or rebleeding have a high risk of infection after gastrointestinal hemorrhage. Systemic antibiotic prophylaxis can prevent bacterial infections in these patients.

▶ Bacterial infections occur frequently in patients with cirrhosis and gastrointestinal bleeding, and such infections are not only intestinal but also respiratory and cutaneous in relation to invasive and inhalation procedures. This important study by Pauwels et al. provides useful guidelines for identification (and treatment) of bleeding patients with cirrhosis and the highest risk of infection. Infection occurred in 18.2% of patients with bleeding cirrhosis classified as Childs-Pugh class A or B (see below). By contrast, infection developed in a striking 52.9% of patients classified as Childs B or C. Treatment with either ciprofloxacin or amoxicillin plus clavulanic acid resulted in a sharply reduced infection rate (13.3%) in a group of predominately Childs-Pugh class C patients (see table below). The authors conclude that Childs-Pugh class C cirrhotic patients with gastrointestinal bleeding are at high risk of infection and prophylactic treatment with systemic antibiotics is very effective in preventing such infections.

TABLE.—Childs-Pugh Classifications of Cirrhosis

	A	B	C
Serum bilirubin mg/dL	< 2.0	2.0–3.0	> 3.0
Serum albumin gm/dL	> 3.5	2.8–3.5	< 2.8
Prothrombin time seconds	Prolonged < 4	Prolonged 4–6	Prolonged > 6
Ascites	Absent	Present in past	Present
Portal systemic encephalopathy	Absent	Present in past	Present

N.J. Greenberger, M.D.

Hepatopulmonary Syndrome

Hepatopulmonary Syndrome With Progressive Hypoxemia as an Indication for Liver Transplantation: Case Reports and Literature Review
Krowka MJ, Porayko MK, Plevak DJ, et al (Mayo Clinic Rochester, Minn; Methodist Hosp, Indianapolis)
Mayo Clin Proc 72:44–53, 1997
5–30

Background.—Hepatopulmonary syndrome (HPS) is a pulmonary vascular complication of liver disease. In patients with HPS, severe hypoxemia from pulmonary vascular dilatation can be very debilitating. Deciding whether liver transplantation should be performed in patients with advanced liver disease and HPS is difficult. Three patients with progressive

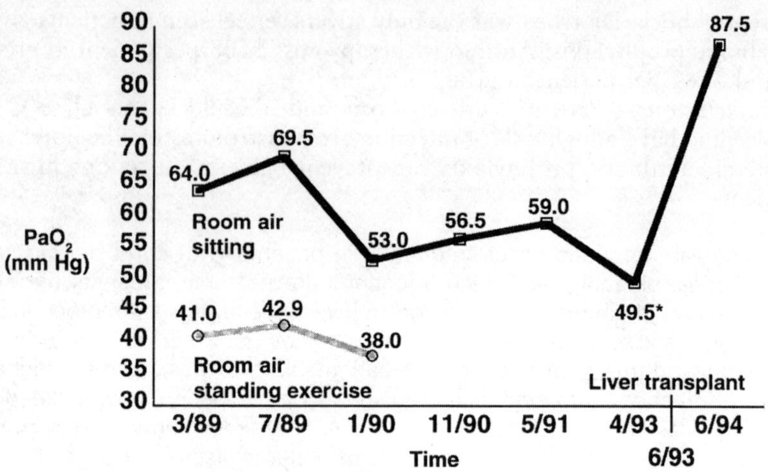

FIGURE 1.—*Case 1*. Diagram showing 4-year progressive deterioration in oxygenation. Liver transplantation resulted in normalization of arterial oxygen tension (PaO₂) while the patient was breathing room air. (Courtesy of Krowka MJ, Porayko MK, Plevak DJ, et al: Hepatopulmonary syndrome with progressive hypoxemia as an indication for liver transplantation: Case reports and literature review. *Mayo Clin Proc* 72:44–53, 1997.)

and severe hypoxemia who had successful liver transplantation and resolution of arterial hypoxemia were described, and the literature was reviewed.

Patients and Outcomes.—The patients were 3 women, aged 23, 28, and 47 years. The severity of HPS was considered an indication for liver transplantation. Hypoxemia was a major factor in recommending liver transplantation because of concerns about the patients' ability to survive the procedure and postoperative course given their deteriorating pulmonary status. The first patient had a period of clinically stable hepatic dysfunction followed by a fairly rapid decrease in synthetic function and quality of life during at least 4 months before liver transplantation (Fig 1). This surgery was recommended because of hepatic dysfunction and deteriorating arterial oxygenation from HPS. Liver transplantation was recommended to the second patient mainly because of debilitating, severe hypoxemia necessitating increasing amounts of supplemental oxygen 24 hours a day with stable hepatic abnormality. Adult respiratory distress syndrome complicated HPS in this patient, but she recovered and subsequently underwent a successful liver transplantation. In the third patient, severity of hypoxemia from HPS was the main reason for transplantation. The degree of hepatic dysfunction appeared minimal clinically. Oxygenation was normal in this patient 4 months after transplantation.

Literature Review.—Eighty-one children and adults with HPS undergoing liver transplantation have been reported in the literature. The post-transplantation mortality rate was 16% and was associated with the severity of hypoxemia. The death rate was significantly higher (30%) among those with a pretransplantation PaO₂ of 50 mm Hg or lower compared with those with a PaO₂ of more than 50 mm Hg.

Conclusions.—In many patients, HPS appears to be reversible after liver transplantation. Progressive hypoxemia may be an indication for liver transplantation. The criteria for patient selection for children and adults may differ. The long-term outcomes of liver transplantation and HPS resolution have yet to be established.

▶ The HPS is defined by 3 criteria: (1) chronic liver disease; (2) intrapulmonary vascular dilatation with shunts; and (3) arterial hypoxemia, which may worsen with increased activity. Pulmonary angiography may reveal diffuse or discrete vascular lesions. This report from the Mayo Clinic provides a detailed literature review of 73 patients with HPS who underwent liver transplantation. A key finding is that patients with a pretransplantation PaO_2 of 50 mm Hg or lower had significantly greater mortality (30%) compared with patients with a PaO_2 of greater than 50 mm Hg (4%). The Mayo Clinic investigators have developed guidelines and now recommend that patients who are candidates for liver transplantation be tested for their response to 100% oxygen. Any patient with a PaO_2 of less than 150 mm Hg while breathing 100% oxygen should undergo pulmonary angiography to determine whether discrete arteriovenous communications are present that could be amenable to embolization therapy.

Kuo and colleagues[1] evaluated several preoperative screening modalities for portopulmonary hypertension, including EKG, chest x-ray, transthoracic echocardiography, and room air arterial blood gases in 50 orthotopic liver transplant candidates. Respiratory alkalosis as evidenced by a PCO_2 of less than 30 mm Hg had excellent sensitivity, specificity, and positive predictive value in identifying patients with portopulmonary hypertension. The mean pulmonary artery pressure in the patients with portopulmonary hypertension was 50.9 ± 3.9 (± 1 SD) mm Hg.

Martinez and associates[2] described 4 patients with portopulmonary hypertension who underwent liver transplantation, 3 of whom died within 1 week. All 4 had pulmonary artery pressures greater than 50 mm Hg (50, 52, 75, and 88 mm Hg). None of the 4 patients responded to vasodilator therapy, including calcium channel blockers, nitroglycerin, prostaglandin, or nitrous oxide, that altered the fixed nature of the pulmonary vascular lesions.

N.J. Greenberger, M.D.

References

1. Kuo PC, Plotken JS, Whiting JF, et al: A multicenter analysis of portopulmonary hypertension: What are the predictive capacities of screening modalities? *Hepatology* 24:429A, 1996.
2. Martinez EJ, Wright RK, Schiff ER, et al: Portopulmonary hypertension and liver transplantation: Why we fail. *Hepatology* 24:184A, 1996.

39 Primary Biliary Cirrhosis

Natural History of Early Primary Biliary Cirrhosis
Metcalf JV, Mitchison HC, Palmer JM, et al (Univ of Newcastle, Newcastle Upon Tyne,England; City Hosps Sunderland NHS Trust, England)
Lancet 348:1399–1402, 1996   5–31

Introduction.—Some patients who are positive for antimitochondrial antibody (AMA), the disease-specific marker for primary biliary cirrhosis (PBC), may initially have normal liver function test results and no liver-related symptoms. A group of 29 such patients were monitored long-term to determine their prognosis and the expected progression of the disease. Previous studies suggest that once symptoms develop, these patients have an outlook similar to that of patients with symptomatic PBC.

Methods.—The patients were identified through an antibody screen or were found to have positive AMA tests during investigations for other diseases. They were assessed yearly at a PBC clinic, and full clinical, biochemical, immunologic, and liver histologic data were reviewed. All surviving patients were interviewed; information on causes of death was sought for the 5 patients who died during follow-up. Initial and follow-up serum samples were tested by enzyme-linked immunosorbent assay for E2 components of the pyruvate dehydrogenase complex and the 2-oxoglutarate dehydrogenase complex.

Results.—None of the deaths during follow-up resulted from liver disease. Median follow-up for the 24 surviving patients was 17.8 years; their median age at the last review was 67. Symptoms of PBC (including pruritus, persistent fatigue, and persistent pain in the right upper quadrant) developed in 22 patients (Table 2), including 2 of the 5 who died. Persistently abnormal liver function had developed in 24 patients. The median time from the first positive AMA test to persistently raised serum alkaline phosphatase values was 5.6 years. Ten patients had repeat liver biopsy samples available; PBC had progressed from Scheuer grade 1 to grade 2 in 2 of these patients and from grade 1 to grade 3 in 2 others. In 9 cases, the initial and follow-up samples were diagnostic of or compatible with PBC; in 1 patient, both biopsy samples were normal despite some positive laboratory findings (Table 1). Enzyme-linked immunosor-

TABLE 2.—Clinical and Laboratory Data

Patient	Pruritis	Fatigue	Pain in Right Upper Quadrant	Serum Alkaline Phosphatase (IU/L)	Serum alanine aminotransferase (IU/L)	Serum Billrubin (μmol/L)	Serum Albumin (g/L)
1	−	++	−	82	17	5	48
2	−	−	−	223	36	6	43
3	+++	++	−	177	32	5	44
4	−	−	−	101	16	5	41
5	++	+++	−	90	35	8	12
6	−	−	−	141	87	2	38
7	+++	++	−	570	76	12	39
8	+++	−	−	1,072	107	13	34
9	+	−	−	197	22	7	39
10	++	+++	−	101	16	8	38
11	−	−	−	390	73	39	30
12	−	++	−	220	15	8	42
13	++	++	−	129	11	8	43
14	++	+	−	326	53	8	45
15	++	+	−	116	21	7	42
16	++	++	++	123	19	9	40
17	−	−	−	288	50	15	35
18	++	−	−	122	11	6	44
19	−	++	−	105	8	6	39
20	−	++	−	110	27	8	45
21	++	++	−	174	20	10	39
22	++	++	++	114	20	8	46
23	−	++	−	108	25	6	38
24	+++	−	++	97	33	15	44
25	++	+	−	129	25	2	42
26	−	−	−	96	9	6	43
27	−	++	−	139	50	10	43
28	+++	+	−	70	33	5	43
29	++	+	−	99	13	6	45

Normal ranges: serum alkaline phosphatase, 40–95 IU/L; serum alanine aminotransferase, 0–35 IU/L; serum bilirubin, 1–17 μmol/L; serum albumin, 35–50 g/L.

(Courtesy of Metcalf JV, Mitchison HC, Palmer JM, et al: Natural history of early primary biliary cirrhosis. *Lancet* 348:1399–1402, 1996, copyright by *The Lancet* Ltd.)

bent assay of baseline serum samples from 27 patients was positive in 21, all of whom had a first biopsy sample compatible with or diagnostic of PBC.

Discussion.—Individuals who are repeatedly positive for AMA but who have normal liver biochemistry and are asymptomatic do have very early PBC. In most cases the disease will slowly progress to classic PBC. Such patients need to be monitored, but potentially toxic treatment may not be advisable.

► This study provides new information about the early natural history of PBC. Furthermore, it confirms the hypothesis that asymptomatic individuals

TABLE 1.—Follow-up Data

Patient	Age at Follow-up	Date of First Abnormality			ELISA	Liver Histology for PBC	
		AMA	Symptom	Abnormal LFT		First Sample	Repeat Sample
1	78*	1977	1981	NA	+	Compatible	Compatible
2	72*	1976	NA	1977	+	Compatible	Diagnostic
3	40	1978	1995	NA	+	Compatible	ND
4	75*	1975	NA	1981	NA	Diagnostic	ND
5	67	1977	1986	NA	+	Diagnostic	ND
6	72	1976	NA	1995	−	Non-specific hepatitis	ND
7	71	1978	1979	1979	+	Diagnostic	ND
8	67	1978	1978	1995	+	Compatible	ND
9	84*	1975	1977	1980	+	Compatible	ND
10	83	1972	1985	1979	−	Non-specific hepatitis	ND
11	82*	1977	NA	1979	+	Diagnostic	Compatible
12	68	1977	1978	1977	+	Diagnostic	ND
13	69	1972	1989	1979	+	Diagnostic	Diagnostic
14	70	1975	1991	1977	+	Diagnostic	ND
15	48	1977	1979	1980	+	Diagnostic	Compatible
16	74	1979	1985	1980	+	Compatible	ND
17	81	1983	1984	1984	NA	Diagnostic	ND
18	77	1981	1990	1984	−	Granulomatous hepatitis	ND
19	62	1981	1983	1995	+	Compatible	ND
20	60	1981	1993	1995	−	Normal	ND
21	64	1982	1984	1984	+	Diagnostic	Diagnostic
22	79	1981	1981	1984	−	Compatible	ND
23	74	1981	1984	1987	+	Compatible	ND
24	49	1984	1987	1995	+	Compatible	Diagnostic
25	61	1982	1982	1985	+	Compatible	Diagnostic
26	60	1982	1984	1991	+	Compatible	ND
27	58	1983	NA	1986	+	Diagnostic	Compatible
28	37	1982	1983	NA	+	Diagnostic	Diagnostic
29	60	1984	1995	1994	−	Normal	

Note: Patients are numbered as in the original study.

*Died.

Abbreviations: AMA, antimitochrondrial antibody; *LFT,* liver function test; *ELISA*, enzyme-linked immunosorbent assay; *PBC*, primary biliary cirrhosis; *NA*, not available; *ND*, not done because not clinically indicated.

(Courtesy of Metcalf JV, Mitchison HC, Palmer JM, et al: Natural history of early primary biliary cirrhosis. *Lancet* 348:1399–1402, 1996, copyright by *The Lancet* Ltd.)

with repeatedly positive tests for antimitochondrial antibody but otherwise normal liver tests do have early PBC that will progress to classic PBC in most cases. However, such patients with neither signs nor symptoms of PBC appear to have much slower progression of the disease than previously reported. The only laboratory measures of prognostic value, i.e., the serum bilirubin, serum albumin, and prothrombin time values, are usually normal in asymptomatic individuals.

For an excellent recent review article on PBC see the paper by Kaplan.[1] For a detailed commentary on the efficacy of ursodeoxycholic acid see the editorial by Lim et al.[2]

N.J. Greenberger, M.D.

References

1. Kaplan MM: Preliminary biliary cirrhosis. *N Engl J Med* 335:1570–1580, 1996.
2. Lim AG, Jazrawi RP, Northfold TC: The ursodeoxycholic acid story in primary biliary cirrhosis. *Gut* 37:301–309, 1995.

40 Hemochromatosis

Long-term Survival in Patients With Hereditary Hemochromatosis
Niederau C, Fischer R, Pürschel A, et al (Heinrich-Heine-Universität Düsseldorf, Germany; Heinz Kalk-Klinik, Bad Kissingen, Germany)
Gastroenterology 110:1107–1119, 1996   5–32

Objective.—A cohort of 251 patients with hereditary hemochromatosis was monitored for a mean of 14.1 years to evaluate the impact of early diagnosis and treatment on the course of disease and on survival. Various factors that might influence outcome were also analyzed.

Methods.—Patients were identified by a review of the records of 2 hospitals for the period 1947–1991. All had clinical, biochemical, and histologic evidence of hereditary hemochromatosis. From 1979 on, a prospective protocol for diagnostic workups and therapeutic procedures was followed. The protocol included liver biopsy, repeated phlebotomies, and another biopsy to confirm iron depletion. At study entry, 109 patients did not have cirrhosis; 62% of these patients had symptoms vs. 95.1% of the 142 cirrhotic patients. Follow-up data were obtained by questionnaires sent to patients and their physicians. Two patients were lost to follow-up, and 69 died during the study. The observed survival curve of the patients with hemochromatosis was compared with their expected survival curve. In addition, various subgroups of patients were compared with each other.

Results.—The mean patient age at study entry was 45.7 years; 89.2% were men, 56.6% had liver cirrhosis, and 47.8% had diabetes mellitus. The cumulative survival rate was 93% at 5 years, 77% at 10 years, 62% at 15 years, 55% at 20 years, 46% at 25 years, and 20% at 30 years. These rates were significantly lower than the expected survival rates in a normal matched population. Patients who were noncirrhotic and without diabetes at the time of diagnosis, however, had survival equivalent to that expected. Multivariate analysis found neither arthritis nor sex and age at diagnosis to have significant prognostic value. Liver biopsies confirmed iron depletion in 185 patients. These patients had received a mean of 84.8 phlebotomies before iron depletion was achieved. More severe iron overload was associated with reduced survival. Cumulative survival increased over the years (Fig 6) as hereditary hemochromatosis without symptoms or cirrhosis was diagnosed in more patients early in the course of disease (Fig 7). Deaths caused by liver cancer were 119 times more frequent than expected, and deaths caused by both cardiomyopathy and diabetes were 14

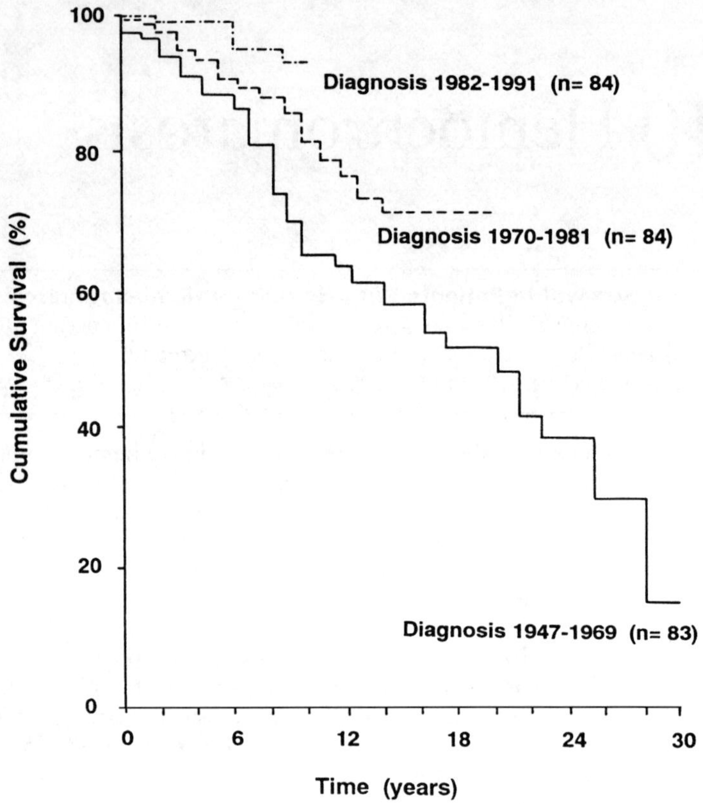

FIGURE 6.—Cumulative survival in 3 subgroups of patients in whom hereditary hemochromatosis was diagnosed in 3 different time periods: patients in whom hereditary hemochromatosis was diagnosed between 1947 and 1969 ($n = 83$) had reduced survival when compared with patients in whom hereditary hemochromatosis was diagnosed between 1970 and 1981 ($n = 84$), and patients in whom hereditary hemochromatosis was diagnosed between 1982 and 1991 had better survival than did the subgroups with earlier diagnosis of hemochromatosis (log-rank test; $P \leq 0.05$). (Courtesy of Niederau C, Fischer R, Pürschel A, et al: Long-term survival in patients with hereditary hemochromatosis. *Gastroenterology* 110:1107–1119, 1996.)

times more frequent than expected in a normal matched population. Liver cancers were associated with the presence of cirrhosis and the amount of mobilizable iron, but not with hepatitis B or C markers.

Conclusion.—The amount and duration of iron excess determine complications and prognosis in patients with hereditary hemochromatosis. Early diagnosis and removal of excess iron can result in normal life expectancy and prevent many complications of the disease.

▶ I selected this paper because it contains a wealth of information on the natural history of hemochromatosis and it underscores the importance of early diagnosis and therapeutic intervention. The data obtained indicate that prognosis and complications of hemochromatosis, probably including the

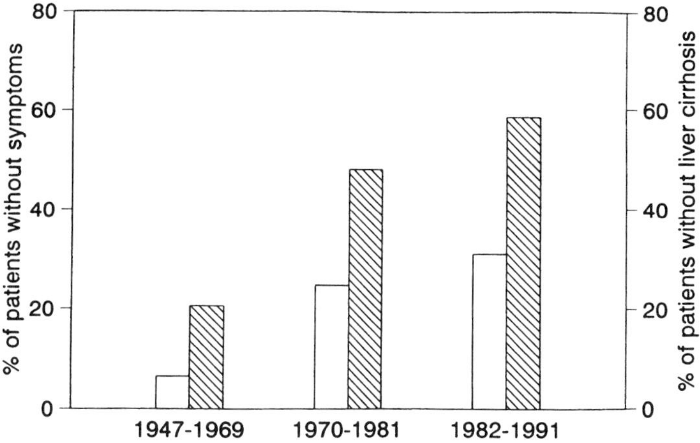

FIGURE 7.—Early diagnoses in 251 patients with hemochromatosis, defined as either absence of symptoms or absence of liver cirrhosis at the time of diagnosis. Data are shown as the percentage of asymptomatic and noncirrhotic patients in whom hereditary hemochromatosis was diagnosed in 3 different time periods as indicated in the figure. *Open bars*, no symptoms; *shaded bars*, no cirrhosis. (Courtesy of Niederau C, Fischer R, Pürschel A, et al: Long-term survival in patients with hereditary hemochromatosis. *Gastroenterology* 110:1107–1119, 1996.)

development of liver cancer, depend on the amount of iron excess and the point at which iron accumulation is interrupted by phlebotomy.

The clinical distinction between patients with hereditary hemochromatosis and those with alcoholic hepatic siderosis continues to be a diagnostic problem. Clinical parameters helpful in distinguishing the 2 disorders include hepatic iron concentration, hepatic iron index, and family studies using HLA typing. An interesting recent study[1] has re-examined the prevalence of alcohol use in hereditary hemochromatosis by using the aforementioned criteria. The main finding is that heavy consumption of alcohol (>80 g ethanol per day) was found in only 15% of 105 homozygous hemochromatosis patients.

N.J. Greenberger, M.D.

Reference

1. Adam PC, Agnew S: Alcoholism in hereditary hemochromatosis revisited. Prevalence and clinical consequences among homozygous siblings. *Hepatology* 23:724–727, 1996.

41 Pyogenic Hepatic Abscess

Pyogenic Liver Abscess: Changes in Etiology, Management, and Outcome
Seeto RK, Rockey DC (San Francisco Gen Hosp; Univ of California, San Francisco)
Medicine 75:99–113, 1996   5-33

Background.—Pyogenic liver abscess (PLA), a potentially life-threatening disorder with a changing clinical spectrum, may be more common than appreciated. Changes in presentation, management, and outcomes of PLA were documented in 1 series of patients seen during a 16-year period.

Methods.—The medical records were reviewed of all patients admitted to two hospitals affiliated with the University of California–San Francisco who had PLA diagnosed between 1979 and 1994. One hundred forty-two of 216 such patients were included in the current analysis.

Findings.—Men and women were equally represented, in contrast to previous reports. Although PLA was most common among older patients, a downward trend in age range was noted. In most patients, no underlying cause was identified. Regardless of cause, single PLA was more common than multiple PLA. Treatment most often consisted of percutaneous drainage combined with IV antibiotics. Seventy-six percent of all patients who underwent such treatment were cured, compared with 65% who were treated with antibiotics alone and 61% who were treated with surgery alone. In the past 5 years, percutaneous drainage plus IV antibiotics was successful in 90% of 50 patients. A subgroup of patients with no or low-level increases in bilirubin and alkaline phosphatase concentrations, single right-sided PLA, and no readily identifiable cause of PLA had a particularly good prognosis. Death from PLA occurred mainly in patients with severe underlying disease processes, such as malignancy.

Conclusions.—Patients with PLA have a nonspecific clinical presentation, emphasizing the need for a high index of suspicion. Although jaundice and marked increases in alkaline phosphatase concentration suggest biliary tract involvement, these findings may not distinguish patients with liver abscess from those with other hepatic processes. Ultrasound and abdominal CT are key in making a diagnosis of PLA and in delineating its cause. The prognosis of PLA, which was once considered fatal, is now excellent.

▶ Pyogenic liver abscess is a condition worthy of revisiting from time to time because it is a serious illness that is occurring more frequently without specific cause in our aging, disease-burdened society. This article provides an excellent bellwether of the current status of the entity. Although it is a long, comprehensive treatment of the topic, it is worth reading. The study was a retrospective multi-institutional review during a time period when contemporary imaging techniques and antibiotics were emerging or were already available. Nonetheless, delay in diagnosis and in initiation of appropriate therapy was the *focus* for the simple reason that the classical signs of fever, chills, and upper abdominal pain occurred in less than half the patients. The authors have a right to strongly recommend percutaneous aspiration and drainage as primary therapy in combination with 3 weeks of appropriate antibiotics given by the IV route in view of the relatively low (11%) mortality. Most of the deaths occurred in patients with serious associated medical illnesses that predisposed them to their episode of PLA.

F.G. Moody, M.D.

Pyogenic Hepatic Abscess: Changing Trends Over 42 Years
Huang C-J, Pitt HA, Lipsett PA, et al (Taichung Veterans Gen Hosp, Taiwan; Johns Hopkins Med Insts, Baltimore, Md; Univ of Michigan, Ann Arbor)
Ann Surg 223:600–609, 1996   5–34

Introduction.—Pyogenic hepatic abscess is a rare and highly lethal infection. A comparison of the cause, diagnosis, bacteriology, treatment, and outcome of patients with pyogenic hepatic abscesses was made of records of 80 patients treated from 1952 to 1972 and 153 patients treated from 1973 to 1993.

Methods.—The cause of each abscess was established for both time periods and assigned to 1 of 6 categories: bile ducts, portal vein, direct extension, blunt or penetrating trauma, hepatic artery, and obscure origin. Patients' charts were also reviewed for clinical features, results of radiography, laboratory data, and microbiological data.

Results.—From 1973 to 1993, there was an increase of 13 to 20 patients per 100,000 hospital admissions for pyogenic hepatic abscess. The most dramatic change in the treatment approach between the 2 time periods was the current use of percutaneous abscess drainage. This was not available before 1973. Before 1973, most patients received antibiotics alone. In the later period, patients were more likely to have an underlying malignancy. Most malignancies (81%) were hepatobiliary or pancreatic cancer. The most likely infecting organisms in the earlier period were *Escherichia coli*, *Klebsiella*, and streptococci. In the later period, patients were significantly less likely to be infected by *E. coli* and more likely to be infected by *Klebsiella*, streptococci, fungi, and mixed bacteria. These dramatic changes may be a reflection of the increased use of in-dwelling biliary stents. The appearance of fungi in abscess cultures is probably a result of the use of broad-spectrum antibiotics in patients with stents who have frequent episodes of cholangitis. In both periods, the anaerobes *Bacteroides*, clostridia, and streptococcal species were about equal. The overall mortality rate decreased from 65% in the first period to 31% in the second period. This reduction was greatest in patients with multiple abscesses (88% vs. 45%). Mortality for single abscesses decreased from 31% to 19%. Increased mortality in both periods was associated with multiple abscesses, an associated malignancy, jaundice, hypoalbuminemia, leukocytosis, bacteremia, and a significant complication. From 1952 to 1972, advanced age, biliary etiology, elevated alanine aminotransferase, and aerobic infection were also associated with increased mortality, compared with no association with increased mortality during the 1973–1993 period. During the latter period, the mortality rate from surgical drainage was lower than that for percutaneous abscess drainage (14% vs. 26%).

Conclusion.—There was an increased incidence of pyogenic hepatic abscesses during the 1973–1993 period, most likely the result of more aggressive approaches to the management of hepatobiliary and pancreatic neoplasms. The bacteriology of these abscesses has changed during the 2 periods, probably because of the use of biliary stents and the frequent use of broad-spectrum antibiotics. Better imaging and the development and use of percutaneous abscess and nonoperative biliary drainage have contributed to the significant reduction in mortality rates (65% vs. 31%). The mortality rate remains high and remains a diagnostic and therapeutic challenge.

▶ This report from Johns Hopkins Medical Institutions on the management of hepatic abscess during a 40-year–plus period provides insight into the changing patterns of the disease and the impact of modern imaging studies on the management of the problem. The decrease in mortality rates between the 2 periods from 65% to 31% is impressive. However, it still remains a highly lethal complication of malignant and benign biliary tract disease. Mixed bacterial, multiple, and fungal abscesses continue to be difficult problems to manage.

F.G. Moody, M.D.

Pyogenic Hepatic Abscess: Results of Current Management
Hashimoto L, Hermann R, Grundfest-Broniatowski S (Cleveland Clinic Found, Ohio)
Am Surg 61:407–411, 1995
5–35

Introduction.—Previously, hepatic abscesses have been treated with operative drainage. However, with the use of CT, CT-guided percutaneous catheter drainage has become a treatment of choice. The treatment and outcome of pyogenic liver abscesses are reviewed in a retrospective analysis.

Methods.—Treatment of pyogenic liver abscesses in 56 patients was retrospectively reviewed. Clinical features, laboratory parameters, disease characteristics, microorganisms isolated, and type of treatment were assessed.

Results.—Fever, chills, and abdominal pain were the most common symptoms, with abdominal tenderness and hepatomegaly present on physical examination. The CT scan was used in the diagnosis of 47 patients, with abscesses observed in 46. Twenty-eight patients had a single abscess, and 28 patients had multiple or loculated lesions. Bacterial cultures were positive in 44 patients. Treatment of hepatic abscess consisted of surgical drainage, nonsurgical treatment (percutaneous drainage or aspiration), or no drainage. Surgical drainage was initially performed on 6 patients, with 1 death and 5 cures. Thirty-eight patients underwent CT-guided percutaneous drainage as initial treatment. Twenty-seven patients were considered cured, 4 patients died, and 8 patients either failed or had a recurrence. Patients who failed percutaneous drainage underwent surgical drainage and were cured. Patients who had a recurrence underwent either repeat drainage or aspiration. Ten patients had aspiration as the initial treatment, with 6 cures, 1 repeat aspiration, and 3 deaths. One patient with advanced pancreatic cancer received antibiotics only without drainage and subsequently died.

Conclusion.—The use of CT scans allowed for diagnosis of hepatic abscess within 4 days. Computed tomographic-guided percutaneous catheter drainage resulted in a success rate of 77%, making it the preferred method of treatment in patients with hepatic abscesses.

▶ Computed tomographic-guided catheter drainage is the preferred treatment for hepatic abscess coupled with appropriate long-term antibiotic drainage. It is not unexpected that *Escherichia coli, Enterococcus, Enterobacter,* and *Klebsiella,* organisms indigenous to the gut, were the predominant organisms found in the abscesses as well as in the blood. The paper's strength is that it points out the numerous and varied causes of hepatic abscesses. Unfortunately, the report is much too casual in its discussion of the details of management of such a complex disease. For example, the need for aggressive antibiotic coverage before percutaneous drainage should be emphasized, and the indications and timing of surgical intervention after cathether drainage should have been discussed. In this regard, I can state that the tendency is to wait too long when only a partial response to catheter drainage is obtained. The tendency to procrastinate is encouraged by the severe nature of the diseases the abscesses are related to. This is an important area for general surgeons to be informed of.

F.G. Moody, M.D.

42 Liver Involvement in Systemic Mastocytosis

Hepatic Involvement in Mastocytosis: Clinicopathologic Correlations in 41 Cases
Mican JM, Di Bisceglie AM, Fong T-L, et al (Natl Inst of Allergy and Infectious Diseases, Bethesda, Md; Natl Inst of Diabetes and Digestive and Kidney Diseases, Bethesda, Md; NIH, Bethesda, Md)
Hepatology 22:1163–1170, 1995　　　　　　　　　　　　　　　5–36

Introduction.—Mastocytosis, a disease of mast cell hyperplasia, may affect the skin only or internal organs such as the bone marrow and gastrointestinal tract. Hepatic involvement can occur, causing elevated serum alkaline phosphatase levels, hepatomegaly, ascites, and portal hypertension. Reported histologic findings include mast cell infiltration, fibrosis, and cirrhosis. Little is known about the prevalence of these findings and their relation to disease category. Hepatic involvement was assessed in a group of adult patients with mastocytosis.

Patients and Findings.—Forty-one patients with mastocytosis were studied, most prospectively. Sixty-one percent had evidence of liver disease. Twenty-four percent had hepatomegaly, and 41% had splenomegaly. More than half had elevated serum alkaline phosphatase, serum aminotransaminases, 5'-nucleotidase, or gamma-glutamyltranspeptidase (GGTP). The alkaline phosphatase levels were related to GGTP levels, hepatomegaly and splenomegaly, and liver mast cell infiltration and fibrosis. Patients with category II or III mastocytosis were more likely to have elevated alkaline phosphatase levels and splenomegaly. Five patients in these disease categories had ascites or portal hypertension and died of mastocytosis complications. At death, 3 of the 5 patients had hypoprothrombinemia.

Thirty-five liver biopsy specimens from 25 patients were analyzed. Patients with category II or III disease had more severe mast cell infiltration. This finding was correlated with hepatomegaly, splenomegaly, alkaline phosphatase level, and GGTP level. Special stains (i.e., toluidine blue and chloroacetate esterase) often were required to see the mast cells. Sixty-eight percent of specimens showed increased portal fibrosis; this finding was associated with mast cell infiltration and portal inflammation. There were

"

no instances of cirrhosis. Twenty-three percent of specimens showed nodular regenerative hyperplasia, portal venopathy, and veno-occlusive disease. In 4 of 8 cases, these changes may have been the cause of portal hypertension or ascites.

Conclusions.—Many patients with mastocytosis have liver disease with mast cell infiltration. Other findings can include nodular regenerative hyperplasia, portal venopathy, or veno-occlusive disease. The liver involvement usually is not severe, except in patients in disease categories II and III. In these patients, hepatic involvement may be a significant cause of morbidity and mortality.

▶ Mastocytosis is a disease with protean manifestations that may involve the skin, liver, spleen, gastrointestinal tract, bones, and bone marrow. Mastocytosis can be categorized by the following classification system[1]: category 1A, indolent disease involving the skin only; category 1B, indolent systemic disease with or without skin involvement; category II, mastocytosis with an associated hematologic disorder; category III, aggressive mastocytosis (lymphadenopathy with eosinophilia); and category IV, mast cell leukemia.

The report by Mican and colleagues provides useful information on liver involvement in mastocytosis. Although liver test abnormalities were seen in more than 50% of the patients, severe liver disease was uncommon; ascites or portal hypertension developed in only 5 patients, and these patients were in disease categories II or III. It is important to remember that mastocytosis can be associated with nodular regenerative hyperplasia, portal venopathy, and veno-occlusive disease. Severe liver disease with ascites carries an ominous prognosis.

That mast cells and their mediator products may play a role in liver fibrogenesis was documented in a recent reported by Farrell and colleagues.[2] These investigators quantified mast cell numbers in percutaneous biopsy specimens from normal livers, and from patients with alcoholic liver disease or primary biliary cirrhosis (PBC). Small numbers of mast cells were found within the portal tracts and sinusoids of normal livers. In chronic liver disease, mucosal markers of mast cells were present that correlated with the increased amount of fibrosis. Interestingly, significantly more mast cells were found in the PBC group compared with the alcoholic group for a given amount of fibrosis. The authors suggest that cholestasis enhances mast cell action, and this in turn facilitates the development of fibrosis.

N.J. Greenberger, M.D.

References

1. Metcalfe DD: Clinical advances in mastocytosis: An interdisciplinary round table discussion. Conclusions. *J Invest Dermatol* 96:64S–65S, 1991.
2. Farrell DJ, Hines JE, Ealls AF, et al: Intrahepatic mast cells in chronic liver disease. *Hepatology* 22:1175–1181, 1996.

43 Neoplasms—Clinical and Radiographic Studies

Hepatocellular Carcinoma in the United States: Prognostic Features, Treatment Outcome, and Survival
Stuart KE, Anand AJ, Jenkins RL (Deaconess Hosp, Boston; Boston Ctr for Liver Cancer)
Cancer 77:2217–2222, 1996   5–37

Background.—Hepatocellular carcinoma (HCC) is the most common lethal malignancy in the world, but it is relatively uncommon in the United States. A large series of American hepatoma patients who presented to the Deaconess Hospital in Boston were reviewed to identify prognostic factors and determine the length of survival.

Study Design.—A retrospective analysis was performed of the hospital Tumor Registry from 1986 to 1995. Age; sex; tumor, node, metastasis staging; serum biochemistry; serum alpha-fetoprotein (AFP); patency of portal vein; cirrhosis; history of alcohol abuse; hepatitis status; hemochromatosis; treatment; and survival were recorded.

Findings.—Three hundred fourteen patients with hepatoma in the registry during this time period were identified. The overall median survival was 10 months. Cirrhosis, history of alcohol abuse, low albumin, high bilirubin, abnormal AFP, portal vein obstruction (PVO), and advanced stage were each associated with significantly shorter survival time. Albumin, AFP, and PVO were independent risk factors by multiple regression analysis. Patients who had surgery had the longest median survival time at 45 months, followed by those who had chemoembolization at 14 months. Those who received systemic chemotherapy alone or were untreated had the shortest survival time of 2–4 months.

Conclusion.—The prognostic factors that influenced survival in this large series of American patients with hepatoma were similar to those among Asian patients, in whom HCC is more common. The prognosis was poor. Understanding the factors that influence prognosis may help in the selection of those patients most likely to benefit from specific types of therapy.

▶ This report about the clinical characteristics of HCC in a single institution in America (i.e., the Deaconess in Boston) provides an important contribution to our understanding of this nefarious disease. It comes as no surprise that alcoholism, poor liver function, and PVO are bad prognostic signs. That surgery provided the longest survival and chemotherapy the shortest suggests that the patient's lesions were self-selected as to possible treatment options. Hepatoma is far less common in the Western than in the Eastern world, but it appears to be no less lethal.

F.G. Moody, M.D.

Hepatic Resection of Hepatocellular Carcinoma in Cirrhotic Livers: Is It Unjustified in Impaired Liver Function?
Wu C-C, Ho W-L, Yeh D-C, et al (Taichung Veterans Gen Hosp, Taiwan)
Surgery 120:34–39, 1996   5–38

Background.—Resection for hepatocellular carcinoma (HCC) is usually considered unjustified in patients with cirrhosis and impaired liver function, because the surgical risk is higher and the long-term prognosis poorer. The value of HCC resection in cirrhotic livers with impaired function based on preoperative indocyanine green clearance testing was investigated.

Methods.—Thirty-six patients with a preoperative indocyanine green 15-minute retention rate of 20% or more (group 1) and 34 patients with a 15-minute retention rate of 10% or less (group 2) were included in the study. The backgrounds and resectional results of these 2 groups were compared retrospectively.

Outcomes.—Patients in group 1 had a significantly lower serum albumin level and a higher serum bilirubin level, a longer prothrombin time, a greater incidence of associated esophageal varices, and a poorer Child's cirrhosis classification than patients in group 2. Although the 2 groups had a comparable tumor diameter, the amount of resected liver in group 2 was larger because the extent of liver resection was greater and the surgical margin wider. The 2 groups did not differ in the amount of operative blood loss and blood transfusion, operative morbidity, or operative mortality. Pathologic features and staging were also similar. The 5-year disease-free and actuarial survival rates were 30.9% and 29.6%, respectively, for group 1 and 45.2% and 33.4%, respectively, for group 2 (Fig 1).

Conclusion.—Liver resection for HCC is justified in selected patients with cirrhosis and impaired liver function when the nontumorous liver parenchyma can be preserved well. Poorer preoperative liver function does not always mean a worse long-term prognosis. Even in a large, centrally located HCC, resection is not absolutely contraindicated in such patients

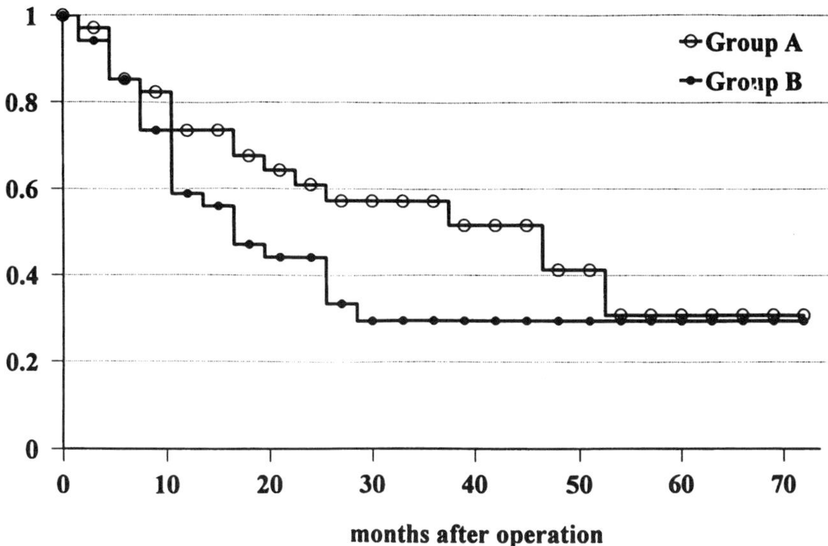

FIGURE 1.—Cumulative disease-free survival rate of patients with hepatocellular carcinoma and corrhosis. Group A vs. group B, $P = 0.16$. (Courtesy of Wu C-C, Ho W-L, Yeh D-C, et al: Hepatic resection of hepatocellular carcinoma in cirrhotic livers: Is it unjustified in impaired liver function? *Surgery* 120:34–39, 1996.)

with cirrhosis. For patients with HCC and more advanced cirrhosis, orthotopic liver transplantation is probably more suitable.

▶ Wu and associates at the Taichung Veterans General Hospital in Taiwan utilize the clearance of indocyanine green dye at 15% to distinguish patients at risk for liver failure after resection of hepatocellular carcinoma in cirrhosis. They found no difference in patients with poor or good functional reserve, provided they reduced the amount of liver resected in the former group. I doubt whether the indocyanine green retention test made much of a difference, because patients with poor excretion had poor liver function in general. Rikkers, Aldrete, and I were interested in quantifying hepatic reserve by indocyanine green clearance in candidates for portacaval shunts but were disappointed in the lack of discrimination power of the test, even when carried out in a dose response manner.[1] The point of view of this group that resection should leave as much noncancerous tissue as possible is well taken.

F.G. Moody, M.D.

Reference

1. Moody FG, Rikkers LF, Aldrete JS; Estimation of the functional reserve of human liver. *Ann Surg* 180:592–598, 1974.

Prognostic Value of Serum Alpha-1-Antitrypsin in Hepatocellular Carcinoma

Pirisi M, Fabris C, Soardo G, et al (Univ of Udine, Italy)
Eur J Cancer 32A:221–225, 1996

5–39

Introduction.—The acute-phase reactant alpha-1-antitrypsin (A1AT) is reported to predict survival in patients with hepatocellular carcinoma (HCC). Because measurement of A1AT is simple, reliable, and inexpensive, it would be a useful prognostic marker of HCC. Seventy-five patients with HCC that developed in the setting of long-standing cirrhosis were retrospectively reviewed to assess the use of serum A1AT in estimating prognosis.

Patients and Methods.—The 75 consecutive patients, 60 men and 15 women, were hospitalized between December 1990 and November 1994. Diagnosis was based on imaging findings, increased alpha-1-fetoprotein levels (>400 µg/L), and/or histopathologic data. Thirty-six patients received supportive treatment, and 39 underwent surgical resection and/or arterial chemoembolism. Fifty-two patients died during follow-up. At the end of the study, 23 surviving patients had been followed for a median of 766 days. The prognostic value of A1AT, measured on admission, was compared with that of other relevant factors using Cox regression analysis with stepwise selection of variables.

Results.—Using a cutoff of 2.20 g/L, representing the 95th percentile of a group of healthy blood donors, patients were divided into 2 groups according to baseline A1AT levels. In 30 patients (group A), serum A1AT concentrations were 2.20 g/L or less; the remaining 45 patients (group B) had A1AT levels of more than 2.20 g/L. Median survival was 518 days in group A vs. 81 days in group B. The difference in survival time between groups was significant, even after patients were stratified for age, sex, tumor size, type of treatment, bilirubin level, alpha-1-fetoprotein level, and Child-Pugh class. Multivariate analysis identified 4 independent predictors of survival from among 17 variables: tumor size, bilirubin level, A1AT level, and blood urea nitrogen (BUN) concentration.

Discussion.—In this group of patients with HCC concurrent with cirrhosis, those with serum A1AT concentrations in the lower-normal range (less than or equal to 2.20 g/L) had a median survival more than 6 times that of patients with higher A1AT levels. The prognostic weight of A1AT was greater than that of tumor size and BUN concentration and almost equal to that of bilirubin concentration. Measurement of serum A1AT levels might provide a useful, inexpensive prognostic marker in HCC.

▶ The search continues for a number that will tell us when a hepatoma has developed in a patient with cirrhosis. Pirisi and associates have provided the best thing, a number that predicts survival. Although the number of patients studied is relatively small for such a complex problem, I suspect that serum A1AT levels will be helpful in managing patients with advanced cirrhosis and may evolve as an inexpensive way to raise suspicion that a neoplasm may have developed within a cirrhotic liver.

F.G. Moody, M.D.

Predictive Score for the Development of Hepatocellular Carcinoma and Additional Value of Liver Large Cell Dysplasia in Western Patients With Cirrhosis
Ganne-Carrié N, Chastang C, Chapel F, et al (Hôpital Jean Verdier, Bondy Cedex, France; Hôpital Saint-Louis, Paris; Hôpital Tenon, Paris; et al)
Hepatology 23:1112–1118, 1996   5–40

Background.—Regular screening of patients with cirrhosis for the early detection of hepatocellular carcinoma (HCC) has allowed small tumors to be identified in Asian patients. In Europe, however, where the annual incidence of HCC is as high as in Asia, ultrasound investigations and serum α-fetoprotein (AFP) determinations detect few resectable tumors. One hundred fifty-one consecutive patients with cirrhosis but no detectable HCC were studied to identify clinical, biological, and histologic parameters associated with a high risk for HCC.

Patients and Methods.—The patients were hospitalized from January 1987 to January 1990 and followed until June 1994 or death. Cirrhosis was confirmed in all cases by liver biopsy; HCC was ruled out by ultrasonography and serum AFP levels of less than 250 ng/mL. The 85 men and 66 women had a mean age of 57 years. Cirrhosis resulted from alcohol in 71 cases, hepatitis C virus (HCV) in 28, alcohol and HCV in 22, and other etiologies in 30 cases. Using the log rank test and the Cox proportional hazards model, 22 variables recorded at entry were assessed for their predictive value for HCC. Screening tests for HCC were performed every 6 months.

Results.—Hepatocellular carcinoma developed in 31 patients during the study period. Clinical and biological variables significantly predictive of HCC in the Cox model were age 50 or older, male, large esophageal varices, prothrombin activity less than 70%, serum AFP level of 15 ng/L or greater, and the presence of anti-HCV antibodies. Relative risks for HCC were 4.4, 2.6, 2.3, 2.2, 2.2, and 2.0, respectively, for age, sex, esophageal varices, prothrombin activity, serum AFP, and anti-HCV antibodies. These 6 variables, coded 0 if absent and 1 if present, were incorporated into an equation that yielded a possible score of 0–22. Low-risk and high-risk groups were distinguished according to scores of less than 11 and greater than 11. The cumulated incidence of HCC at 3 years was 0% in the low-risk group and 24% in the high-risk group. A subgroup of high-risk patients with liver large-cell dysplasia were at very high risk for HCC (3-year cumulative incidence 72%).

Discussion.—In a study population representative of Western countries, 6 clinical and biological variables identified patients with cirrhosis who are at high risk for HCC. The score's predictive value was confirmed by prospective follow-up of 49 patients with non–biopsy-proven cirrhosis. Liver biopsy specimens showing large-cell dysplasia identifies a subgroup at very high risk who will benefit from intensive screening or preventive measures.

▶ The identification of predictive criteria for patients at risk for HCC provides a way to screen for early and potentially resectable lesions. I was surprised to learn from this report that the annual incidence of HCC is as high in Europe as in Japan and is associated with cirrhosis in more than 80% of cases. Age, male sex, large varices, and decreased synthetic liver function, along with an elevated AFP level, appear to be the most sensitive variables. Clearly, these individuals should have a biannual ultrasound for the purpose of early detection of a hepatoma, which in our country might best be treated by a liver transplant in such patients.

F.G. Moody, M.D.

Current Perspectives on Repeat Hepatic Resection for Colorectal Carcinoma: A Review

Wanebo HJ, Chu QD, Avradopoulos KA, et al (Brown Univ, Providence, RI)
Surgery 119:361–371, 1996   5–41

Background.—Sixty-five percent to 85% of the patients who undergo initial hepatectomy for colorectal cancer metastases have recurrences. About half of them have liver metastases. In 20% to 30% of these patients, the only organ involved is the liver. The presence of diffuse liver disease or extrahepatic extension often limits the opportunity for resection, which is possible in only 10% to 25% of such patients. The rationale, indications, and outcomes of further resection of hepatic metastases from colorectal cancer were reviewed.

Methods and Findings.—Major liver resection studies were reviewed. The analysis included 28 series. The mean interval between the first and second liver resections ranged from 9 to 33 months. In the two largest series, this interval was about 17.5 months. In a series of 10 or more patients, the median survival rate was 19 months, which is similar to the survival rate in single resection series. The French Association study, which included 1,626 patients who underwent one and 144 patients who underwent two resections, reported 5-year survival rates of 25% and 16%, respectively. The recurrence rate after repeated resection exceeded 60%. Half of the recurrences were located in the liver. Possible favorable prognostic factors were no contiguous structure involvement at the time of primary tumor resection, complete removal of macroscopic disease at repeated hepatectomy, hepatic lesions of less than 6 cm in diameter at initial hepatic resection, and solitary recurrences.

Conclusions.—Repeated hepatic resection in patients with colorectal metastases appears to be safe and effective in carefully selected patients. The procedure is associated with a low surgical mortality, and survival

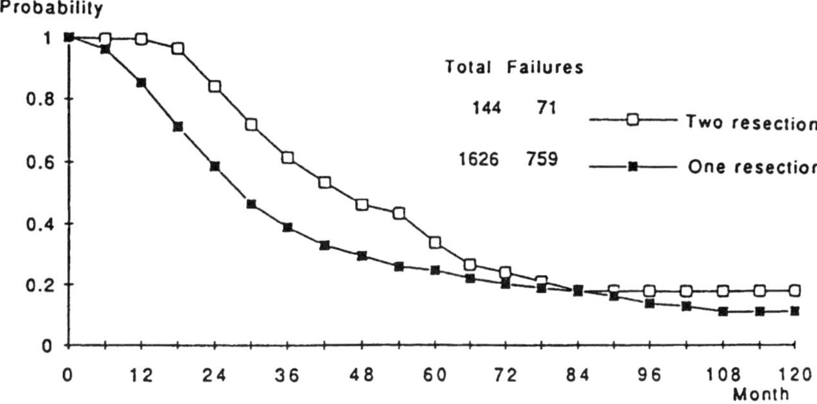

FIGURE 1.—Survival rates as measured from time of initial hepatic resection in patients who underwent single and repeated liver resections. (From Nordlinger B, Jacek D, Guigust M, et al: Surgical resection of hepatic metastases: Multicentric study by the French Association of Surgery, In Nordlinger B, Jaeck D (eds): *Treatment of Hepatic Metastases of Colorectal Cancer.* New York, Springer-Verlag, 1992 pp 129–146. Courtesy of Wanebo HJ, Chu QD, Avradopoulos KA, et al: Current perspectives on repeat hepatic resection for colorectal carcinoma: A review. *Surgery* 119:361–371, 1996.)

rates are similar to those in patients undergoing initial hepatic resections (Fig 1). The prognostic factors favoring repeated resection, although variable, include no extrahepatic tumor extension and complete liver metastases resection.

▶ A second hepatectomy for recurrent metastatic colon cancer appears to be marginally therapeutic, but by collative analysis the authors may be on to something here. Although the surgical approach has a high mortality rate (25%), of those who survive, 25% do so for 5 years. Obviously, this approach is not for the timid or, in fact, for the overly bold, because careful selection appears to be the secret to success. Hopefully, measures to prevent colon cancer will start to decrease the prevalence of this all-too-common, preventable disease.

F.G. Moody, M.D.

Prevention of Second Primary Tumors by an Acyclic Retinoid, Polyprenoic Acid, in Patients With Hepatocellular Carcinoma

Muto Y, for the Hepatoma Prevention Study Group (Gifu Univ, Japan; Tokyo Women's Med College; Gifu Municipal Hosp, Japan, et al)
N Engl J Med 334:1561–1567, 1996   5–42

Background.—The long-term prognosis for patients with primary hepatoma is dependent on tumor recurrence and the development of second primary tumors, both of which occur at a high rate despite surgical resection and ethanol injection therapy. Efforts to develop synthetic compounds for cancer chemoprevention yielded an acyclic retinoid, poly-

TABLE 2.—Incidence of Treatment Failure

Type of Treatment Failure	Polyprenoic Acid Group (N = 44)*	Placebo Group (N = 45)*	P Value†
Disease recurrence	5 (11)	2 (4)	0.23
Early (<6 mo)	5 (11)	2 (4)	0.23
Late (≥6 mo)	0	0	—
Distant metastasis	0	0	—
Second primary tumor	7 (16)	20 (44)	0.004
All	12 (27)	22 (49)	0.04

*Values are numbers of patients (%).
†By the chi-square test without Yates' correction.

(Reprinted by permission of *The New England Journal of Medicine* from Muto Y, for the Hepatoma Prevention Study Group: Prevention of second primary tumors by an acyclic retinoid, polyprenoic acid, in patients with hepatocellular carcinoma. *N Engl J Med* 334:1561–1567. Copyright 1996, Massachusetts Medical Society. All rights reserved.)

prenoic acid, that inhibits hepatocarcinogenesis in rats and induces differentiation and apoptosis in human hepatoma–derived cell lines. In phase I trials, polyprenoic acid (25–600 mg/day) was well tolerated by healthy subjects and patients with liver cirrhosis. A prospective study tested the effects of the compound on recurrence and second primary hepatomas after curative treatment.

Methods.—The randomized, controlled study included 89 patients who were free of disease after surgical resection or percutaneous ethanol injection therapy. Forty-five were allocated to placebo and 44 to polyprenoic acid (two 150-mg capsules twice daily, a dose found to be effective in laboratory studies and safe in the phase I trial). Treatment was started within 8 weeks of surgery or ethanol injection and continued for 12 months. The remnant liver was studied by US every 3 weeks for the development of new hepatomas.

Results.—During a median follow-up of 38 months, at least 1 histologically confirmed hepatoma developed in 34 patients (Table 2). The proportion of patients with a second hepatoma was significantly lower in the active treatment group (27%) than in the placebo group (49%). Although the 2 groups were comparable in the incidence of disease recurrence, polyprenoic acid significantly reduced the rate of second primary hepatomas over time relative to placebo (16% vs. 44%) (Fig 2). When polyprenoic acid was compared with placebo by the proportional hazards model, the estimated relative risk of a second primary hepatomas was 0.31. Only 1 patient in the active treatment group withdrew because of toxic effects.

Conclusion.—Oral polyprenoic acid was safe and effective when administered for the prevention of second primary hepatomas in patients clinically free of disease after curative surgical resection of the original tumor or ethanol injection.

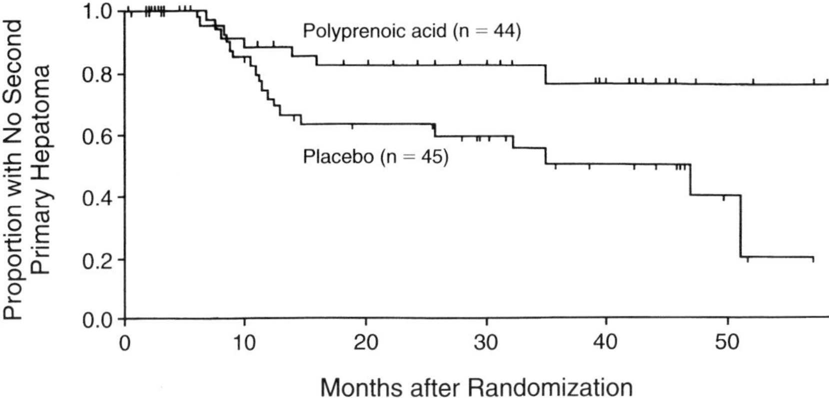

FIGURE 2.—Kaplan-Meier estimates of the proportion of patients without second primary hepatomas in the two study groups. The treatment period lasted for 12 months, beginning with month 0. $P = 0.04$ for the comparison between groups by the log-rank test. *Tick marks* indicate patients who withdrew or were excluded from the study. (Reprinted by permission of *The New England Journal of Medicine* from Muto Y, for the Hepatoma Prevention Study Group: Prevention of second primary tumors by an acyclic retinoid, polyprenoic acid, in patients with hepatocellular carcinoma. *N Engl J Med* 334:1561–1567. Copyright 1996, Massachusetts Medical Society. All rights reserved.)

▶ The study demonstrates that oral polyprenoic acid prevents second primary hepatomas after surgical resection of the original tumor. The clinical presentation of hepatocellular carcinoma is highly variable, and diagnosis is still often made at an advanced stage of disease. The introduction of improved imaging techniques has provided opportunities to detect hepatomas when they are small focal lesions and more likely to be amenable to surgical resection. Solmi et al. utilized US to prospectively study 360 patients with chronic liver disease (254 had cirrhosis). Hepatoma was diagnosed in 24 of 360 patients (6.6%) during a mean follow-up period of 56 months. In 18 of the 24 cases, hepatic lesions were unifocal and smaller than 3 cm. By contrast, in a retrospective study of 2,170 cirrhotics without serial US follow-up, unifocal tumors smaller than 3 cm in size were detected in only 15%. The use of chemopreventive agents such as polyprenoic acid appears to be most appropriate in patients with small hepatomas after resection.

N.J. Greenberger, M.D.

Reference

1. Solmi L, Primeriano AMM, Gandolfi L: Ultrasound follow-up of patients at risk for hepatocellular carcinoma: Results of a prospective study on 360 cases. *Am J Gastroenterol* 91:1189–1194, 1996.

Intraoperative Ultrasonogaphy in Detection of Hepatic Metastases From Colorectal Cancer

Rafaelsen SR, Kronborg O, Larsen C, et al (Odense Univ, Denmark)
Dis Colon Rectum 38:355–360, 1995

5–43

Background.—Recent studies have reported that 25% of patients with limited liver metastases from colorectal carcinoma and no evidence of spread elsewhere can be cured. The accuracy of intraoperative ultrasonography (IOUS) in the diagnosis and location of liver metastases was compared with measurements of liver enzymes, preoperative ultrasonography (PUS), and surgical exploration.

Methods.—A total of 295 consecutive patients (148 males, 147 females) admitted to the hospital for elective surgery for colorectal carcinoma were studied by IOUS, as well as PUS and measurement of liver enzymes. At surgery, the liver was inspected and palpated by the surgeon and findings regarding metastases were recorded before the results of PUS were known and prior to IOUS. The size and location of liver metastases detected by IOUS were recorded. Biopsy was performed on all doubtful lesions before resection. Patients were examined 3 months postoperatively with conventional ultrasonography. If the examination was negative, the patient was considered cured. If the ultrasonography was positive, previous negative findings were considered as false negatives. The sensitivity and the specificity of each diagnostic method were compared.

Results.—There were no complications of IOUS; the usual duration of the study was 8 to 10 minutes. Curative operations were performed in 216 patients and palliative procedures in 79. Sixty-four of the 295 patients (21.7%) had a total of 204 liver metastases. The sensitivity of IOUS in detecting metastases (62/64) was significantly superior to the findings at surgery (54/64) and to the findings on PUS (45/64). The sensitivity of IOUS was significantly superior to the other diagnostic methods ($P <$ 0.0001). The differences in specificity were not significantly different. Intraoperative ultrasound was significantly superior to both PUS and surgical exploration in the detection of small and deeply seated metastases, and it was also significantly superior to PUS in identifying metastatic lesions in the posterior segments of the liver (II, VII, and VIII) and in segments IV and V. In addition, IOUS was superior to surgical exploration in detecting metastases in segments IV, V, and VIII. Intraoperative ultrasound was superior to liver function abnormalities in 29 patients who had fewer than 4 metastatic lesions.

Conclusions.—Intraoperative ultrasonography is a safe and quickly performed procedure that is superior to preoperative ultrasonography and surgical exploration in the detection of liver metastases from colorectal carcinoma. Its use may result in the identification and treatment of patients who may potentially be cured by surgery and in the prevention of unnecessary liver surgery.

▶ Intraoperative ultrasound is better than preoperative ultrasound, the surgeon's eyes and hands, or liver enzyme analysis in detection of liver metastases from colorectal cancer. The authors in this controlled trial have gone to great lengths to blind the respective observers. My own philosophy (and personal practice) is to perform intraoperative ultrasonography of the liver in all cases of intra-abdominal malignancy. In fact, I use this technique whenever I can to keep up my skills in its usage.

F.G. Moody, M.D.

Intrahepatic Cholangiocarcinoma: Results of Aggressive Surgical Management
Cherqui D, Tantawi B, Alon R, et al (Université Paris XII)
Arch Surg 130:1073–1078, 1995
5–44

Introduction.—Locoregional extension is usually advanced at the time of diagnosis in patients with intrahepatic cholangiocarcinoma (ICC). The results of 19 patients with ICC who underwent aggressive surgical management are reported.

Methods.—Four of the 19 patients had a history of chronic alcoholism. All patients except 1 were symptomatic: 9 had right upper quadrant pain, and 5 each had obstructive jaundice, abdominal mass, or weight loss. Five patients were considered to have unresectable disease. Fourteen of 19 patients underwent liver resections. Of these 14 patients, 6 underwent right or left hepatectomies and 8 had extended right or left hepatectomies. One patient underwent orthotopic liver transplantation (OLT) after exploratory laparotomy. Another patient received OLT after limited recurrence following partial liver resection. The 15 patients who underwent liver resection or OLT underwent analysis of diagnostic evaluation, treatment, pathologic findings, and outcome.

Results.—Patients were diagnosed with liver tumor using ultrasonography and dynamic CT or MRI. Five patients with jaundice had diffuse dilation of the intrahepatic bile ducts. Segmental dilatation was observed in 3 patients without jaundice. Nine patients with large and/or central tumors located in the vicinity of the inferior vena cava or main hepatic veins and underwent total vascular exclusion of the liver. One patient died of sepsis and liver failure 20 days after extended right hepatectomy with bile duct reconstruction. Six patients had 9 postoperative complications: 4 biliary leaks, 2 pleural effusions, 1 pneumonia, and 2 wound infections. Three patients underwent postoperative adjuvant celiac radiotherapy, and 4 patients with postoperative recurrence received chemotherapy. All patients had typical adenocarcinoma. The actuarial 1- and 2-year survival rates, respectively, were 58% and 32%. In 5 patients, the operation was considered curative. The overall median survival was 14 months in the whole series. Median survival was 27 months in patients with curative resections and 9 months in those with palliative resections. The patients who underwent OLT were alive and free of disease at 25 and 31 months after transplantation, respectively.

Conclusion.—Aggressive surgical management of patients with ICC is recommended. Complex liver resection procedures are the first choice and (OLT) should be considered selectively.

▶ There is no doubt that ICCs can be resected with a low mortality rate and prolonged survival, but they should be limited to institutions such as this where liver resections and transplantation are done almost on a daily basis. The use of transplantation in this disease is questionable in view of the uniform rate of early recurrence in the face of immunosuppression. One cannot argue with the success they have achieved in 2 selected cases. The cases illustrated by the CT scans reveal the remarkable challenges that the surgeons faced in this unique series of patients.

F.G. Moody, M.D.

44 Surgical Issues

Retrograde Right Hepatic Trisegmentectomy
Yanaga K, Kawahara N, Taketomi A, et al (Kyushu Univ, Fukuoka, Japan)
Surgery 119:592–595, 1996   5–45

Background.—The conventional approach to right hepatic trisegment-ectomy can be difficult or dangerous in patients with a centrohepatic or huge liver mass. The technique described modifies the procedure so that right-sided liver tumors with hilar distortion can be removed safely. Seven of 20 patients who underwent right trisegmentectomy of the liver between December 1987 and March 1995 required the retrograde technique because of distortion of the hepatic hilar anatomy. In 3 cases, the entire right lobe and the medial segment were replaced by tumors.

Technique.—The retrograde modification involves division of inflow pedicles that supply the medial segment and come off to the right of the umbilical portion of the Glissonian sheath. Care is taken to avoid dissection of the left side of the umbilical fissure and devascularization of the lateral segment. The liver is divided to the right of the falciform ligament, and the right hepatic hilar structures are identified and divided. After longitudinal division of the caudate process, roots of the middle and right hepatic veins are identified within parenchyma and divided.

Results.—All 7 patients survived and none had liver failure. Additional procedures (portal vein thromboembolectomy, portal vein thrombectomy, partial hepatectomy, and portal vein replacement) were required in 4 cases. The portal vein procedures were able to be performed when retraction of the medial segment toward the operator provided access to the right inflow pedicle. Postoperative complications (subphrenic abscess and intra-abdominal bleeding) occurred in 2 patients. The degree of transient postoperative liver dysfunction in this series of patients was comparable with that reported for conventional right hepatic trisegmentectomy.

Discussion.—The technique of retrograde right hepatic trisegmentectomy consists of inflow control of the medial segment, inflow occlusion of the right lobe, completion of parenchymal division, and detachment from the inferior vena cava and the posterior structures. Although successful in these patients, the technique should not be viewed as a replacement for the standard operation or performed in cases of suspected invasion of the retrohepatic inferior vena cava by cholangiocarcinoma or metastatic adenocarcinoma.

▶ Yanaga and his associates from Kyushu University remind us that even very bulky neoplasms of the right lobe of the liver, which involve the medial segment of the left lobe, can be safely resected. Obviously, this is not a procedure for the nonspecialist or the timid, but as described, it appears to offer a way to approach what appears to be unresectable lesions.

F.G. Moody, M.D.

Portal Triad Clamping or Hepatic Vascular Exclusion for Major Liver Resection: A Controlled Study

Belghiti J, Noun R, Zante E, et al (Univ Paris VII)
Ann Surg 224:155–161, 1996

5–46

Background.—Blood loss during liver resection is reduced by portal triad clamping (PTC) or under hepatic vascular exclusion (HVE). The operative course of patients undergoing major liver resection under PTC or HVE were compared.

Methods.—Fifty-two noncirrhotic patients undergoing major liver resections were enrolled in the prospective, randomized study. Twenty-four had PTC and 28 had HVE. Intraoperative and postoperative courses were analyzed.

Findings.—Eight patients were crossed over to the other group during resection. Fourteen percent in the HVE group had hemodynamic intolerance. Pedicular clamping was inefficient in 4 patients in the PTC group. Three of these patients had involvement of the cavohepatic intersection, and 1 had persistent bleeding from tricuspid insufficiency. The 2 groups were similar in intraoperative blood loss and postoperative enzyme level reflecting hepatocellular injury. After HVE, the mean durations of surgery and of clampage were significantly increased. Postoperative abdominal collections and pulmonary complications were 2.5-fold greater after HVE but not significantly so. The mean length of stay after surgery was longer after HVE.

Conclusion.—Portal triad clamping and HVE are equally effective in decreasing blood loss in patients undergoing major liver resections. Hepatic vascular exclusion is associated with unpredictable hemodynamic intolerance and increased postoperative complications and hospitalization. Thus, it should be restricted to lesions involving the cavohepatic intersection.

▶ The authors are to be complimented upon choosing a randomized prospective protocol to answer the question of whether HVE is superior to PTC, a much simpler technique. They have shown that HVE does not only reduce blood loss, but it increases postoperative morbidity and postoperative stay.

It is the procedure of choice, however, when resecting centrally located lesions. I doubt that there are many choices that can challenge their conclusions, which required accession of 52 patients into a controlled trial over a 3-year period for a major hepatic resection.

F.G. Moody, M.D.

Laparoscopic Partial Hepatectomy and Left Lateral Segmentectomy: Technique and Results of a Clinical Series
Kaneko H, Takagi S, Shiba T (Toho Univ, Tokyo)
Surgery 120:468–475, 1996   5–47

Background.—In recent years, the introduction of new laparoscopic instruments has made laparoscopic hepatectomy more feasible. A new technique for performing partial hepatectomy and left lateral segmentectomy by laparoscopy was applied in 11 patients.

Methods.—Treatment was indicated by an isolated metastatic lesion, hepatocellular carcinoma, hemangioma, Wilson's disease, and hemochromatosis. A microwave tissue coagulator was used with an US surgical aspirator to divide hepatic parenchyma without pneumoperitoneum. Branched vessels and ducts were clipped and transected, and, in some patients, the largest vessels were suture ligated. The left hepatic vein was transected using the endoscopic linear stapler for left lateral segmentectomy. After liver resection, the argon beam coagulator was used to secure hemostasis in the plane of transection. Left lateral segmentectomy was performed in 3 patients and partial hepatectomy in 8.

Outcomes.—Ten of the 11 procedures were performed uneventfully. In 1 patient, conversion to open hepatectomy was needed because of excessive bleeding. Blood losses were notably different compared with open hepatectomy. There were no postoperative complications, and postoperative pain was minimal.

Conclusions.—Laparoscopic hepatectomy appears to reduce postoperative pain and recovery time compared with open hepatectomy. Although the laparoscopic technique may not supplant the open procedure, it may be the best treatment in certain patients.

▶ Laparoscopic technology has advanced to the point where the surgeons at Toho University in Tokyo have been able to perform segmental liver resections in a timely manner and with a high level of safety. Note that they did not use a pneumoperitoneum but lifted the anterior abdominal wall away from the liver for access. Laparoscopic US allowed them to define the extent of the lesion, and a microwave tissue coagulator, ultrasonic dissector, and argon beam coagulator were used to remove it. They show schematics as well as colored pictures to illustrate the use of this technology, which adds further attestation to the relative affluence of their surgical unit.

F.G. Moody, M.D.

Dorsocranial Liver Resection and Direct Hepatoatrial Anastomosis for Hepatic Venous Outflow Obstruction: Long-term Outcome and Functional Results

Vogt PR, Andersson LC, Jenni R, et al (Univ Hosp, Zurich, Switzerland; Royal London Hosp)
Am J Gastroenterol 91:539–544, 1996

5–48

Background.—The occlusion of the major hepatic venous outflow in patients with Budd-Chiari syndrome can be partial or complete, and may result in reversible liver damage. Prognosis is generally poor, but there have been recent improvements in surgical treatment. A new surgical procedure consists of dorsocranial liver resection and direct hepatoatrial anastomosis that aims to re-establish blood flow from the hepatic veins and alleviate liver dysfunction. Long-term outcome in patients with Budd-Chiari syndrome after dorsocranial liver resection and direct hepatoatrial anastomosis was investigated.

Methods.—Dorsocranial liver resection with direct hepatoatrial anastomosis was performed in 16 patients with Budd-Chiari syndrome and various preoperative signs and symptoms (Fig 1). In 10 patients, the inferior vena caval vein was occluded.

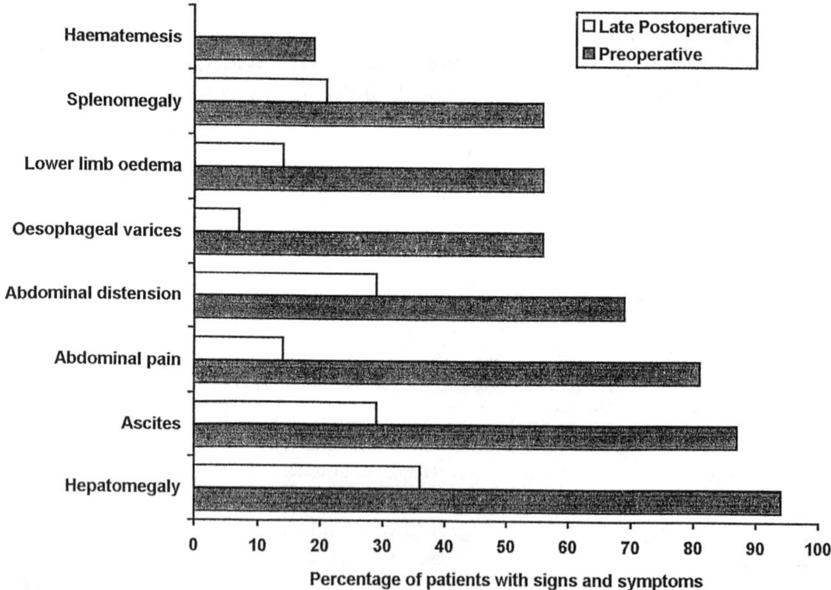

FIGURE 1.—Hepatic venous outflow obstruction. Percentage of patients with preoperative ($n=16$) and late postoperative ($n=14$) signs and symptoms. (Courtesy of Vogt PR, Andersson LC, Jenni R, et al: Dorsocranial liver resection and direct hepatoatrial anastomosis for hepatic venous outflow obstruction: Long-term outcome and functional results. *Am J Gastroenterol* 91:539–544, 1996.)

Technique.—The right atrium is opened and the incision is extended into the inferior vena cava and liver parenchyma (Fig 2). The surgeon resects the liver parenchyma while preserving the liver capsule. The right atrium is sutured to the liver capsule. This creates a combined orifice of all hepatic parenchyma and liver veins. An expandable metallic stent is placed in the intrahepatic and infrahepatic vena cava if there is severe stenosis or obstruction of the inferior vena cava.

Results.—The operative mortality rate was 12.5% and the late mortality rate was 14%. During a mean follow-up of 7.2 years, reoperation was required in 3 patients; 2 of these patients had veno-occlusive disease. Clinical improvement was noted postoperatively. The incidence of preoperative vs. postoperative signs and symptoms was as follows: hematemesis, 19% vs. 0%; splenomegaly, 56% vs. 21%; lower limb edema, 56% vs. 14%; esophageal varices, 56% vs. 7%; abdominal pain, 81% vs. 14%; ascites, 87% vs. 29%; and hepatomegaly, 94% vs. 36% (Fig 1). The mean serum bilirubin concentration decreased from 40.2 to 27.1. The serum albumin level was unchanged. In 10 of 12 survivors, a patent hepatoatrial anastomosis was observed. The survival rate was 74.2% at 5 and 10 years.

Discussion.—In the majority of these patients, dorsocranial liver resection and direct hepatoatrial anastomosis resulted in a complete cure. This

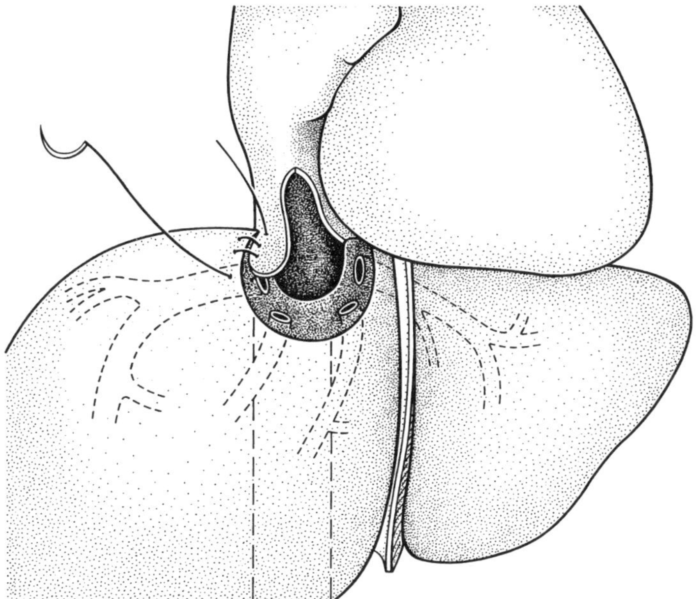

FIGURE 2.—Schematic representation of the surgical technique. The liver parenchyma, containing the orifices of all major hepatic veins, is resected. The right atrium and inferior vena cava are anastomosed to the liver capsule. (Courtesy of Vogt PR, Andersson LC, Jenni R, et al: Dorsocranial liver resection and direct hepatoatrial anastomosis for hepatic venous outflow obstruction: Long-term outcome and functional results. *Am J Gastroenterol* 91:539–544, 1996.)

procedure recreates an adequate hepatic runoff, moderates liver dysfunction, and prevents complications from portal hypertension. This procedure may be especially appropriate when the inferior vena cava is occluded; it can prevent or delay liver transplantation.

▶ It is unlikely that this operation, although apparently successful in relieving the complications of hepatic venous occlusive disease, will be applied extensively elsewhere. Although the procedure designed by Senning is a logical approach to the pathology responsible for the syndrome, it nonetheless is complex, requiring cardiopulmonary bypass and induced cardiac arrest (fibrillation). The article fails to identify the control population alluded to in the summary and to provide details of the preoperation therapy used in the study group. It is unlikely that the issue of efficacy will be resolved by a controlled trial because the entity is so diverse in origin and is fortunately relatively uncommon.

F.G. Moody, M.D.

45 Clinical Hepatology: Profile of an Urban Practice

Clinical Hepatology: Profile of an Urban, Hospital-based Practice
Byron D, Minuk GY (Univ of Manitoba, Canada)
Hepatology 24:813–815, 1996   5–49

Background.—Although liver failure is one of the major causes of death from disease among adults in North America, there is a lack of physicians with specific training in hepatology. Certain common misperceptions of the field make it less attractive to undergraduate and postgraduate students considering specialties. In general, hepatology is perceived as a specialty without diversity, dealing mainly with middle-aged alcoholic men with alcohol-induced liver disease. The nature and dynamics of an urban, hospital-based, outpatient, clinical liver practice were defined, providing information for medical students to make more informed career decisions.

Methods.—A total of 1,226 charts were reviewed retrospectively. Patients referred between July 1, 1987 and January, 1994 were included.

Findings.—Referrals for evaluation and care of patients with liver disease are rapidly increasing in frequency. Most referred patients in this series were aged 25–45 years, and the distribution of women and men was equal. Referrals were most often from general practitioners and internists. Patient turnover was common. Fifty-six percent of referred patients were no longer being followed up. Forty-seven percent of the patients had acute and chronic viral hepatitis; 11%, nonalcoholic steatohepatitis; 6%, drug-induced liver disease; 5%, alcoholic liver disease; 4%, primary biliary cirrhosis; 3%, primary sclerosing cholangitis; 3%, autoimmune chronic hepatitis; and 3%, "cryptogenic" cirrhosis. The remaining 20% had liver disease of miscellaneous or undiagnosed causes (Fig 4).

Conclusions.—Contrary to popular belief, most patients with liver disease (seen in this urban, hospital-based practice) are not middle-aged alcoholics. Rather, they are young adults with a variety of hepatobiliary disorders.

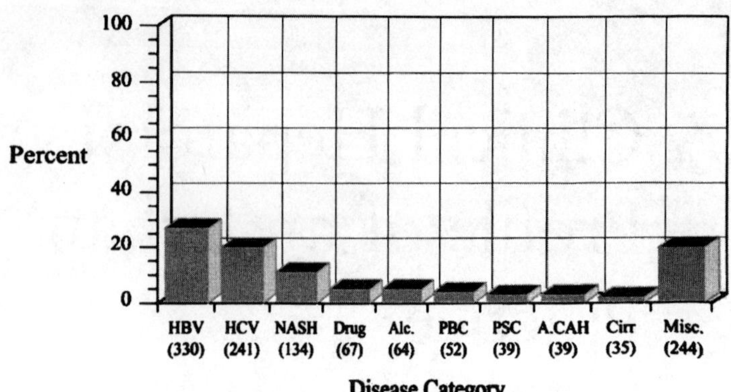

FIGURE 4.—Principal cause of liver disease in 1,226 patients attending an urban, hospital-based, outpatient liver clinic. *Abbreviations: NASH,* nonalcoholic steatohepatitis; *Alc,* alcohol-induced liver disease; *PBC,* primary biliary cirrhosis; *PSC,* primary sclerosing cholangitis; *A-CAH,* autoimmune chronic hepatitis; *Cirr,* cryptogenic cirrhosis; *Misc,* miscellaneous. (Courtesy of Byron D, Minuk GY: Clinical hepatology: Profile of an urban, hospital-based practice. *Hepatology* 24:813–815, 1996.)

▶ The perception that liver disease is associated with alcohol abuse continues to be disconcerting to the public and has stigmatized patients as well as the field of hepatology. Although alcohol abuse remains a major cause of liver disease in the United States, recent reports such as this article by Byron and Minuk and the editorial by Bach[1] indicate that alcoholic liver disease is no longer the mainstay of many contemporary hepatology practices. To illustrate, diagnostic information accumulated for 1,000 patients seen during 1995 by a faculty liver disease practice[1] indicated that hepatitis C accounted for the greatest number of referrals (45%), followed by primary biliary cirrhosis (22%), hepatitis B (7%), autoimmune chronic hepatitis (7%), hepatitis (7%), cryptogenic cirrhosis (3%), and alcoholic liver disease (only 3%).

The reports by Byron and Minuk and Bach should not be extrapolated to define an urban referral practice of hepatology. As Bach[1] emphasizes, the population of the practice, the catchment area, and the interests of the physicians within the practice will obviously influence the makeup of the profile. It seems clear, however, that the recognition of chronic viral hepatitis C facilitated by sensitive and specific diagnostic tests has uncovered a large reservoir of patients with chronic liver disease. Nevertheless, alcoholic liver disease remains a major health problem and is the second most common diagnosis among liver transplant recipients.

N.J. Greenberger, M.D.

Reference

1. Bach N: The significance of alcoholic liver disease in contemporary clinical hepatology (editorial). *Hepatology* 24:959–960, 1996.

PART SIX

THE GALLBLADDER AND BILIARY TRACT

Introduction

You will want to read this section carefully, because it will answer several very important questions related to the use of laparoscopic and retrograde endoscopic manipulations of the biliary tree in gallstone disease. For example, is laparoscopic ultrasonography as sensitive as operative (video) cholangiography in detecting the presence of a stone in the common bile duct? Possibly in some cases, but it is obviously very user dependent. Intravenous cholangiography is useful for detection of patients who would benefit from an endoscopic retrograde cholangiopancreatography; however, the patient must be at risk clinically for having a common duct stone.

Large population-based studies for a state (North Carolina) and a country (Scotland) reveal the efficacy and safety of laparoscopic surgery when its use is meaned out for all users. Studies of this type reveal that there is a prolonged learning curve and that there are situations (anatomical and pathologic) in which bile duct injury may occur. Surprisingly, these factors are involved in only a third of bile duct injury cases. Users beware. Bile duct injuries can occur for unexplained reasons and appear to have the same incidence rates in laparoscopic and open surgery. It is interesting that if a small incision is used for an open cholecystectomy, the morbidity (length of stay) is the same as when done laparoscopically. Furthermore, it is cheaper because the operating time is less.

It is now clear that surgeons who do this type of work should become proficient in clearing the duct of shadows by the transcystic route at the time of laparoscopic cholecystectomy and not leave the task to their endoscopic colleagues. However, at the slightest hint of a problem postoperatively, an endoscopic retrograde study should be done, because it will not only be diagnostic but may be therapeutic if a stone is present or a clip has slipped off from the cystic duct stump.

Frank G. Moody, M.D.

46 Radiologic Considerations

Imaging of the Common Bile Duct During Laparoscopic Cholecystectomy: Sonography Versus Videofluoroscopic Cholangiography
Teefey SA, Soper NJ, Middleton WD, et al (Washington Univ, St Louis, Mo)
AJR 165:847–851, 1995   6–1

Introduction.—Intraoperative evaluation during open cholecystectomy has included laparoscopic sonography and cholangiography; however, videofluoroscopy can further enhance the detection of bile duct calculi and delineating ductal anatomy because of its ability to show real-time video images of the injection of contrast material. During laparoscopic cholecystectomy, the accuracies of laparoscopic sonography and laparoscopic videofluoroscopic cholangiography were compared in detecting common bile duct stones and in identifying ductal anomalies.

Methods.—Laparoscopic sonography and laparoscopic videofluoroscopic cholangiography were performed on 95 patients who had laparoscopic videofluoroscopic cholecystectomy. The sonographs were conducted by a gastrointestinal surgeon using a linear-array transducer, in which the real-time video images of the studies were relayed to a remote viewing site for interpretation by an experienced radiologist. The laparoscopic cholangiograms were also performed by a gastrointestinal surgeon using a standard C-arm digital fluoroscopy unit, in which the real-time video images of the injection of contrast material were recorded using a standard videocassette recorder and relayed to a remote viewing site for interpretation by an experienced radiologist. The evaluation included the number of successful studies, the time required to complete the study, complications, the ability to completely visualize the common bile duct, cystic duct, ductal anomalies, maximum diameter of the common bile duct, and stones or debris.

Results.—Laparoscopic videofluoroscopic cholangiography was successfully performed in 90 of 95 patients, and laparoscopic sonography was successfully performed in 93 of 95 patients. Laparoscopic cholangiography took a mean of 14 ± 6 minutes to perform, whereas laparoscopic sonography took a mean of 8 ± 3 minutes to perform. The common bile duct was completely visualized in 84 of 93 patients with sonography, whereas cholangiography visualized the common bile duct in 86 of 90 patients. The cystic duct was shown in 87 of 93 patients with sonography, whereas cholangiography revealed the cystic duct in 80 of 90 patients. No ductal anomalies were seen in any of the 93 patients using sonography, whereas cholangiography showed ductal variants in 13 of 90 patients. Common bile duct stones were seen in 12 of 93 patients using sonography (Fig 1) whereas 5 of 90 patients were found to have common bile duct stones with cholangiography. In 2 of 93 patients, sonography altered operative management.

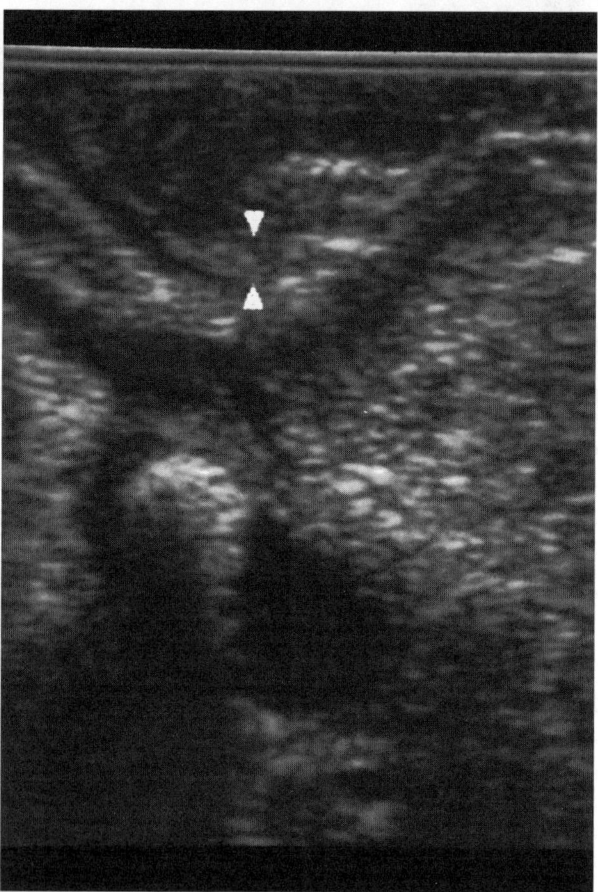

FIGURE 1.—Choledocholithiasis. Axial sonographic image of anterolateral aspect of pancreas shows obstructing 10-mm stone in distal part of common bile duct detected with laparoscopic sonography. *Triangle-shaped cursors* are centered on duodenum. Pancreatic head is located to right (*P*). (Courtesy of Teefey SA, Soper NJ, Middleton WD, et al: Imaging of the common bile duct during laparoscopic cholecystectomy: Sonography versus videofluoroscopic cholangiography. *AJR* 165:847–851, 1995.)

Conclusion.—In visualizing the common bile duct and cystic duct and in detecting common bile duct stones, laparoscopic sonography is as accurate as laparoscopic videofluoroscopic cholangiography. However, regarding the detection of ductal anomalies, data are limited to determine whether laparoscopic sonography is as accurate as laparoscopic cholangiography.

▶ Although laparoscopic ultrasonographic scanning appeared to offer little advantage over videofluoroscopic cholangiography in this study, it may be a useful adjunct to the latter when access to the bile duct cannot be obtained. I was impressed with the quality of the image generated by the Tetrad scanner as shown in Figure 1.

F.G. Moody, M.D.

Intravenous Infusion Cholangiography for Investigation of the Bile Duct: A Direct Comparison With Endoscopic Retrograde Cholangiopancreatography
Bloom ITM, Gibbs SL, Keeling-Roberts CS, et al (Stepping Hill Hosp, Stockport, England)
Br J Surg 83:755–757, 1996
6–2

Background.—The optimal method of identifying bile duct stones is controversial. Endoscopic retrograde cholangiopancreatography (ERCP) has been used increasingly frequently, but it is invasive, expensive, and associated with significant morbidity and mortality. A newer technique of slow IV infusion cholangiography (IIC) has been developed and has been reported to be safe, simple, and inexpensive. The accuracy of constant IIC was compared with that of ERCP in the investigation of the bile duct.

Methods.—Intravenous infusion cholangiography was performed in 111 consecutive patients with cholelithiasis but no jaundice and at high risk of bile duct calculi, using a 2-hour infusion of meglumine iotroxate. Within 24 hours of IIC, ERCP was also performed. The films from both procedures were interpreted by an independent radiologist.

Results.—Both procedures were successful and interpretable in 100 of the patients. There were no adverse reactions to IIC. Three patients experienced mild acute pancreatitis after ERCP, which resolved but lengthened the hospital stay. With ERCP as the gold standard, IIC had a sensitivity of 89% and a specificity of 99%.

Conclusions.—Intravenous infusion cholangiography is sensitive and specific in the evaluation of possible bile duct stones in patients without jaundice. The following investigation protocol is recommended. Patients with a low risk for bile duct stones should not undergo preoperative evaluation, and high-risk patients should undergo IIC. Patients with detected calculi or equivocal IIC results should then undergo preoperative

ERCP. This protocol will reduce the incidence of unnecessary ERCP, thereby reducing morbidity, mortality, and costs.

▶ The authors put forth a practical approach to bile duct stones in association with gallstones in high-risk patients. An IV infusion cholangiogram had a sensitivity of 89% and a specificity of 99%. This safe, relatively cheap (compared to ERCP) test deserves wider usage in this age of cost containment.

F.G. Moody, M.D.

47 Gallstones, Cholecystitis and Related Problems

Pathophysiology of Gallstones

7α-Dehydroxylating Bacteria Enhance Deoxycholic Acid Input and Cholesterol Saturation of Bile in Patients With Gallstones

Berr F, Kullak-Ublick G-A, Paumgartner G, et al (Univ of Munich; Med College of Virginia, Richmond)
Gastroenterology 111:1611–1620, 1996   6–3

Background.—Many patients with cholesterol gallstones (CGs) have excessive deoxycholic acid (DCA) in the bile acid pool with cholesterol supersaturation of bile. Whether this is caused by increased conversion of cholic acid (CA) to DCA by intestinal bacteria was studied.

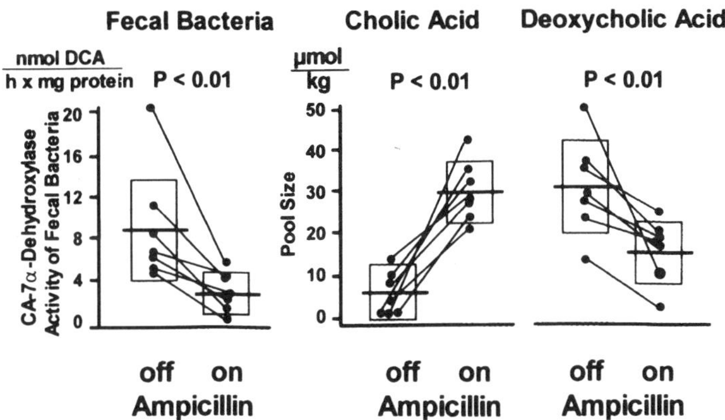

FIGURE 5.—Effect of intake of ampicillin (500 mg 4 times daily for 5 weeks) in 7 patients with DCA excess on CA-7α-dehydroxylase activity of mixed fecal anaerobic bacteria (**left panel**) and on the pool sizes of CA and DCA (**right panel**). Suppression of the CA dehydroxylating anaerobic intestinal microflora (**left panel**) reverts the bile acid metabolism to normal in patients with DCA excess (**right panel**). *Abbreviations:* DCA, deoxycholic acid; CA, cholic acid. (Courtesy of Berr F, Kullack-Ublick G-A, Paumgartner G, et al: 7α-Dehydroxylating bacteria enhance deoxycholic acid input and cholesterol saturation of bile in patients with gallstones. *Gastroenterology* 111:1611–1620, 1996.)

TABLE 5.—Effect of Ampicillin Intake on Patients With Deoxycholic Acid Excess

	Before ampicillin	Receiving ampicillin
Bile acid kinetics (n = 7)		
CDCA		
Pool size ($\mu mol \cdot kg^{-1}$)	17 ± 10	22 ± 10
Synthesis rate		
($\mu mol \cdot kg^{-1} \cdot day^{-1}$)	5.3 ± 2.0	5.6 ± 2.5
FTR (day^{-1})	0.36 ± 0.18	0.28 ± 0.12
CA		
Pool size ($\mu mol \cdot kg^{-1}$)	4.7 ± 5.6	30.5 ± 7.5*
Synthesis rate		
($\mu mol \cdot kg^{-1} \cdot day^{-1}$)	7.3 ± 1.7	11.6 ± 3.3
FTR (day^{-1})	0.70 ± 0.19	0.39 ± 0.11
DCA		
Pool size ($\mu mol \cdot kg^{-1}$)	30 ± 11	15 ± 8†
Input rate		
($\mu mol \cdot kg^{-1} \cdot day^{-1}$)	8.0 ± 1.8	4.4 ± 3.3‡
FTR (day^{-1})	0.31 ± 0.17	0.28 ± 0.10
Composition of duodenal bile (n = 6)		
Bile acid pattern (%)		
CDCA	29 ± 5	38 ± 14
CA	26 ± 5	40 ± 3*
DCA	39 ± 6	19 ± 15†
Lithocholic acid	3 ± 2	0.4 ± 0.8
Others	3 ± 2	3 ± 2
Bile acid concentration ($mmol/L$)	51 ± 22	55 ± 41
Total lipid content (g/dL)	3.93 ± 1.87	4.53 ± 3.21
Cholesterol saturation index	1.33 ± 0.22	0.92 ± 0.12*

Note: Results are expressed as mean ± SD.
*$P < 0.01$.
†$P < 0.02$.
‡$P = 0.06$ by Wilcoxon matched pair signed rank test.
Abbreviations: CDCA, ^{13}C-deoxycholic acid; *CA*, cholic acid; *DCA*, deoxycholic acid; *FTR*, fractional turnover rate.
(Courtesy of Berr F, Kullack-Ublick G-A, Paumgartner G, et al: 7α-Dehydroxylating bacteria enhance deoxycholic acid input and cholesterol saturation of bile in patients with gallstones. *Gastroenterology* 111:1611–1620, 1996.)

Methods.—Ten patients with CGs and DCA excess and 10 with low DCA were assessed. Cholic acid and DCA kinetics, ileal absorption of ^{75}Se-homotaurocholic acid (^{75}Se-HCAT), and CA-7α-dehydroxylation activity of the fecal microflora were compared. In 7 patients, the effects of ampicillin therapy on DCA excess were determined.

Findings.—The mean pool sizes of CA were 5.8 and 34 µmol/kg in the DCA excess and low DCA groups, respectively. The corresponding pool sizes of DCA were 28 and 11 µmol/kg, and DCA inputs were 8.8 and 3.5 µmol·kg⁻¹·day ⁻¹. The excretion of ^{75}Se-HCAT was similar in the 2 groups. However, patients with DCA excess had a threefold increase in CA-7α-dehydroxylation activity and a 1,000-fold higher level of fecal 7α-dehydroxylating bacteria. Treatment with ampicillin reduced CA-7α-dehydroxylation activity and DCA pool size, expanded the CA pool to normal size, and decreased cholesterol saturation of bile (Fig 5, Table 5).

Conclusions.—In a subgroup of patients with CGs, the CA pool is largely replaced by DCA. The intestinal microflora appear to play an important role in the cause of CG in some patients. Increased DCA formation seems to significantly increase the amount of cholesterol secreted into bile, associated with an increase in the cholesterol saturation index.

▶ In healthy adults, DCA constitutes 20% or less of the bile acid pool and the DCA:CA ratio is less than 1.0. However, enrichment of the bile acid pool with more DCA than CA occurs in 20% to 30% of patients with CGs. In such patients with gallstones, CA is rapidly dehydroxylated to DCA, most of which is absorbed, enters the bile acid pool, and changes the DCA:CA ratio to 1.5 or more.

This study sought to determine the mechanism of increased DCA formation in a select group of patients with CGs. The investigators have demonstrated that the increased DCA formation in their patients is the result of a 1,000-fold increase in the titers of intestinal bacteria with 7-α dehydroxylate activity. These findings suggest an important role for the intestinal microflora in the pathogenesis of CGs in selected patients. Note the effect of ampicillin in suppressing the CA dehydroxylating activity of the intestinal microflora resulting in a reversion, albeit temporary, of bile acid metabolism to normal in patients with an excess of DCA in their bile acid pool. As the authors point out, the study rekindles interest in the role of intestinal microflora in producing excess DCA in CG disease, a hypothesis first proposed over 20 years ago.[1]

N.J. Greenberger, M.D.

Reference

1. Low-Bear TS, Pomore EW: Can colonic bacterial metabolites predispose to cholesterol gallstones? *BMJ* 1:438–440, 1975.

A New Subgroup of Lectin-bound Biliary Proteins Binds to Cholesterol Crystals, Modifies Crystal Morphology, and Inhibits Cholesterol Crystallization
Busch N, Lammert F, Marschall H-U, et al (Aachen Univ of Technology, Germany)
J Clin Invest 96:3009–3015, 1995   6–4

Background.—Biliary proteins that inhibit or promote cholesterol crystallization are thought to play an important role in the pathogenesis of cholesterol gallstones. A new subgroup of 4 biliary glycoproteins (GPs) that adsorb to cholesterol crystals was reported.

Methods and Findings.—Various GP mixtures were extracted from abnormal human gallbladder bile using lectin affinity chromatography on concanavalin A, lentil, and *Helix pomatia* columns. These mixtures were added to supersaturated model bile. The same 4 GPs were isolated from the cholesterol crystals harvested, independent of the protein mixtures added. The molecular masses of these GPs were 16, 28, 63, and 74 kd,

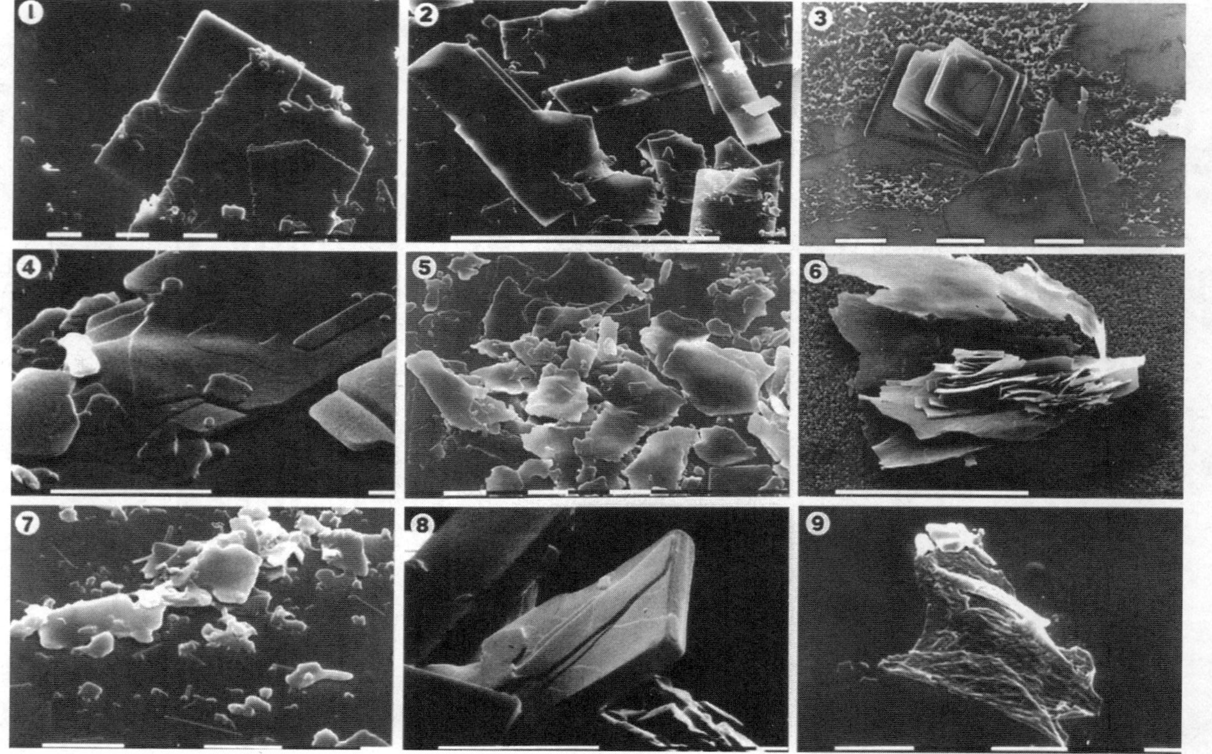

FIGURE 3.—Representative scanning electron micrographs of the characteristic classes of cholesterol crystals. **1,** euhedral triclinic crystal plate; **2,** regular aggregates; **3,** compact microliths; **4,** polycyclic crystal plates; **5,** random aggregates; **6,** cluster of radially arranged polycyclic plates; **7,** random aggregates and rodlike structures showing augmentations at 1 end representing evolving crystal plates; **8,** a compact triclinic crystal plate; and **9,** amorphous concrement. In the presence of lectin-bound proteins, structures 1–3 and 8 were found most frequently. In controls, structures 4–6 were predominant. *Bars* represent 100 μm in 2 and 6, and 10 μm in all other micrographs. (Courtesy of Busch N, Lammert F, Marschall H-U, et al: A new subgroup of lectin-bound biliary proteins binds to cholesterol crystals, modifies crystal morphology, and inhibits cholesterol crystallization. *J Clin Invest* 96:3009–3015, 1995. Reproduced from *The Journal of Clinical Investigation* by copyright permission of The American Society for Clinical Investigation.)

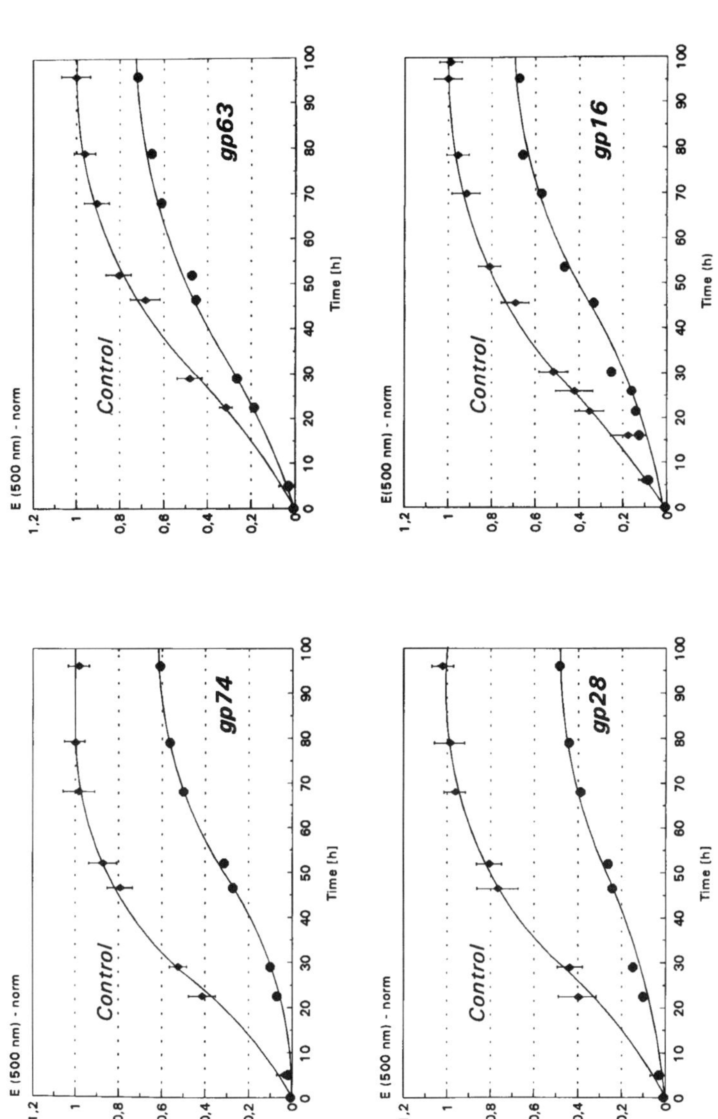

FIGURE 5.—Comparative effect of the isolated glycoproteins (10 μg/mL) on cholesterol crystal growth curves in model bile. Crystal concentrations are proportional to the absorbance of the samples measured at 500 nm. Graphs were normalized by setting the plateau of each individual control of the independent experiments to unity [Extinction (E) (500 nm) − norm]. Control curves are given as mean ± SD ($n = 3$). Each experimental curve is given as a mean ($n = 2$). Differences between control and experimental curves were statistically significant: $P = 0.001$ for GP28, GP63, and GP74; $P < 0.05$ for GP16. Growth curve indices were calculated from measured values for each glycoprotein: GP74; $I_g = 0.56$, $I_c = 0.61$; GP63: $I_g = 0.67$, $I_c = 0.73$; GP16: $I_g = 0.63$, $I_c = 0.69$; GP28: $I_g = 0.39$, $I_c = 0.46$. (Courtesy of Busch N, Lammert F, Marschall H-U, et al: A new subgroup of lectin-bound biliary proteins binds to cholesterol crystals, modifies crystal morphology, and inhibits cholesterol crystallization. *J Clin Invest* 96:3009–3015, 1995. Reproduced from *The Journal of Clinical Investigation* by copyright permission of The American Society for Clinical Investigation.)

respectively. After protein purification using preparative SDS-PAGE, their influence on cholesterol crystallization in model bile was assessed at 10 μg/mL. Glycoprotein 63 reduced crystal growth by 76%; GP16, by 65%; GP74, by 55%; and GP28, by 40%. Scanning electron microscopic studies provided further evidence that the inhibiting effect on cholesterol crystallization is mediated by protein-crystal interaction. Significantly more ordered structures were associated with crystals grown in the presence of inhibiting proteins. Compared with control values, the incidence of triclinic crystals and regular aggregates was shifted from 30% to 70% (Figs 3 and 5).

Conclusions.—These new biliary proteins bind to cholesterol crystals, modify crystal morphology, and inhibit cholesterol crystallization. They are the most potent biliary inhibitors of cholesterol crystallization reported to date.

▶ This elegant study describes 4 novel biliary GPs that are the most potent biliary inhibitors of cholesterol crystallization reported thus far. The inhibitory effect on cholesterol crystallization is mediated by protein-crystal interaction and was demonstrated by scanning electron microscopic studies. The irregular aggregates and the clusters of crystals that predominated in the populations grown *without* inhibitor proteins suggest that such aggregates may form a nidus for the deposition of biliary mucus, pigment, and precipitates of calcium, bilirubinate, and carbonate. These observations are an important contribution to our understanding of cholesterol gallstone pathogenesis.

N.J. Greenberger, M.D.

Gallbladder Emptying and Gallstone Formation: A Prospective Study on Gallstone Recurrence
Pauletzki J, Althaus R, Holl J, et al (Univ of Munich)
Gastroenterology 111:765–771, 1996   6–5

Introduction.—Patients with gallstones have been shown to have a smaller fractional gallbladder emptying, compared with healthy controls. A signal-transduction defect in gallbladder smooth muscle in patients with cholesterol stones is thought to cause this impairment in gallbladder motility. The effect of gallbladder emptying on the formation of recurrent stones was evaluated prospectively to determine the role of impaired gallbladder motility in this process.

Methods.—Fifty-four patients were evaluated for gallstone recurrence after lithotripsy and findings were compared with those of 24 healthy controls. Patients and controls underwent sonographic assessment of gallbladder emptying before lithotripsy and a mean of 1.8 years after gallstone disappearance. Patients were observed for gallstone recurrence for a median of 2.6 years (range, 0.6–4.1 years).

Results.—Compared with healthy controls, patients with gallstones had fasting volumes that were one-third larger. Between-group ejection volumes were similar because patients with gallstones had residual volumes that were more than double those of normal controls. The ejection rate was decreased by one third in patients with gallstones. After lithotripsy, stone-free patients and controls had similar fasting volumes, but stone-free patients had moderately increased residual volumes and significantly decreased ejection fraction and ejection rate. Recurrent stones formed in 16 of 54 patients at a range of 0.5–2.6 years after successful initial therapy. Compared with patients without later recurrence of gallstones, patients with recurrence had distinctly decreased gallbladder emptying. Patients who formed recurrent stones had marked reductions in ejection volume, ejection fraction, and ejection rate. Patients with recurrence had an enlarged (by one third) residual volume of the gallbladder. The residual volume of patients with recurrence was 250% greater, compared with normal controls. Patients with good gallbladder emptying had a much lower risk of recurrence, compared with patients with impaired gallbladder emptying. In the first 3 years of follow-up, 13% of patients with an ejection fraction greater than 60% and 53% of patients with ejection fraction less than 60% had recurrent stones. The major determinant of gallstone recurrence was the ejection fraction.

Conclusion.—The presence of gallbladder stones is correlated with a reversible enlargement of fasting and residual volumes of the gallbladder. Thirteen percent and 53% of patients with good and poor gallbladder emptying, respectively, formed recurrent stones. Gallbladder emptying was a major determinant of gallstone recurrence in patients who underwent biliary lithotripsy.

▶ The gallstone busters at the Klinikum Grosshadern have made an important observation. Patients who have the highest recurrence rate of gallstones have the lowest ejection fraction as an index of gallbladder dysmotility. This finding adds further credence to the hypothesis that a disturbance in gallbladder emptying is an important event in cholesterol gallstone formation.

F.G. Moody, M.D.

Total Protein Content of Human Gallbladder Bile: Relation to Cholesterol Gallstone Disease and Effects of Treatment With Bile Acids and Aspirin
Sahlin S (Karolinska Inst Danderyd Hosp, Stockholm)
Eur J Surg 162:463–469, 1996   6–6

Background.—The nucleation time of cholesterol monohydrate crystals may be a better variable than cholesterol saturation for discriminating between patients with and without cholesterol gallstones. Several researchers have suggested that gallbladder mucin may play an important role as a nucleating substance. However, there has been no major breakthrough for any specific protein fraction or other substances. The total protein content of gallbladder bile was measured and related to cholesterol gall-stone formation.

Methods.—One hundred two consecutive patients were enrolled in the prospective study. Seventy-three were undergoing cholecystectomy for cholesterol gallstones and 29 for adenomyomas or cholesterolosis in the gallbladder wall. Treatment with the gallstone solvents chenodeoxycholic acid (CDCA), ursodeoxycholic acid (UDCA) or aspirin was given to 30 patients will gallstones.

Findings.—Total protein content differed only in the group treated with UDCA, which had significantly less protein than the other groups. Bile with and without crystals did not differ. Protein content was positively correlated with biliary cholesterol concentration and saturation. Total protein content in bile was unaffected by aspirin.

Conclusion.—Patients with and without cholesterol crystals have similar total protein concentrations in gallbladder bile, suggesting that the total protein content in bile does not affect the formation of cholesterol crystals nor, subsequently, gallstones. The UDCA-treated group was the only one with significantly less protein, indicating that the mode of action of UDCA differs from that of CDCA.

▶ This study presents some interesting data for those interested in cholelithogenesis and protein content in bile. The ingestion of UDCA, but not CDCA or aspirin, was associated with a decreased protein concentration in bile. The protein contents of bile with and without cholesterol crystals were similar. This raises the question of the presumed role of glycoprotein as a nidation factor in human bile. Hopefully, this study will provoke further studies of bile composition under a variety of circumstance, including patients who have their normal gallbladders removed prophylactically or in association with other procedures such as radical pancreaticoduodenectomy for pancreatic neoplasms.

F.G. Moody, M.D.

Ursodeoxycholic Acid Reduces Protein Levels and Nucleation-promoting Activity in Human Gallbladder Bile
van Erpecum KJ, Portincasa P, Eckhardt E, et al (Univ Hosp Utrecht, The Netherlands; St Antonius Ziekenhuis, Nieuwegein The Netherlands; Univ Hosp, Amsterdam)
Gastroenterology 110:1225–1237, 1996   6–7

Background.—In selected patients, ursodeoxycholic acid (UDCA) can prevent gallstone formation. Whether reduced concentrations and nucleation-promoting activity of various proteins contribute to this benefit was determined.

Methods.—Twenty-six patients with symptomatic cholesterol gallstones undergoing elective cholecystectomy were studied. Thirteen patients were treated with UDCA, 10 mg/kg per day, at bedtime for 3 weeks. The remaining 13 patients served as the control group.

Findings.—Treatment with UDCA greatly reduced the total protein concentration in gallbladder bile and the concanavalin A–binding fraction. There were also significant reductions in gallbladder bile α1-acid glyco-protein, haptoglobin, Ig A, Ig G, γ-glutamyl transpeptidase, and amino-peptidase N. However, Ig M, mucin, and β-glucuronidase were not de-creased. The most marked reductions were in proteins of canalicular membrane origin. Gallbladder bile total protein was associated with the cholesterol saturation index but not the bile salt hydrophobicity index. Treatment with UDCA also significantly reduced the crystallization-pro-moting activity of the concanavalin A-binding fraction.

Conclusion.—Treatment with UDCA reduces the concentrations of var-ious proteins and their nucleation-promoting activity in the gallbladder bile of patients with cholesterol gallstones. The effects of UDCA on nu-cleation-promoting proteins may be associated with the efficacy of UDCA in preventing cholesterol gallstone formation.

▶ The advent of laparoscopic cholecystectomy has slowed the pace of studies directed toward understanding the pathogenesis of gallstones. This is one of the negative effects of this new effective therapy, because it detracts from the knowledge required to prevent cholesterol crystallization in patients at risk, a potentially preventable pathologic process that leads to cholesterol gallstones. This multiinstitutional study from the Netherlands sheds further light on how UDCA, when taken orally, can prevent gallstones. The results clearly show that the secretion of a variety of mucoproteins are attenuated after ingestion of UDCA, several of which may contribute to the nucleation-promoting activity in the bile of patients in whom cholesterol gallstones develop.

F.G. Moody, M.D.

Bowel Habits After Cholecystectomy

Bowel Habit After Cholecystectomy: Physiological Changes and Clinical Implications
Fort JM, Azpiroz F, Casellas F, et al (Autonomous Univ, Barcelona)
Gastroenterology 111:617–622, 1996   6–8

Background.—A 2-year prospective study estimated that persistent di-arrhea develops in approximately 8% of patients undergoing elective cholecystectomy; the true incidence could be higher because milder cases may not be reported. To elucidate the pathophysiology of postcholecys-tectomy diarrhea, the effects of cholecystectomy on both transit time and bowel habit were examined.

Methods.—Five experimental groups of patients were included in the study: 29 patients before and 1 month after uncomplicated cholecystec-tomy, 22 patients 4 years after cholecystectomy, 14 patients with post-cholecystectomy diarrhea, and 2 control groups consisting of 5 patients

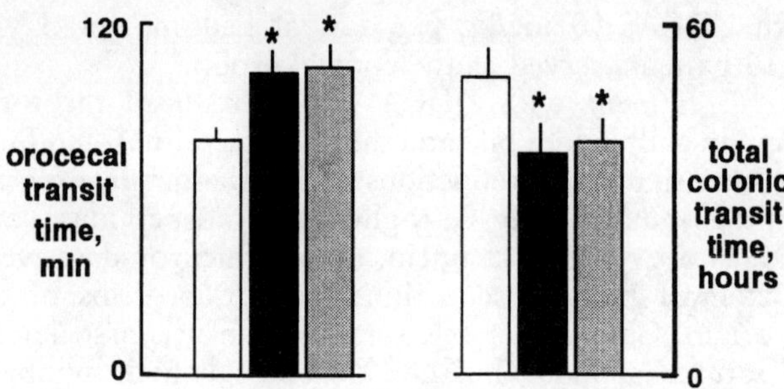

FIGURE 1.—Effect of cholecystectomy on orocecal and total colonic transit time. One month after cholecystectomy (*solid bars*), patients had slower orocecal and faster colonic transit than before cholecystectomy (*open bars*). Transit times in patients 4 years after cholecystectomy (*shaded bars*) were more similar than transit times after 1 month. Values are expressed as means ± SE. *$P \leq 0.05$ vs. before cholecystectomy. (Courtesy of Fort JM, Azpiroz F, Casellas F, et al: Bowel habit after cholecystectomy: Physiological changes and clinical implications. *Gastroenterology* 111:617–622, 1996.)

with acute infectious diarrhea and 13 patients before and 1 month after other elective surgery. A modified radiopaque pellet method was used to measure colonic transit, and the standard lactulose breath H_2 test was used to measure orocecal transit.

Results.—Colonic transit was substantially accelerated (51 hours before vs. 38 hours after) and orocecal transit was slightly delayed (80 minutes before vs. 103 minutes after) 1 month after cholecystectomy as opposed to before (Fig 1). Four years after cholecystectomy, similar colonic and orocecal transit times were measured. Patients with postcholecystectomy di-

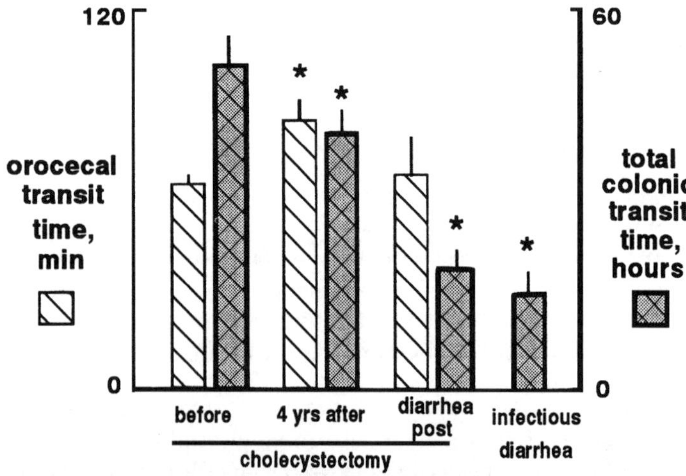

FIGURE 3.—Orocecal transit time and total colonic transit time in patients with postcholecystectomy diarrhea. Colonic transit was in the range of transit times of patients with infectious diarrhea, markedly faster than in patients before cholecystectomy and 4 years after cholecystectomy. In contrast to the latter, orocecal transit was not prolonged in patients with postcholecystectomy diarrhea. Values are expressed as means ± SE. *$P \leq 0.05$ vs. before cholecystectomy. (Courtesy of Fort JM, Azpiroz F, Casellas F, et al: Bowel habit after cholecystectomy: Physiological changes and clinical implications. *Gastroenterology* 111:617–622, 1996.)

arrhea and patients with acute infectious diarrhea showed similar acceleration in colonic transit time (Fig 3). Gut transit was not affected by surgery per se. Postcholecystectomy diarrhea occurred in 12% of this study population.

Conclusions.—These data suggest that cholecystectomy shortens gut transit time by accelerating passage of the fecal bolus through the colon, with marked acceleration in the right colon. Cholecystectomy may cause an increase in colonic bile output and a shift in bile acid composition toward the more diarrheogenic secondary bile acids. A substantial fraction of patients having cholecystectomy were aware of a change in bowel function after surgery, although all did not consider the change to have a significant effect on their lives (a few patients who had previously suffered from constipation considered the effect positive.)

▶ This study clearly demonstrates that cholecystectomy induces persistent changes in gut transit and that these changes effect a noticeable modification of bowel habits. The major change is accelerated transit in the right colon. This colonic effect is apparently due to an increase in colonic bile acid input, which in turn is related to increased enterohepatic cycling of bile acid cycles after removal of the gallbladder.

The authors also conducted a phone survey of 148 patients who underwent cholecystectomy 4 years previously; in this survey 47 patients (32%) had noted a change in bowel habits, i.e., either an increase in defecation frequency or decreased stool consistency. Further, in 18 patients (12%) the diarrhea was severe enough, i.e., 3 or more watery movements per day, to be classified as postcholecystectomy diarrhea. This finding is in accord with previous surveys[1] that have reported that persistent diarrhea develops in approximately 8% of patients undergoing elective cholecystectomy. In this setting, treatment with a bile acid sequestering agent such as cholestyramine is often effective in ameliorating troublesome diarrhea.

N.J. Greenberger, M.D.

Reference

1. Ros E, Zambon D: Post cholecystectomy symptoms: A prospective study of gall stone patients before and two years after surgery. *Gut* 28:1500–1504, 1987.

48 Laparoscopic Cholecystectomy and Related Issues

Randomised, Prospective, Single-blind Comparison of Laparoscopic Versus Small-incision Cholecystectomy
Majeed AW, Troy G, Nicholl JP, et al (Univ of Sheffield, England)
Lancet 347:989–994, 1996   6–9

Background.—The size of the incision made for open cholecystectomy has been getting smaller in the past 10 years, which makes the procedure safer. Before small-incision procedures became established in surgical practice, however, laparoscopically assisted removal of the gallbladder was introduced. This procedure rapidly became popular despite safety concerns. Previous trials of these two techniques did not account for the effects of patients' and health care providers' beliefs, which may affect study results. The current prospective, randomized, single-blind comparison of laparoscopic and small-incision cholecystectomy was designed to eliminate such bias.

Methods.—Two hundred patients were randomly assigned to one or the other procedure in the operating room. Anesthetic technique and pain-control methods were standardized. Both types of procedures were performed by four experienced surgeons. Identical wound dressings were applied so that care providers were unaware of the procedure type.

Findings.—The median length of laparoscopic cholecystectomy was 65 minutes, which was significantly longer than the median 40 minutes required for the small-incision surgery. The two groups did not differ significantly in postoperative recovery, length of hospitalization, time until return to work, or time until full activity.

Conclusions.—Laparoscopic cholecystectomy offers no advantages over small-incision cholecystectomy in postoperative recovery, hospital stay, or time until back to work or full recovery. It also takes longer to perform. Thus, laparoscopic cholecystectomy may be more expensive than the small-incision procedure.

▶ The authors have made an effort to conduct a well-controlled randomized trial of mini cholecystectomy (small incision) vs. laparoscopic cholecystectomy. One could argue about why the patients who underwent laparoscopic cholecystectomy stayed in the hospital for 3 days and could possibly quibble about other facets of the trial, but the results are clear; laparoscopic cholecystectomy took considerably longer to perform without any apparent beneficial effects. I imagine that this outcome related to the operating surgeons being careful to not molest the peritoneal cavity by placing their hands within it. Compression and stretching of the intra-abdominal viscera are likely the reason for a slower recovery in patients undergoing open cholecystectomy.

F.G. Moody, M.D.

Bile Duct Injuries, 1989–1993; A Statewide Experience
Russell JC, for the Connecticut Laparoscopic Cholecystectomy Registry (Connecticut Society of American Board Surgeons)
Arch Surg 131:382–388, 1996   6–10

Background.—Laparoscopic cholecystectomy (LC) has supplanted open cholecystectomy (OC) in the treatment of symptomatic cholelithiasis. Despite the obvious advantages of LC, however, it appears to be associated with an increase in the incidence of major bile duct injuries (MBDIs). This association was further investigated.

Methods and Findings.—The medical records of 30,211 patients undergoing OC or LC in Connecticut hospitals were reviewed. Forty-seven cases of MBDI were confirmed. The incidence of MBDI increased from 0.04% in 1989 to 0.24% in 1991, then declined to 0.11% in 1993. The increase was attributed to the greater number of cholecystectomies and the initial increased risk of LC-related injury. The decrease in LC MBDI between 1990 and 1993 was significant. The difference between LC and OC was no longer significant by 1993. Acute cholecystitis and gallstone pancreatitis raised the risk of MBDI during LC, the odds ratios being 3.3 and 3.6, respectively. The LC MBDIs tended to be ductal excision or transections and frequently were not diagnosed during surgery. Intraoperative recognition and repair were facilitated by cholangiography during surgery. Eighty-nine percent of the patients had definitive management of MBDI at their hospital of origin. Five percent of that group needed further intervention.

Conclusion.—Surgery for acute cholecystitis and gallstone pancreatitis increases the risk for MBDI. Outcomes depend on ductal anatomy, the timing of injury recognition, and the method of repair. Most patients are treated successfully at the hospital of origin. Long-term outcomes are good. Late bile duct strictures seem to be rare.

▶ Doctors participating in the Connecticut Laparoscopic Cholecystectomy Registry have established that they now have reached a point in their learning curve where bile duct injury is at the level of open cholecystectomy. Patients with complex gallstone disease (gallstone pancreatitis and acute cholecystitis) are at risk for this complication. Intraoperative cholangiography was helpful in early recognition of injury. One major injury per 1,000 operations will likely be adopted as the standard of care.

F.G. Moody, M.D.

Incidence and Nature of Bile Duct Injuries Following Laparoscopic Cholecystectomy: An Audit of 5913 Cases
Richardson MC, Bell G, Fullarton GM, et al (Gartnavel Gen Hosp, Glasgow, Inverclyde Royal Hosp, Greenock, Scotland)
Br J Surg 83:1356–1360, 1996   6–11

Background.—The apparent increase in the incidence of bile duct injury associated with laparoscopic cholecystectomy has raised concern worldwide. However, the true incidence and mechanism of iatrogenic ductal injury remain unclear. Biliary ductal injuries associated with the introduction of laparoscopic cholecystectomy in the west of Scotland were audited prospectively during a 5-year period.

Methods and Findings.—Forty-eight surgeons performing laparoscopic cholecystectomy in 19 hospitals contributed data between September 1990 and September 1995. Complete data were available for 98.3% of 5,913 laparoscopic cholecystectomies attempted. Thirty-seven laparoscopic bile duct injuries occurred during the study period. The annual incidence peaked at 0.8%, declining to 0.4% in the last year of the audit. In the practices of 22 surgeons, injuries occurred after a median personal experience of 51 procedures. Twenty of the 37 injured patients had major bile duct injuries, for an incidence of 0.3%. The mechanisms underlying laparoscopic ductal injury included tenting, confluence, and diathermy injuries as well as the classical and variant classical types. In 18 patients, ductal injuries were noticed intraoperatively and repaired, yielding good clinical outcomes in 17. Only 13 of the 37 patients had contributory factors such as severe inflammation, aberrant anatomy, and poor visualization.

Conclusions.—In the introductory period of laparoscopic cholecystectomy use, the overall bile duct injury rate is higher than that associated with open cholecystectomy (though the incidence of major ductal injury is similar). The later downward trend seen in the current study suggests a prolonged learning curve. A better understanding of the mechanism of injury may help to further reduce the occurrence of this complication.

▶ The Scottish surgeons who participated in this trial provide a strong statistical view of the incidence of bile duct injury in association with laparoscopic cholecystectomy. Major bile duct injuries occurred in 0.3% of cases. It is of interest that the data suggest a prolonged learning curve, which implies that if one does a large number of such procedures, a major injury will ultimately occur. Their experience delineates "contributing factors" (anatomical and pathological) that occurred in about a third of those injured.

F.G. Moody, M.D.

Technical Difficulties and Complications During Laparoscopic Cholecystectomy: Predictive Use of Preoperative Ultrasonography
Santambrogio R, Montorsi M, Bianchi P, et al (Ospedale San Paolo, Milan, Italy; Universita di Milano, Italy; Osp Fatebenefratelli e Oftalmico, Milan, Italy)
World J Surg 20:978–982, 1996   6–12

Background.—Although the rate of technical problems and incidence of postoperative complications associated with laparoscopic cholecystectomy (LC) are low, they can result in significant morbidity. The role of preoperative US findings in predicting potential intraoperative difficulties and complications was investigated.

Methods.—One hundred forty-three patients with symptomatic cholelithiasis underwent US assessment the day before LC. Gallbladder (GB) volume, GB wall thickness, GB neck position, GB stone mobility, stone maximum size, and GB adhesions were assessed. One hundred one patients initially had uncomplicated symptomatic cholelithiasis, and 42 had acute cholecystitis.

Findings.—On the basis of the US findings, surgery was predicted to be easy in 38% of the patients, difficult in 49%, and very difficult in 13%. The correlation with the surgeon's intraoperative judgment was good. Stone mobility, presence of adhesions, and procedure difficulty were significantly correlated. The predictive US assessment was associated significantly with some intraoperative technical steps and with intraoperative bleeding.

Conclusions.—Preoperative US is a useful screening tool to help predict technical problems in LC. However, in a significant number of patients, the concordance between the preoperative US classification and surgical findings was not satisfactory.

▶ It is encouraging to learn that a test as cheap and noninvasive as ultrasonography of the gallbladder can yield useful information toward safety of its removal when diseased. The authors are obviously surgeons, because they categorize the anticipated difficulty of the procedure as easy, difficult, or very difficult. Keep in mind that it is the easy cholecystectomy that is vulnerable to bile duct injury, because the bile duct may be small and quite mobile. Elisabeth Vincent-Hamelin, M.D., of the University of San Carlos Hospital, in Madrid, provides additional US criteria that would enhance the predictive value of US, and, in her invited commentary, she suggests that one use more than one criterion for this purpose. I agree with her on this point and with her recommendation that the authors should more precisely define operative difficulty.

F.G. Moody, M.D.

The Impact of Laparoscopic Cholecystectomy on the Management and Outcome of Biliary Tract Disease in North Carolina: A Statewide, Population-based, Time-series Analysis
Rutledge R, Fakhry SM, Baker CC, et al (Univ of North Carolina, Chapel Hill)
J Am Coll Surg 183:31–45, 1996   6–13

Introduction.—The surgical community has undergone a revolution in basic ideology with the introduction of laparoscopic cholecystectomy (LC). Few randomized trials have been large and comprehensive enough to be able to make generalized conclusions regarding LC in comparison with open cholecystectomy (OC). A statewide population-based database was used to determine the effects of LC on biliary surgery.

Methods.—A complete population-based, time-series analysis of all patients admitted for biliary tract disease from all 157 nonfederal hospitals in North Carolina from 1988 through 1993 was performed using the statewide hospital discharge database.

Results.—From 1989 to 1993, there was a 74% drop in the number of OCs performed (14,083 vs. 3,731). This decline was correlated with a rapid rise in LCs from 1990 to 1993. In that period, the rate of LCs rose from 0.1% to 67% of all cholecystectomies performed (Fig 1). Increased use of LC was not associated with an overall rise in the rate of cholecystectomy; the total yearly rate of all cholecystectomies actually decreased in North Carolina after 1990. The rate of bile duct repairs rose from 13 in 1988 to 36 in 1992. There was a significantly strong association between the rate of LCs and rate of bile duct repairs. Regardless of age or type of gallbladder disease, patients undergoing LC had significantly lower hospital charges and component charges, compared with patients undergoing

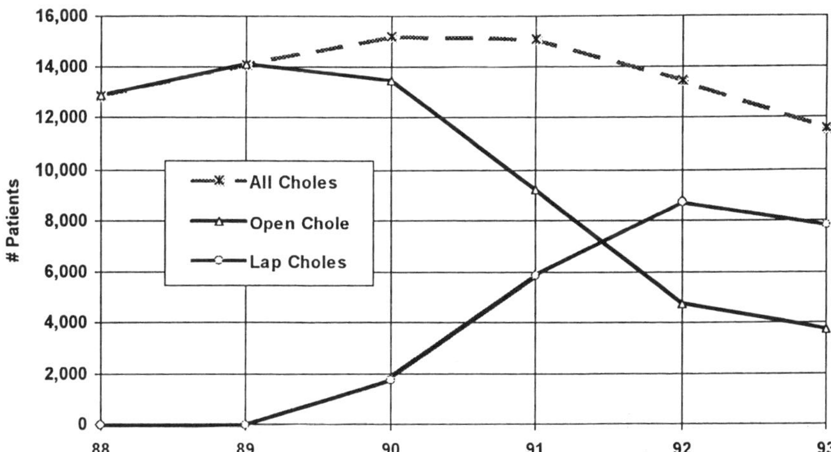

FIGURE 1.—Rates of laparoscopic and open cholecystectomy, shown by year. *Abbreviations: Chole,* cholecystectomy: *Lap,* laparoscopy; #, number. (From Rutledge R, Fakhry SM, Baker CC, et al: The impact of laparoscopic cholecystectomy on the management and outcome of biliary tract disease in North Carolina: A statewide, population-based, time-series analysis. *J Am Coll Surg* 183:31–45, 1996. By permission of the *Journal of the American College of Surgeons.*)

OC. Patients undergoing LC had significantly shorter hospital stays than patients undergoing OC. Compared with older and non–board certified surgeons, surgeons who were younger and board certified adopted LC more quickly. Surgeons from large hospitals were quicker to adopt LC than surgeons from smaller hospitals.

Conclusion.—From 1988 though 1993, LCs in North Carolina went from being nonexistent to the "gold standard" approach for managing patients with cholelithiasis. Use of LC was positively correlated with shorter hospital stays and lower charges.

▶ This geographically defined, population-based study likely reflects what is happening nationwide. Laparoscopic cholecystectomy is gradually replacing OC as the treatment of gallstones for cholelithiasis. There are no surprises in this comprehensive report from North Carolina. The mortality for the procedure was marginally less for the laparoscopic approach, but this could have been the result of selection of lower risk groups. The 27% decrease in cost for LC, however, appeared to be directly related to a significant decrease in length of hospital stay, as has been the experience elsewhere. It was heartening to learn that the bile duct injury rate, as judged by yearly rate of bile duct repairs, has returned to an acceptable rate (0.36%) as experience has been gained with the laparoscopic approach; and as the authors currently point out, LC is the standard approach to almost all complications of gallstone disease.

F.G. Moody, M.D.

A Cost-minimization Analysis of Laparoscopic Cholecystectomy Versus Open Cholecystectomy

Berggren U, Zethraeus N, Arvidsson D, et al (Uppsala Univ, Sweden; Stockholm School of Economics)

Am J Surg 172:305–310, 1996

6–14

Background.—Previous cost analyses of open and laparoscopic cholecystectomy have assessed charges but have not considered the costs nor lost production associated with each procedure. The costs of open and laparoscopic cholecystectomy were compared in a cost-minimization analysis.

Methods.—Data were obtained from clinical studies, Swedish national registers, local patient statistics, and hospital accounting systems. Both direct and indirect costs were determined. A clinical decision model was used.

Findings.—Laparoscopic cholecystectomy was less costly than the open procedure. The cost savings achieved with the former technique was approximately $310 per patient (in 1994), provided at least 68 patients were operated on annually. When only hospital expenses were calculated, open cholecystectomy was less costly (Fig 1).

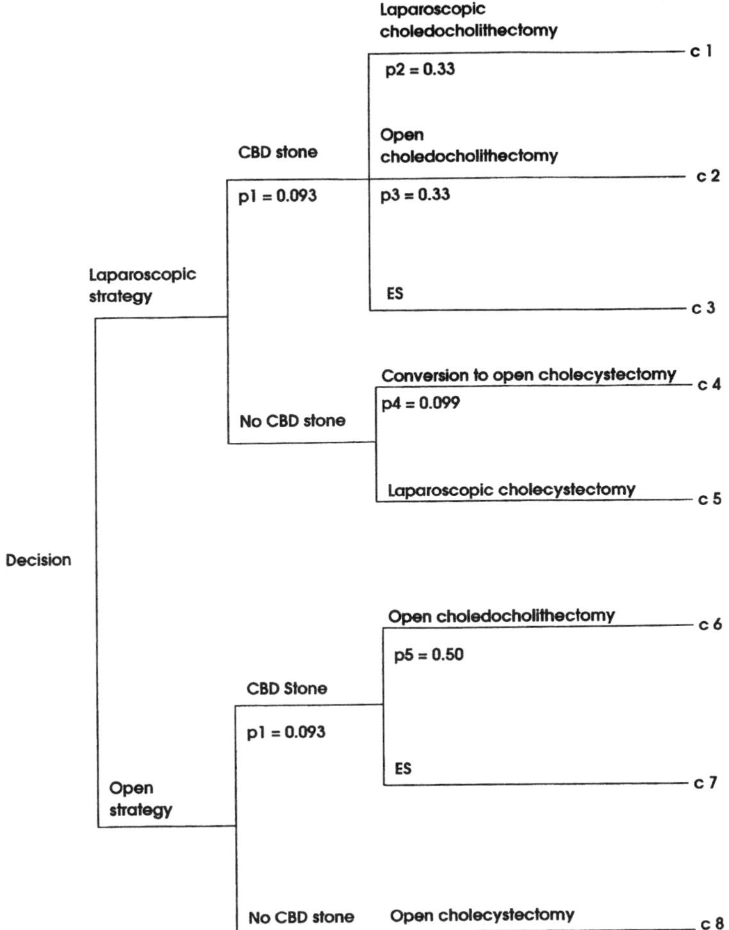

FIGURE 1.—A clinical decision model showing relevant clinical options for treating gallstones. There are 8 different cost end points, c1–c8. *Abbreviations: CBD,* common bile duct; *ES,* endoscopic sphincterotomy. (Reprinted by permission of the publisher, from Berggren U, Zethraeus N, Arvidsson D, et al: A cost-minimization analysis of laparoscopic cholecystectomy versus open cholecystectomy. *Am J Surg* 172:305–310, Copyright 1996, by Excerpta Medica Inc.)

Conclusions.—When indirect costs are considered in economic analyses of open and laparoscopic cholecystectomy, the laparoscopic procedure is less expensive. This is because patients are able to return to work in a shorter period.

▶ Swedish physicians and surgeons are decades ahead of their U.S. counterparts in rationalizing health care as to its costs. In this communication, they compare the relative cost to society of laparoscopic vs. open cholecystectomy. The former saved them (the people through their government) 2,400 Swedish kronor (approximately $400). To achieve this savings, the operating unit had to perform 68 cases. It is of interest that the hospital-based costs were cheaper for the open procedure because of the incremental up-front costs of the technology and larger operating times associated with the laparoscopic approach.

F.G. Moody, M.D.

49 Endoscopic Biliary Tract Procedures and Related Problems

Complications of Endoscopic Biliary Sphincterotomy

Complications of Endoscopic Biliary Sphincterotomy
Freeman ML, Nelson DB, Sherman S, et al (Hennepin County Med Ctr, Minneapolis, Minn; Minneapolis Veterans Affairs Med Ctr, Minn; Indiana Univ, Indianapolis)
N Engl J Med 335:909–918, 1996   6–15

Background.—Endoscopic sphincterotomy is often used to treat bile duct stones and other problems. Risk factors for complications associated with this procedure were investigated prospectively.

Methods and Findings.—Complications occurring within 30 days of endoscopic biliary sphincterotomy in 2,347 consecutive patients treated at 17 centers in the United States and Canada from 1992 through 1994 were documented. Ten percent of the patients had complications. Pancreatitis occurred in 5.4% and hemorrhage in 2% of the whole group (Table 1). Fifty-five patients died within 30 days of the procedure, 10 from causes directly or indirectly associated with the procedure. In a multivariate analysis, suspected dysfunction of the sphincter of Oddi, cirrhosis, difficulty cannulating the bile duct, achieving access to the bile duct by "precut" sphincterotomy, and the use of a combined percutaneous-endoscopic procedure were significantly related to complications. The complication rate was greatest when the indication for the procedure was suspected dysfunction of the sphincter of Oddi and lowest when it was bile duct stone removal within 30 days of laparoscopic cholecystectomy. Endoscopists performing more than 1 sphincterotomy per week had lower complication rates than those doing fewer procedures.

Conclusions.—The complication rate associated with endoscopic biliary sphincterotomy varies greatly. It is mainly related to endoscopic technique. Clinicians should be aware of these findings when interpreting other research findings, making treatment decisions, and informing patients of the risks of sphincterotomy.

TABLE 1.—Complications of Endoscopic Biliary Sphincterotomy in 2,347 Patients

TYPE OF COMPLICATION	PATIENTS WITH COMPLICATIONS	PATIENTS WITH SEVERE COMPLICATIONS	PATIENTS WITH FATAL COMPLICATIONS
		number (percent)	
Pancreatitis	127 (5.4)	9 (0.4)	1 (<0.1)
Hemorrhage	48 (2.0)	12 (0.5)	2 (0.1)
Perforation	8 (0.3)	5 (0.2)	1 (<0.1)
Cholangitis	24 (1.0)	2 (0.1)	1 (<0.1)
Cholecystitis	11 (0.5)	3 (0.1)	1 (<0.1)
Miscellaneous*	25 (1.1)	8 (0.3)	5 (0.2)
Any†	229 (9.8)	38 (1.6)	10 (0.4)

*Miscellaneous complications included cardiopulmonary complications (in 6 patients); complications of combined percutaneous access (in 3 patients: bile leak in 1 and intrahepatic bleeding in 2); ductal perforations by guide wires (in 3); stent malfunctions (in 3); ileus (in 3); papillary obstruction (in 2); diarrhea induced by antibiotics (in 2); indeterminate abdominal fluid collections (in 2); and infection of a pancreatic pseudocyst (in 1). The deaths in this category were caused by cardiopulmonary events (arrhythmia in 1 patient, aspiration pneumonia in 1, and acute chest syndrome in sickle cell disease in (1) or were stent-related (in 2).

†Some patients had more than 1 complication.

(From Freeman ML, Nelson DB, Sherman S, et al: Complications of endoscopic biliary sphincterotomy. *N Engl J Med* 335:909–918, 1996. Reprinted by permission of The *New England Journal of Medicine*, Copyright 1996, Massachusetts Medical Society. All rights reserved.)

▶ Endoscopic biliary sphincterotomy (EBS) has become a well-established procedure to remove bile duct stones and for other biliary and pancreatic problems. Approximately 150,000 such procedures are performed annually in the United States. This study is a major contribution to our understanding of the complications of EBS. The key findings in the study bear re-emphasis.

• Dysfunction of the sphincter of Oddi was the most frequent patient-related risk factor for complications

• Pancreatitis was more frequent in young patients

• Difficulty in cannulating the bile duct and the use of "precut" sphincterotomy were the most important technique-related risk factors for complications

• Precutting techniques used in 4.7% of sphincterotomies carried an inordinately high complication rate of 24.3%

• Experience and the volume of procedures proved to be important; endoscopists who performed more than one EBS per week had lower complication rates than endoscopists who performed a smaller number of procedures

In high-risk elderly patients, complication rates after EBS as high as 19% have been reported.[1] The value of an endoprosthesis rather than EBS in such patients has now been evaluated. Chopra et al.[1] compared the value of an endoprosthesis insertion with conventional endoscopic duct clearance by EBS for management of choledocholithiasis in elderly or debilitated patients. For immediate bile duct drainage, endoprosthesis insertion proved a safe and effective alternative to EBS with 72-hour complication rates of 7% and 16%, respectively. However, the long-term complication rate of endoprosthesis insertion was higher.

N.J. Greenberger, M.D.

Reference

1. Chopra KB, Peters RA, O'Toole PA, et al: Randomized study of endoscopic biliary prosthesis versus duct clearance for bile duct stones in high-risk patients. *Lancet*, 348:791–793, 1996.

Postsurgical Bile Leaks

Postsurgical Bile Leaks: Endoscopic Obliteration of the Transpapillary Pressure Gradient Is Enough

Bjorkman DJ, Carr-Locke DL, Lichtenstein DR, et al (Brigham and Women's Hosp, Boston; Univ of Utah Health Sciences Ctr, Salt Lake City)
Am J Gastroenterol 90:2128–2133, 1995   6–16

Background.—Biliary surgery is sometimes complicated by postoperative bile leaks. This uncommon but well-documented complication is seen more often after laparoscopic procedures. One effective treatment for bile

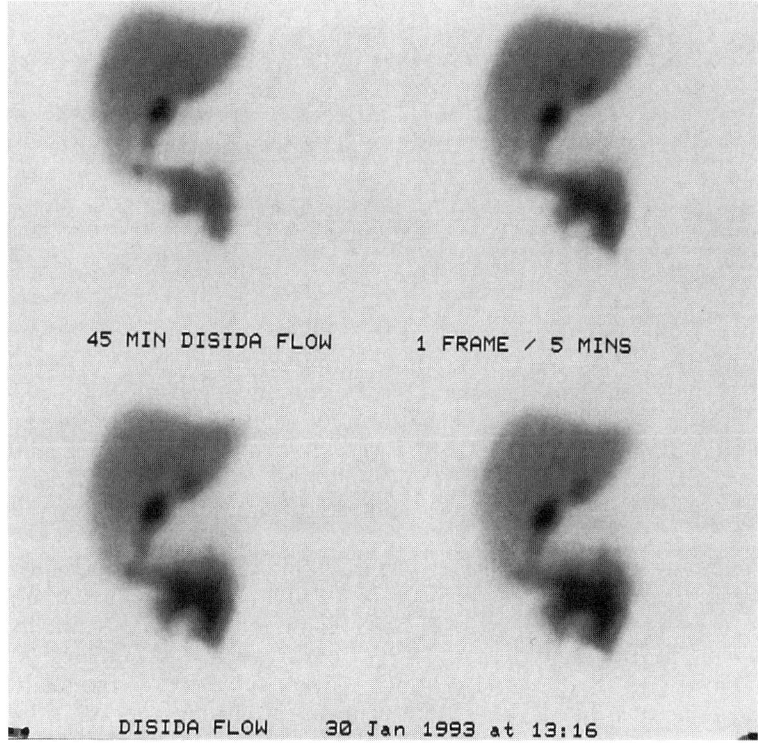

FIGURE 1.—Sequential 2-minute images of a DISIDA scan over 30 minutes from a patient with a bile leak showing liver uptake but no visualization of the bile duct or bowel. During the time of the scan, there is increasing activity outside the bowel. (Courtesy of Bjorkman DJ, Carr-Locke DL, Lichtenstein DR, et al: Postsurgical bile leaks: Endoscopic obliteration of the transpapillary pressure gradient is enough. *Am J Gastroenterol* 90(12):2128–2133, 1995.)

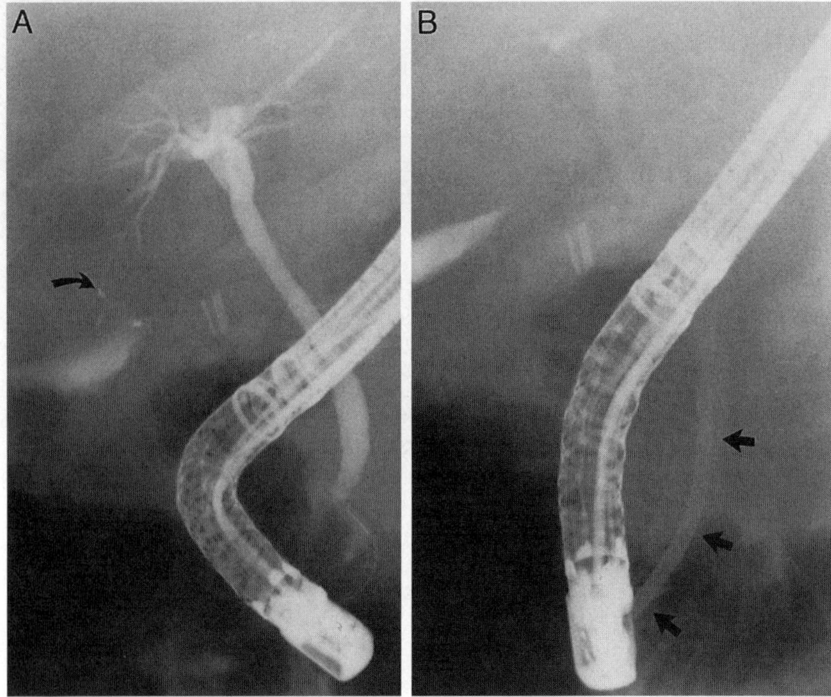

FIGURE 4.—Endoscopic retrograde cholangiography demonstrating (A) bile leak from a duct of Luschka (*arrow*) in the gallbladder bed and (B) its treatment by insertion of a 10-Fr 2-cm endoprosthesis (*arrows*). (Courtesy of Bjorkman DJ, Carr-Locke DL, Lichtenstein DR, et al: Postsurgical bile leaks: Endoscopic obliteration of the transpapillary pressure gradient is enough. *Am J Gastroenterol* 90(12):2128–2133, 1995.)

leaks is endoscopic therapy with a long biliary endoprosthesis traversing the site of the leak. However, equalizing biliary and duodenal pressures with a short transpapillary stent may be equally effective.

Methods.—Thirty-one patients seen consecutively with postoperative bile leaks during a 52-month period were studied to determine the value of endoscopic obliteration of the transpapillary pressure gradient. Treatment consisted of long endoprostheses, sphincterotomy, or short transpapillary stents.

Findings.—All 25 patients in whom a bile leak was documented responded to endoscopic treatment (Figs 1 and 4). For all treatment modalities, the clinical success rates, the need for radiologic drainage, the length of hospitalization, and the incidence of pancreatitis were similar.

Conclusion.—Endoscopic treatment is very successful in the treatment of postoperative bile leaks. The mechanism of healing appears to be the equalization of bile duct and duodenal pressure, permitting bile flow into the duodenum. Endoscopically placing short transpapillary stents without sphincterotomy is a temporary, effective, and technically simple way to equalize pressure and should be considered primary treatment for most postoperative bile leaks.

▶ I find myself in total agreement with the authors of this paper. Bile leaks after laparoscopic or open cholecystectomy are best treated initially by transpapillary stenting. This report is extremely relevant because of the frequency of laparoscopic cholecystectomy and high incidence of bile leaks (about 2%) from the cystic duct or ducts of Luschka. It is important to emphasize that endoscopic cholangiography should be used early in patients who complain of pain or have unexplained symptoms after laparoscopic cholecystectomy. Bile leaks are usually associated with only mild gastrointestinal complaints early in their course unless the bile duct is compromised. In this latter instance, jaundice and fever often bring the patient rather quickly to medical attention.

F.G. Moody, M.D.

Endoscopic Laser Lithotripsy of Common Duct Stones

Endoscopic Intracorporeal Laser Lithotripsy of Difficult Common Bile Duct Stones With a Stone-recognition Pulsed Dye Laser System
Schreiber F, Gurakuqi GC, Trauner M (Karl Franzens Univ, Graz, Austria)
Gastrointest Endosc 42:416–419, 1995   6–17

Introduction.—The automated stone recognition laser system provides discharge interruption if the laser fiber does not make contact with a stone's surface. This advance in technology eliminates the need for direct visual control during intracorporeal lithotripsy (ISWL) while it protects against mucosal damage or common bile duct wall injury, caused by uncontrolled energy application. The effectiveness and safety of this technique were evaluated in 16 patients with bile duct stones not suitable for conventional endoscopic maneuvers.

Methods.—The mean patient age was 70 years. The mean number of stones was 4, and the mean stone diameter was 22 mm. Patients either had too large a stone mass, too great a number of stones, or stone location that was too difficult for routine endoscopic treatment. One patient was treated by the trans-hepatic route. Intracorporeal laser lithotripsy was performed on the other 15 patients after they were mildly sedated. A mean of 6800 discharges were applied with a constant repetition frequency of 10 Hz and a constant power setting of 100 mJ. The mean number of sessions was 1.7. The mean duration was approximately 53 minutes. Laser fibers were inserted into the diagnostic endoscopic retrograde cholangiopancreatography catheter or into a balloon extractor catheter for better visualization. This approach made it possible to locate nearly 70% of all discharges onto the stone mass, as indicated by a beeping tone of the laser.

Results.—Without direct visual control, fragmentation by ISWL via the peroral route was achieved in all 15 patients (Fig 1 and Fig 2). Total bile

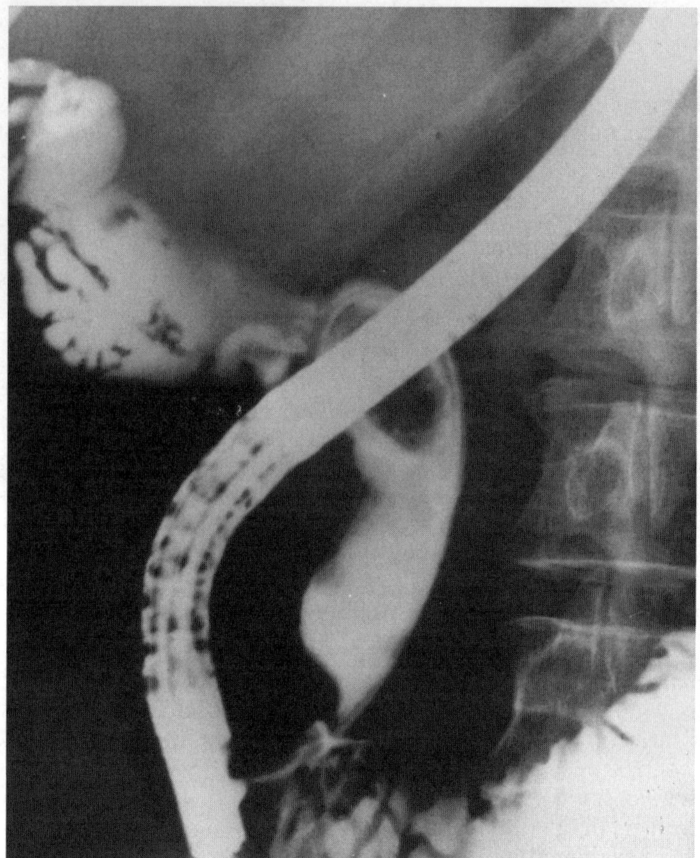

FIGURE 1.—Common bile duct stone before disintegration. (Courtesy of Schreiber F, Gurakuqi GC, Trauner M: Endoscopic intracorporeal laser lithotripsy of difficult common bile duct stones with a stone-recognition pulsed dye laser system. *Gastrointest Endosc* 42:416–419, 1995.)

duct clearance was achieved in 13 patients after extraction of fragments by basket and/or extraction balloon. Small fragments remained in 2 patients with huge stone volumes. These fragments passed spontaneously through the papilla by the time of endoscopic retrograde cholangiopancreatography at 4-week follow-up. One patient had a slight hemobilia during the second ISWL session and 1 patient experienced cholangitis. Both complications resolved with conservative management.

Conclusion.—The stone recognition laser system with ISWL was a highly effective and safe technique in this cohort of patients with difficult common bile duct stones. This maneuver expands the endoscopist's capabilities in the treatment of patients with difficult common bile duct stones.

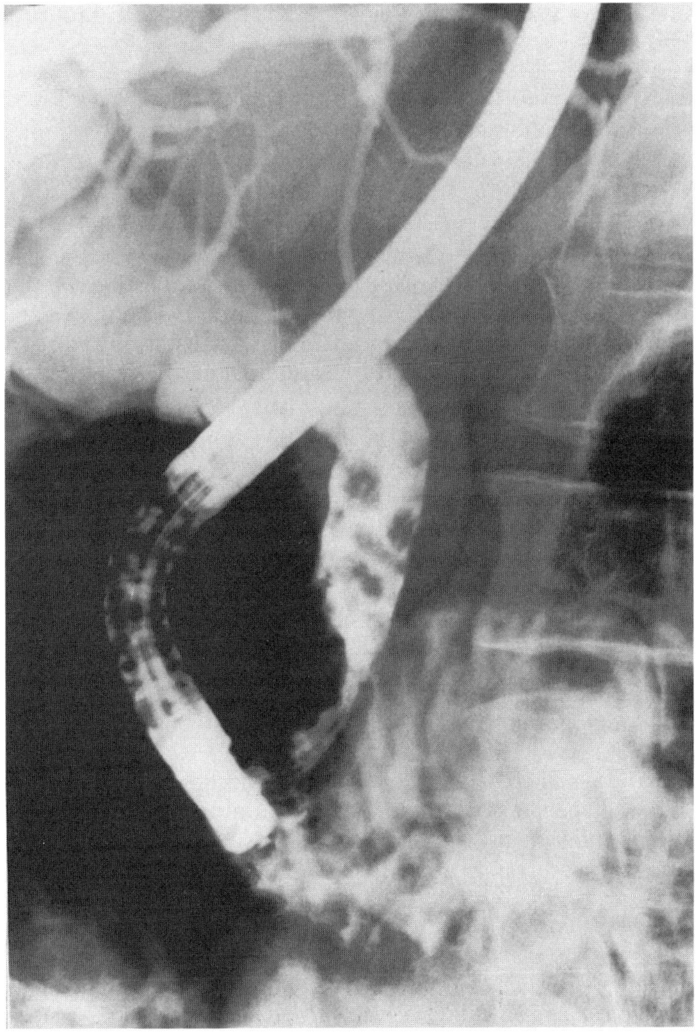

FIGURE 2.—Common bile duct stone after disintegration by laser-induced intracorporeal lithotripsy. (Courtesy of Schreiber F, Gurakuqi GC, Trauner M: Endoscopic intracorporeal laser lithotripsy of difficult common bile duct stones with a stone-recognition pulsed dye laser system. *Gastrointest Endosc* 42:416–419, 1995.)

▶ An occasional common duct stone is too large for extraction through the papilla of Vater, even after a generous sphincteroplasty. The current report suggests that ISWL can add another option to a variety of intracorporeal techniques used to solve this problem. Advances in technology have improved the safety and success of this laser technique, and the article describes in exquisite detail the intricacies of this *"Star Wars"* technology.

F.G. Moody, M.D.

Comparison of ERCP and Magnetic Resonance Cholangiopancreatography

Magnetic Resonance Cholangiography: Comparison With Endoscopic Retrograde Cholangiopancreatography

Soto JA, Barish MA, Yucel EK, et al (Boston Univ)
Gastroenterology 110:589–597, 1996   6–18

Introduction.—Magnetic resonance cholangiography (MRC) is a newer imaging technique for noninvasive imaging of the biliary tract. Three-dimensional fast spin-echo (3D FSE) MRC permits even higher quality images. The sensitivity and specificity of 3D FSE MRC was compared with that of direct cholangiography for evaluation of the biliary tree in 46 patients.

Methods.—During a 1-year period, 15 male and 31 female patients were examined prospectively with 3D FSE MRC at 1 institution. All patients underwent direct cholangiography within 24 hours of MRC. The images were examined in blinded fashion by 2 experienced radiologists.

Results.—Diagnostic quality MRC images could be obtained in 96% of these patients. Sensitivity for the detection of bile duct dilatation was 96%; for biliary strictures, 90%; and for intraductal abnormalities, 100%. The site of obstruction was periampullary in 19 patients: sphincter of Oddi dysfunction in 12 patients, choledocholithiasis with impacted stone in 6 patients and distal common bile duct polyp in 1 patient. Magnetic resonance cholangiography demonstrated a normal bile duct in 16 of 17 patients for a specificity of 94%.

Conclusions.—Three-dimensional fast spin-echo MRC has a very high sensitivity and specificity for noninvasive examination of the biliary tract. Its efficacy justifies its use in routine, noninvasive diagnosis of biliary tract disease.

▶ Diagnostic imaging of the biliary ductal system usually begins with a noninvasive modality such as US or CT scanning. The information provided by these studies often leads to direct cholangiographic studies employing invasive tests such as endoscopic retrograde cholangiopancreatography (ERCP) or percutaneous transhepatocholangiography (PTC). The findings presented here indicate that MRC has excellent sensitivity and specificity in the evaluation of the biliary tract and is a particularly attractive procedure because it is noninvasive. In addition to excellent diagnostic capabilities in biliary tract disease evaluation, the normal and abnormal pancreatic duct can also be visualized with the same technique. Magnetic resonance cholangiography might also decrease the total cost for managing patients with biliary and pancreatic disease by eliminating the need for multiple consecutive invasive studies. One drawback compared to ERCP and PTC is that MRC does not offer any opportunities for therapeutic intervention.

N.J. Greenberger, M.D.

Miscellaneous

Cost-effective Management of Complicated Choledocholithiasis: Laparoscopic Transcystic Duct Exploration or Endoscopic Sphincterotomy
Liberman MA, Phillips EH, Carroll BJ, et al (Naval Med Ctr, San Diego, Calif; Cedars-Sinai Med Ctr, Los Angeles)
J Am Coll Surg 182:488–494, 1996   6–19

Background.—At least 10% of the patients who undergo laparoscopic cholecystectomy (LC) have common bile duct stones. Endoscopic sphincterotomy (ES) is used most commonly to treat common bile duct stones in patients undergoing LC, although laparoscopic transcystic common bile duct exploration (LTCBDE) has been used increasingly. The outcomes and cost of these 2 approaches to choledocholithiasis were compared in patients also undergoing LC in a retrospective study.

Methods.—The records of 76 patients undergoing LC plus ES (in 17 patients) or LC plus LTCBDE (59 patients) were reviewed in detail to determine complications and data on costs of hospitalization and complications. The patients were divided into 3 groups for analysis: those who underwent LC plus LTCBDE (group 1); those who underwent LC plus ES (group 2); and those who underwent LC plus emergency LTCBDE (group 3).

Results.—The groups were similar in age and comorbid illnesses. The average length of hospital stay was 6.1 days in group 1, 12.4 days in group 2, and 6.9 days in group 3. Conversion to an open procedure was required in 1 patient in group 1, 1 patient in group 2, and no patients in group 3. The complication rate was 12% in group 1, 41% in group 2, and 10% in group 3. The average cost was $13,151 and $14,732 with professional reimbursement in group 1, $18,712 or $21,125 with professional reimbursement in group 2, and $13,564 or $15,150 with professional reimbursement in group 3.

Conclusions.—Laparoscopic transcystic common bile duct exploration is associated with a significantly shorter hospital stay and significantly lower total costs compared with ES in patients also undergoing LC. Therefore, LTCBDE is recommended as the initial approach for clearing common bile duct stones, with postoperative ES or open surgery used when LTCBDE fails to remove all calculi.

▶ Laparoscopic cholecystectomy plus LTCBDE is superior to LC plus ES to the tune of $5,561. When professional fees are added, the toll goes up to $6,393. I wonder how Einstein would have viewed these numbers for treating the tiny mass of a small stone lodged in the common bile duct. It is clear that most stones can be retrieved or flushed from the bile duct after dilatation of the cystic duct at the time of laparoscopic cholecystectomy, and that procedure should be mastered by all general surgeons who treat gallstone disease.

F.G. Moody, M.D.

50 Bile Duct Strictures

The Long-term Outcome of Hepaticojejunostomy in the Treatment of Benign Bile Duct Strictures
Tocchi A, Costa G, Lepre L, et al (Univ of Rome)
Ann Surg 224:162–167, 1996   6–20

Background.—Benign stricture of the common bile duct is a serious complication of upper abdominal surgery. If left untreated, it can lead to repeated cholangitis, biliary cirrhosis, hepatic failure, and death. The long-term results of biliary enteric anastomoses for primary benign biliary strictures were assessed.

Methods and Findings.—Between 1975 and 1989, 84 patients with benign bile duct strictures underwent hepaticojejunostomy, choledochojejunostomy, and intrahepatic cholangiojejunostomy. The mean age was 54 years. In the short term, 21.4% had complications. The 30-day operative mortality was 2.2%. Long-term outcomes were excellent or good in 83% of the patients. Ten patients had anastomotic strictures requiring further treatment. Early and late outcomes were not associated with demographic or clinical features at initial assessment nor with the etiologic or pathologic characteristics of the stricture. The best outcomes were associated with high biliary enteric anastomoses and degree of common bile duct dilation independent of bile duct stricture location.

Conclusions.—High biliary enteric anastomosis is a safe, durable, and highly effective treatment for benign strictures of the bile duct. Transanastomotic tube stenting is not needed. Patients in poor condition and with anastomotic strictures appear to benefit more from endoscopic and percutaneous transhepatic dilation.

▶ Reports about the long-term outcomes after bile duct repair are always welcome. What Tocchi and his associates have shown is that a Roux limb hepaticojejunostomy gives good long-term results even when the stricture in the bile duct is high. A dilated proximal biliary tree provides an especially favorable situation. I agree that transstricture intubation should be reserved for the high-risk patient and balloon dilation for those with a biliary enteric anastomosis.

F.G. Moody, M.D.

51 Primary Sclerosing Cholangitis

Natural History and Prognostic Factors in 305 Swedish Patients With Primary Sclerosing Cholangitis
Broomé U, Olsson R, Lööf L, et al (Huddinge Hosp, Stockholm; Karolinska Hosp, Stockholm; Sahlgrenska Hosp, Göteborg, Sweden; et al)
Gut 38:610–615, 1996   6–21

Introduction.—A chronic biliary destructive disease of unknown etiology, primary sclerosing cholangitis can be highly variable, with some rapidly progressing to premature death from liver failure whereas others are asymptomatic for years. Liver transplantation has achieved excellent results, and prognostic models need to be developed to classify patients for the timing of liver transplantation. Previous studies on this have had conflicting results. The outcome of patients with primary sclerosing cholangitis is described, and the prognostic significance of histologic, biochemical, and clinical findings at the time of diagnosis is evaluated.

Methods.—The study included 305 patients with primary sclerosing cholangitis who were monitored a median of 63 months retrospectively. In this group, 79 had a liver transplant or died. Multivariate analysis was used to evaluate the prognostic significance of biochemical, clinical, and histologic findings at the time of diagnosis (Table 2).

Results.—From the time of diagnosis to death or liver transplantation, the median survival was 12 years. At the time of diagnosis, 134 (44%) were asymptomatic, and cholangiocarcinoma was found in 24 (8%) of these patients. In the asymptomatic group, the estimated survival rate was significantly higher and reached 16 years (Fig 1). During the study period, 29 (22%) of the asymptomatic patients became symptomatic. Independent predictors of a bad prognosis were age, serum bilirubin concentration, and histologic state (Fig 2). A prognostic model could be constructed from these variables.

Conclusion.—Inflammatory bowel disease was closely associated with primary sclerosing cholangitis and had a prevalence of 81% in this study population. The finding that symptoms developed in 22% of the asymp-

TABLE 2.—Clinical and Biochemical Features in 305 Patients With Primary Sclerosing Cholingitis Who Were Asymptomatic or Symptomatic at the Time of Diagnosis

	All Patients (n = 305)	Patients Symptomatic at Time of Diagnosis (n = 171)	Patients Asymptomatic at Time of Diagnosis (n = 134)	P Value (Comparison Symptomatic and Asymptomatic Patients)
Age at diagnosis (yr) (mean (SD))	39 (14)	41 (13.3)	37 (14.6)	$P<0.05$
Male (%)	195 (64)	98 (57)	97 (72)	$P<0.001$
IBD (%)	249 (81)	126 (74)	123 (92)	$P<0.001$
Extra hepatic involvement of the biliary tree (%)	222 (72)	138 (80)	84 (63)	$P<0.001$
Follow-up (months) (SD)	63 (47)	59 (48)	69 (46)	$P<0.05$
Death or transplantation (%)	79 (26)	62 (36)	17 (13)	$P<0.001$
Cirrhosis (%)	67 (22)	50 (29)	17 (13)	$P<0.01$
Bilirubin (<21 µmol/L) (mean (SEM))	39 (3.55)	57 (5.86)	16 (1.12)	$P<0.001$
Alkaline phosphatase (<4.2 µkat/L) (mean (SEM))	13 (0.78)	20.7 (1.19)	14 (0.8)	$P<0.001$
Aspartate aminotransferase (<0.80 µkat/L) (mean (SEM))	2.1 (0.15)	2.5 (0.24)	1.7 (0.15)	$P<0.01$
Albumin (35–46 g/L) (mean (SEM))	38 (0.47)	37 (0.60)	40 (0.72)	$P<0.01$

Abbreviation: *IBD*, inflammatory bowel disease.
(Courtesy of Broomé U, Olsson R, Lööf L, et al: Natural history and prognostic factors in 305 Swedish patients with primary sclerosing cholangitis. *Gut* 38:610–615, 1996.)

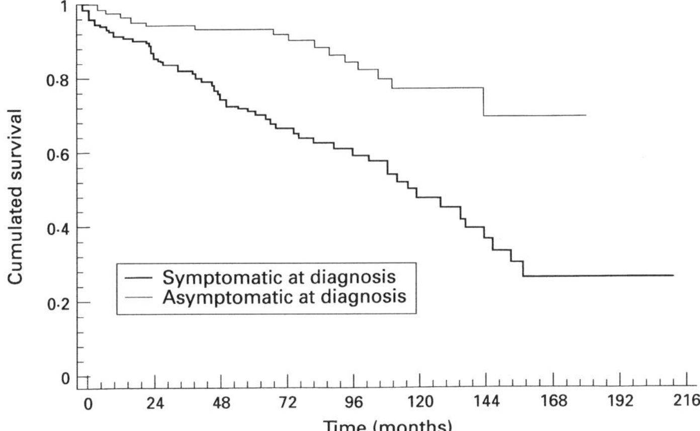

FIGURE 1.—Kaplan-Meier estimated survival curves of patients with symptomatic and asymptomatic primary sclerosing cholangitis ($P < 0.001$). (Courtesy of Broomé U, Olsson R, Lööf L, et al: Natural history and prognostic factors in 305 Swedish patients with primary sclerosing cholangitis. *Gut* 38:610–615, 1996.)

tomatic patients and that 13% died or had a liver transplant emphasizes the progressive nature of this disease.

▶ This study describes the natural history and outcome for 305 patients of Swedish descent with primary sclerosing cholangitis (PSC). One hundred thirty-four (44%) of the patients were asymptomatic at the time of diagnosis and, not surprisingly, had a significantly higher survival rate with a median follow-up time of 63 months. The independent predictors of a bad prognosis were age, serum bilirubin concentration, and liver histologic changes. Cholangiocarcinoma was found in 24 patients (8%).

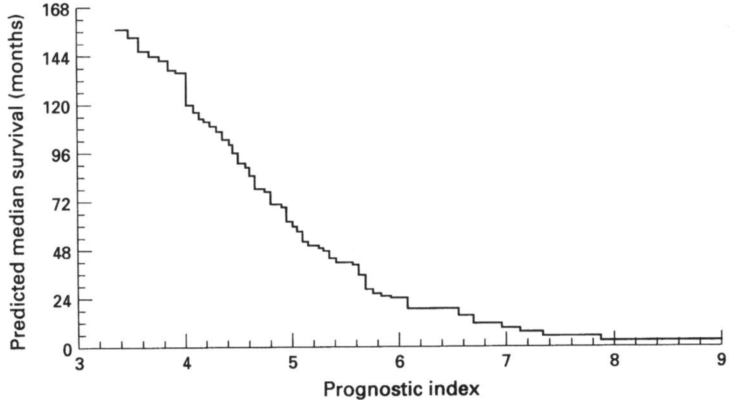

FIGURE 2.—Graph of estimated median survival plotted against the prognostic index. (Courtesy of Broomé U, Olsson R, Lööf L, et al: Natural history and prognostic factors in 305 Swedish patients with primary sclerosing cholangitis. *Gut* 38:610–615, 1996.)

Earlier studies that suggested PSC as a risk factor for the development of colorectal cancer in patients with ulcerative colitis (UC) were limited by small sample size, referral bias, and retrospective analysis. Two recent studies[1, 2] have examined this association and come to somewhat different conclusions. Loftus et al.[1] determined the relative risk and cumulative incidence of colorectal neoplasia in 178 patients with PSC. The increased risk of colorectal cancer relative to the U.S. population was demonstrated only during person-years in which UC coexisted with PSC. Clinically, the absolute risk approximated 20% 10 years after the diagnosis of PSC. The authors concluded that "if PSC is an additional risk factor for neoplasia in ulcerative colitis, the clinical significance of the risk seems to be low."

Brentnall et al.[2] prospectively monitored 20 patients with PSC and UC and 25 patients with UC by colonoscopic surveillance via extensive mucosal biopsy sampling. Nine of 20 patients with PSC and UC (45%) had dysplasia as compared with 4 of 25 patients with UC alone (16%). These investigators concluded that patients with PSC and UC have a markedly increased risk for colonic neoplasia and need colonoscopic surveillance with extensive biopsy sampling.

N.J. Greenberger, M.D.

References

1. Loftus EV, Sandborn WJ, Tremaine WJ, et al: Risk of colorectal neoplasia in patients with primary sclerosing cholangitis. *Gastroenterology* 110:432–440, 1996.
2. Brentnall TA, Haggett RC, Rabinovitch RS, et al: Risk and natural history of colonic neoplasia in patients with primary sclerosing cholangitis and ulcerative colitis. *Gastroenterology* 110:331–338, 1996.

Features of Autoimmune Hepatitis in Primary Sclerosing Cholangitis: An Evaluation of 114 Primary Sclerosing Cholangitis Patients According to a Scoring System for the Diagnosis of Autoimmune Hepatitis
Boberg KM, Fausa O, Haaland T, et al (Rikshospitalet, Oslo, Norway)
Hepatology 23:1369–1376, 1996   6–22

Introduction.—Chemical, biochemical, and histologic features of autoimmune hepatitis (AIH) have been described in some patients with primary sclerosing cholangitis (PSC). There is no consensus on diagnostic criteria for AIH, but The International Autoimmune Hepatitis Group has suggested a set of descriptive criteria and a scoring system based on a selection of clinical, biochemical, serologic, and histologic criteria. To evaluate the features of AIH in patients with PSC, 114 well-defined patients with PSC were scored according to the proposed numerical scoring system for the diagnosis of AIH.

Methods.—The proposed scoring system assigns a score for these parameters: gender, ratio of elevation of serum alkaline phosphatase vs. aminotransferase, serum immunoglobulins, serum autoantibodies, viral

TABLE 1.—Distribution of Scores Among Patients With Primary Sclerosing Cholangitis Evaluated According to a Scoring Table Constructed for the Diagnosis of Autoimmune Hepatitis

Parameters	Score	Definite AIH (n = 2)	Probable AIH (n = 38)	Not AIH (n = 74)
Gender				
Female	2	1	21	14
Male	0	1	17	60
Serum biochemistry				
Ratio of elevation of serum alkaline phosphatase vs. aminotransferase				
>3.0	−2			25
<3.0	2	2	38	49
Serum γ-globulin or IgG (times upper normal limit)				
>2.0	3	1	4	1
1.5–2.0	2	1	4	8
1.0–1.5	1		21	28
<1.0	0		9	34
Autoantibodies				
ANA, SMA, or LKM-1				
>1:80	3	2	7	1
1:80	2		4	3
1:40	1		4	3
<1:40	0		23	64
Antimitochondrial antibody				
Positive	−2			2
Negative	0	2	38	71
Viral markers				
IgM Anti-HAV, HBsAg, or IgM anti-HBc positive	−3			
Anti-HCV positive by ELISA or RIBA	−2			
HCV RNA positive by PCR	−3			
Positive test indicating active infection with any other virus	−3			
Seronegative for all of the above	3	2	38	74
Other causative factors				
History of recent hepatotoxic drug usage or parenteral exposure to blood products				
Yes	−2			
No	1	2	38	74
Alcohol (average consumption)				
Male <35 g/d; female <25 g/d	2	2	38	72
Male 35–50 g/d; female 25–40 g/d	0			2
Male 50–80 g/d; female 40–60 g/d	−1			
Male >80 g/d; female >60 g/d	−2			
Genetic factors				
Other autoimmune diseases in patient or first-degree relative	1	1	14	15
HLA B8-DR3 haplotype or DR4 allotype	1	1	19	24
Histology				
Chronic active hepatitis with piecemeal necrosis				
With lobular involvement and bridging necrosis	3	1	8	2
Without lobular involvement and bridging necrosis	2	1	10	11
Rosetting of liver cells	1	1	4	1
Marked/predominantly plasma cell infiltrate	1		1	
Biliary changes	−1	2	27	54
Any other changes (e.g., granulomas, siderosis and copper deposits) suggestive of a different cause	−3		13	41
No significant histological changes	0		9	10

Abbreviations: ANA, antinuclear antibody, *SMA,* smooth muscle antibody; *LKM-1,* liver-kidney microsome-1; *anti-HAV,* hepatitis A antibody; *HBsAg,* hepatitis B surface antigen; *anti-HBc,* antibody to hepatitis B core; *ELISA,* enzyme-linked immunosorbent assay; *RIBA,* recombinant immunoblot assay; *HCV,* hepatitis C virus; *PCR,* polymerase chain reaction.
From Boberg KM, Fausa O, Haaland T, et al: Features of autoimmune hepatitis in primary sclerosing cholangitis: An evaluation of 114 primary sclerosing cholangitis patients according to a scoring system for the diagnosis of autoimmune hepatitis. *Hepatology* 23:1369–1376, 1996. Courtesy of Johnson PJ, McFarlane IG: Meeting report: International Autoimmune Hepatitis Group. *Hepatology* 18:998–1005, 1993.

markers, history of drug and alcohol intake, genetic factors, histology, and response to therapy. "A definite" diagnosis of AIH requires an aggregate score greater than 15 before treatment and greater than 17 after treatment. Scores of 10–15 before treatment and 12–17 after treatment indicate "probable" AIH.

Results.—Two of 114 patients with PSC had scores greater than 15 points, satisfying the diagnostic criteria for "definite" AIH. Thirty-eight patients with PSC who scored between 10 and 15 points could be categorized as having "probable" AIH. In 68 and 24 patients with PSC, respectively, the serum level of immunoglobulin G was increased and positive titers of antinuclear antibodies or smooth muscle antibodies were observed. In 35 patients with PSC, there were positive scores for histologic features similar to those of AIH. The total score for histology was negative in 72 patients with PSC because of the presence of biliary changes. Twenty-five patients with PSC had serum levels of alkaline phosphatase relative to aminotransferase high enough for a negative score for this value (Table 1).

Conclusion.—The scoring system may need to be modified because of the number of patients with PSC with a high score from the scoring table for the diagnosis of AIH. Increasing the negative score for histologic biliary changes would help the scoring system discriminate between AIH and PSC.

▶ Primary sclerosing cholangitis and AIH may have overlapping clinical features. In this regard, the presence of elevated levels of circulating immunoglobulins, positive tests for non–organic-specific antibodies, histologic findings of periportal inflammation and piecemeal necrosis, and response to corticosteroid have been described in patients with endoscopic retrograde cholangiopancreatography findings characteristic of PSC.[1] In some reports, such patients have been given a diagnosis of autoimmune cholangiopathy. The report by Boberg et al. presents a refinement of a scoring system for discriminating between PSC and AIH. Table 1 provides detailed information on a large number of patients with PSC and illustrates the spectrum of clinical features that may be encountered.

N.J. Greenberger, M.D.

Reference

1. Johnson PJ, McFarlane IG: Meeting report: International Autoimmune Hepatitis Group. *Hepatology* 18:998–1005, 1993.

52 Miscellaneous

Percutaneous Cholecystectomy in Critically Ill Patients

The Efficacy of Percutaneous Cholecystostomy in Critically Ill Patients
Hultman CS, Herbst CA, McCall JM, et al (Univ of North Carolina, Chapel Hill)
Am Surg 62:263–269, 1996   6–23

Background.—Percutaneous cholecystostomy (PC) is an effective biliary decompression method used for clinically stable patients with acute cholecystitis who are not good candidates for surgery. Its use has also been proposed for critically ill patients with acute cholecystitis. The efficacy of PC in such patients was investigated retrospectively.

Methods and Findings.—The medical records of 33 critically ill patients who underwent PC for suspected acute cholecystitis were reviewed. Patient age ranged from 5 to 87 years, with a mean of 52 years. The procedure was technically successful in all patients. No direct mortality or major complications occurred. Increased mortality was associated with failure to improve within 24 hours. Twenty-two patients improved, 17 survived, and eight needed surgery. In two patients, definitive surgery was delayed by PC. Cholelithiasis was correlated with surgery but not with an increased death rate. Favorable prognostic indicators of survival were gallbladder dilation, pericholecystic fluid, and absence of a pulmonary artery catheter. Factors predicting improvement were gallbladder nonvisualization on hepatobiliary scan, positive bile cultures, and initial drainage of 100 cc or less. Changes in antibiotic therapy were prompted by nine positive bile cultures in five patients. The cost of PC was lower than that of open cholecystostomy.

Conclusions.—Critically ill patients with acute cholecystitis benefit from PC. This procedure is safe, cost-effective, and minimally invasive. A general surgeon should be involved to ensure that patients who do not improve within 24 hours receive early surgical treatment and to provide definitive long-term care for patients with cholelithiasis.

▶ This article adds further testimony to the effectiveness of PC. The authors have not only shown that it helps to define the status of the biliary tree in critically ill patients within an intensive care unit, but that it is also safe and inexpensive. They make an important point that could be easily overlooked—

375

patients who appear to be candidates for the procedure should be seen by a general surgeon.

F.G. Moody, M.D.

Choledochal Cysts

Complete Excision of the Intrapancreatic Portion of Choledochal Cysts
Ando H, Kaneko K, Ito T, et al (Nagoya Univ, Japan; Aichi Prefectural Colony, Kasugai, Japan; Nagoya First Red Cross Hosp, Japan)
J Am Coll Surg 183:317–321, 1996

6–24

Introduction.—The treatment of choice for patients with choledochal cysts has been excision of the dilated extrahepatic bile duct. Intramural dissection between the outer and inner layers, leaving part of the cyst in the pancreas, is recommended by many authors because of risk of injury to the pancreas. Other authors recommend performing a partial cyst excision and leaving behind the intrapancreatic portion of the cyst. A different technique based on precise local anatomy, which completely removes the intrapancreatic portion of the choledochal cyst, was compared retrospectively with the 2 conventional techniques.

Methods.—Records of 104 patients who underwent choledochal cyst excision between 1977 and 1995 were reviewed retrospectively. The mean patient age at operation was 6.7 years. Twelve patients underwent partial cyst excision above the pancreas, and 17 patients underwent intramural dissection. With the new technique, the outer plane of the epicholedochal plexus is dissected, exposing the narrow distal segment connecting the cyst to the pancreatic duct. Seventy-five patients underwent complete excision of the intrapancreatic cyst using the new technique.

Results.—There were·no complications in the 75 patients who underwent complete excision of the intrapancreatic cyst. The mean blood loss was 126.0 mL for patients undergoing the new technique and 119.7 mL for those undergoing intramural dissection. Nine, 1, and 1 patients, respectively, who underwent the new technique, partial excision, and intramural dissection experienced postoperative hyperamylasemia (difference not significant). All patients were asymptomatic and the hyperamylasemia resolved within a few days. One patient experienced pancreatic fistula after intramural excision. Two patients undergoing partial excision and 1 patient who underwent intramural dissection had pancreatic stones several years after surgery.

Conclusion.—The findings indicate why complete excision of the intrapancreatic cyst is needed. The formation of pancreatic stones in the residual cyst in the pancreas is a late complication. The new technique may be considered safe and reliable for complete removal of the intrapancreatic portion of choledochal cysts.

▶ I agree with the authors' approach. A meticulous division of the epicholedochal plexus is essential for mobilization of the duodenum and the pancreas from the distal aspect of the cyst. It is not necessary to trace the cyst down to the duct of Wirsung but only to the point where the cyst neck narrows, which usually is at the true intrapancreatic portion of the bile duct. Transection at this level allows the dilated distal bile duct to be turned in upon itself after its lumen has been carefully inspected to rule out evidence of neoplastic degeneration.

F.G. Moody, M.D.

Oriental Cholangiohepatitis

Biliary Access Procedure in the Management of Oriental Cholangiohepatitis
Gott PE, Tieva MH, Barcia PJ, et al (Tripler Army Med Ctr, Honolulu, Hawaii)
Am Surg 62:930–934, 1996   6–25

Introduction.—Oriental cholangiohepatitis (OCH), or recurrent pyogenic cholangitis, is endemic to coastal southeast Asia but is seen with increasing frequency in Western populations because of Asian immigration. Patients with OCH form multiple biliary strictures and ducts are filled with pigmented, friable stones. The left lobe of the liver is most likely to be affected earlier and more severely during the disease course. Biliary stasis contributes to bacterial colonization and overgrowth, with resultant development of multiple intrahepatic abscesses. Treatment of OCH has traditionally aimed at eradicating the disease. Extensive procedures have been performed to achieve intraoperative stone extraction or liver resection, when possible. These approaches are associated with significant morbidity, mortality, and recurrence. A combined approach of surgical access to the biliary tree with cutaneous choledochoenteric conduit and interventional

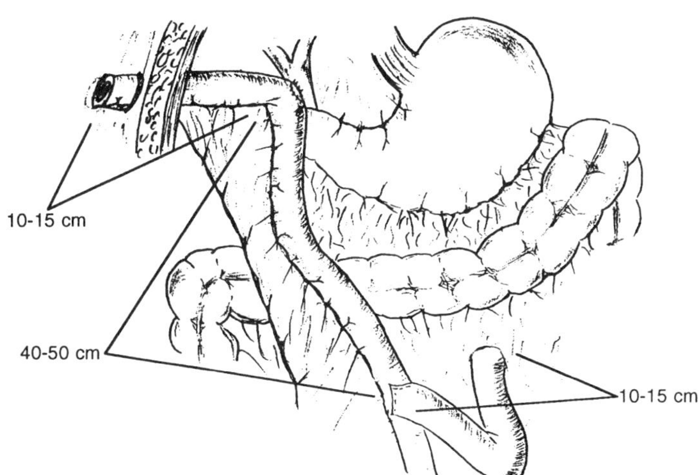

FIGURE 4.—Roux-en-Y choledochojejunostomy with cutaneous stoma. (Courtesy of Gott PE, Tieva MH, Barcia PJ: Biliary access procedure in the management of oriental cholangiohepatitis. *Am Surg* 62:930–934, 1996.)

radiology was used to remove intrahepatic stones and dilate biliary strictures in the treatment of OCH.

Methods.—Records of 10 patients treated for OCH since 1986 were reviewed retrospectively at Tripler Army Medical Center. This hospital is located in Honolulu and serves the military community in Hawaii and the Pacific basin, as well as beneficiaries of the Trust Territories of Micronesia.

Results.—All patients had a history of recurrent bouts of cholangitis that ranged from a few weeks to nearly 30 years. Five patients had undergone previous cholecystectomy and other biliary tract surgeries. One patient was treated using endoscopic sphincterotomy and stone extraction and did not receive further surgical treatment. Another patient gave a history of cholecystectomy in 1963, but the gallbladder was present on exploration. She had extensive adhesions of the duodenum to the porta hepatis that prevented completion of the planned access procedure. She was subsequently treated by endoscopic retrograde cannulation of the pancreatic duct. The remaining 8 patients underwent the Roux-en-Y choledochojejunostomy with a lateral cutaneous stoma.

> *Surgical Technique.*—For this procedure, a 60-to 70-cm segment of bowel is used for the Roux-en-Y limb. A side-to-side choledochojejunostomy is made 10–15 cm from the termination of the jejunal limb. The blind limb is then brought through the abdominal wall in the right upper quadrant to allow straight access to the biliary tree (Fig 4). With lateral placement of the stoma, the interventional radiologist's hands and instruments will not interfere with the fluoroscopy beam. Gross stones are removed, but a complete clearance of the common bile duct or hepatic radicles is not attempted. The abdomen is closed and the stoma is matured in a turn-back fashion. The cutaneous stoma allows subsequent treatment of residual stones and strictures. When the radiologic treatment is completed, the stoma is mobilized, closed, and left buried in the subcutaneous tissue for future access.

Discussion/Conclusion.—Any immigrant from Southeast Asia with biliary tract disease should be suspected of having OCH, particularly in the presence of recurrent disease. The diagnostic procedure of choice is noncontrast CT scan. The combined approach of providing biliary access and use of interventional radiology for eradication of the intrahepatic stones and strictures is effective in treating OCH without the need for hepatic resection. This approach achieves adequate biliary drainage and resolution of the associated hepatic abscesses and subsequent recovery of liver parenchyma.

▶ The surgeons at Tripler have teamed up with their interventional radiology colleagues to effectively treat the complex problem of oriental cholangiohepatitis utilizing an exteriorized choledochojejunostomy (see Fig 1). The key to success, as they point out, is total clearance of stone from the intrahepatic biliary tree. The availability of balloons for dilating strictures, baskets for retrieving stones, and contact and mechanical lithotripsy for reducing their size makes this technique feasible. The next step will be to find a way to gain a retrograde approach without a formal surgical intervention. Unfortunately, the transpapillary route is usually not adequate for this purpose.

F.G. Moody, M.D.

Introduction

The surgical treatment of gallstone pancreatitis has been influenced in a positive and beneficial way by laparoscopic cholecystectomy, and at issue is the role of the timing of the procedure and the role of endoscopic cholangiography and stone retrieval. There is now general agreement that one should be very conservative as regards a direct approach to the pancreatic gland, except in established infected pancreatic necrosis. The use of early endoscopic evaluation still is not resolved in the type of patients that we see in the United States who have a small bile duct stone burden. The trend is toward earlier cholecystectomy by a laparoscopic approach and visualization of the bile duct by dynamic video-cholangiography. If a stone is present, it is retrieved through the cystic duct. There is some evidence than in older patients, it might be safer to perform early endoscopic cholangiography and stone retrieval before laparoscopic cholecystectomy.

Progress is also being made in the surgical management of chronic pancreatitis. Resection of the pancreatic head with duodenal preservation is associated with a high success rate as regards pain relief, but patients must be treated before addiction. Pylorus-preserving pancreaticoduodenectomy is also equally successful under these conditions. What seems to help most however, with or without surgery, is to get the patient to give up smoking and drinking alcohol. It is of interest that simple transendoscopic stenting will provide relief of jaundice in chronic pancreatitis and that the distal stricture will recede in half the patients. This clearly is a good temporizing measure in patients with high-grade jaundice, offering time for assessment. Also, a distal 70% pancreatectomy can be safely performed laparoscopically, because proximal (Whipple) pancreaticoduodenectomies have been performed this way. Note that it took two highly expert laparoscopic surgeons to achieve this task.

Neoplasms of the pancreas still present a difficult challenge. If one is fortunate enough to see patients with nodular intraductal neoplasms, these patients' long-term outcomes will be excellent. There is increasing evidence that one should be aggressive in the approach to cystic neoplasms. They should be resected when encountered. Be sure to read the results of the national survey of patterns of pancreatic care in the United States. It reveals that abdominal pain is a common complaint in pancreatic cancer, that it is a disease of older people, and that the lowest mortality rates are obtained with surgery in institutions that treat the most patients with the disease. It appears that not much progress has been made in overall survival, although the mortality rate has dropped to 6% with resection in the time period 1985 to 1990. Although early detection appears to be the only hope for improving the cure rate, advances in this regard are slow to emerge. Magnetic resonance may help; immunohistochemical identification of tumor markers in pancreatic ductal aspirates may help; but fine-needle aspiration of suspected masses, either percutaneous or at the time of exploration, appears to offer the best near-term aid in early detection. Finally, aggressive surgical approaches still should be attempted in apparently incurable cases, because an occasional remarkable survival will occur. We must learn how to identify the patients whose lives will be prolonged and made more comfortable by extirpation of their tumor even when it appears hopeless.

Frank G. Moody, M.D.

53 Acute Pancreatitis

Gabexate for Prevention of ERCP Pancreatic Damage

Gabexate for the Prevention of Pancreatic Damage Related to Endoscopic Retrograde Cholangiopancreatography

Cavallini G, Tittobello A, Frulloni L, et al (Università di Verona, Italy; Ospedale S Raffaele, Milan, Italy)
N Engl J Med 335:919–923, 1996

7–1

Background.—Levels of pancreatic enzymes and pancreatitis are increased in patients undergoing endoscopic retrograde cholangiopancreatography (ERCP). In a multicenter, double-blind trial, gabexate was compared with placebo.

Methods and Findings.—Four hundred thirty-five adults scheduled for ERCP and, in some cases, endoscopic sphincterotomy, were randomly assigned to gabexate in a 1-g IV infusion beginning 30–90 minutes before endoscopy and continuing for 12 hours or a placebo. Pancreatic enzyme levels were increased in 66% of the patients after ERCP. The frequency of this increase was similar in the active treatment and placebo groups. During the 24 hours of observation, placebo recipients had higher mean serum amylase values than gabexate recipients. Six percent of those in the gabexate group and 14% in the placebo group had abdominal pain. Eight percent of placebo recipients had acute pancreatitis, compared to only 2%

TABLE 2.—Incidence of Hyperenzymemia, Pain, and Acute Pancreatitis in the Treatment Groups

VARIABLE	GABEXATE GROUP (N = 208)	PLACEBO GROUP (N = 210)	TOTAL (N = 418)
	no. of patients (%)		
Hyperenzymemia	134 (64)	142 (68)	276 (66)
Pain	12 (6)*	29 (14)	41 (10)
Acute pancreatitis	5 (2)†	16 (8)	21 (5)

*P = 0.009 for the comparison with the placebo group.
†P = 0.03 for the comparison with the placebo group.

(From Cavallini G, Tittobello A, Frulloni L, et al: Gabexate for the prevention of pancreatic damage related to endoscopic retrograde cholangiopancreatography. *N Engl J Med* 335:919–923, 1996. Reprinted by permission of The *New England Journal of Medicine*, Copyright 1996, Massachusetts Medical Society. All rights reserved.)

of the gabexate recipients (Table 2). Adverse events, all of which resolved, occurred in 2 patients receiving gabexate and 6 receiving placebo. Two patients receiving placebo died of acute pancreatitis, 1 of whom had pancreatitis before ERCP. One patient given gabexate died of a myocardial infarction.

Conclusions.—In these patients undergoing ERCP, prophylaxis with gabexate decreased pancreatic damage. Patients in the active treatment group had reductions in the extent but not the frequency of increased enzyme levels and in the frequency of pancreatic pain and acute pancreatitis.

▶ Endoscopic retrograde cholangiopancreatography (ERCP) has been reported to cause pancreatitis in 2% to 10% of patients. The data provided in the report by Cavallini, et al. (see Table 2) are in accord with previous studies. Note the incidence of elevated enzymes (68%), abdominal pain (14%), and acute pancreatitis (8%) in the 210 patients who received a placebo before ERCP. By contrast, prophylactic treatment with gabexate, a protease inhibitor, given before ERCP reduced pancreatic damage as reflected by a significant decrease in abdominal pain (6%) and acute pancreatitis (2%). These findings can be contrasted with several other studies, which reported negative results with aprotinin, glucagon, calcitonin, nifedipine, somatostatin, and octreotide.

Thus, gabexate appears to reduce pancreatic damage resulting from endoscopic and therapeutic maneuvers involving the papilla of Vater. As the authors point out, further studies should be done to identify patients at greatest risk for acute pancreatitis. One such subgroup appears to be patients in whom the indication for ERCP is sphincter of Oddi dysfunction.

N.J. Greenberger, M.D.

Surgery for Biliary Acute Pancreatitis

Outcome After Surgery for Biliary Pancreatitis
Runkel NS, Buhr HJ, Herfarth C (Univ of Heidelberg, Germany)
Eur J Surg 162:307–313, 1996

7–2

Background.—Surgery for biliary pancreatitis was traditionally delayed until after the acute attack was resolved. However, earlier surgery has been advocated more recently. The few studies comparing the results of early vs. delayed operations have had contradictory findings. The results of early and delayed operations were compared in a 10-year retrospective study.

Methods.—One hundred six patients were treated for biliary pancreatitis between 1980 and 1990. Of those, 81 were treated surgically and 25 were treated nonoperatively. The timing and type of surgical treatment were noted and the relationship between those variables and postoperative morbidity and mortality and the long-term result was analyzed.

Results.—Of the 81 patients who underwent surgery, the operation was performed within 72 hours of the onset of symptoms in 37 patients, was delayed (performed between days 3 and 14) in 27 patients, and was elective (performed more than 14 days after symptom onset) in 17 patients. Early operations occurred in patients with the most severe acute pancreatitis. All the patients underwent cholecystectomy and cholangiography. Pancreatic surgery was more extensive in patients undergoing early operations. There was an overall postoperative morbidity rate of 42%. The morbidity rate was 60% after early surgery and 25% after delayed and elective surgery. The mortality rate was 16% after early surgery and 6% after delayed and elective surgery. Complications were associated with early operation, more invasive pancreatic surgery, and a number of clinical factors. In stepwise logistic regression analysis, only patient age and pancreatic surgery significantly and independently predicted postoperative morbidity.

Conclusions.—Early pancreatic surgery can have harmful effects. Therefore, the delay of operation until after the clinical remission of pancreatitis is recommended.

▶ The timing of cholecystectomy in biliary pancreatitis remains a relevant topic for ongoing discussion in view of rapid advances in less invasive management of gallstone disease. Runkel and his associates in Heidelberg report an experience that precedes the laparoscopic cholecystectomy era at a period of time in which their institution approached the involved pancreas aggressively. They have modified their approach on the basis of the morbidity associated with a direct approach to the pancreas by necrosectomy. They now recommend early endoscopic papillotomy with stone retrieval. Possibly, this is the way to proceed in a population with a high stone burden. Most centers in the United States still pursue the hospitalization, bowel rest, resolution of pancreatitis approach with laparoscopic cholecystectomy with preoperative cholangiogram in 3–5 days. The majority of patients will have passed their stone and be clinically recovered from their pancreatitis. Those who fail to recover rapidly require early papillotomy with stone clearance followed by laparoscopic cholecystectomy when the pancreatitis has declared itself and resolved. Only a few (about 5%) patients will have severe necrotizing pancreatitis and infections or find complications that require a surgical intervention.

F.G. Moody, M.D.

Safe Laparoendoscopic Approach to Biliary Pancreatitis in Older Patients

McGrath MF, McGrath JC, Gabbay J, et al (Cedars Sinai Med Ctr, Los Angeles; Univ of California, Los Angeles)
Arch Surg 131:826–833, 1996   7–3

Introduction.—The current approach to biliary pancreatitis (BP) is laparoendoscopic. Most patients undergo primary upper endoscopic procedures (ERC/ES) or laparoscopic cholecystectomy (LC). Treatment outcomes for older and younger patients with BP were compared.

Methods.—A retrospective review of patients with a discharge diagnosis of BP during a 4-year period was conducted. Data collected included: age, sex admission laboratory values (including Ranson criteria), treatment strategies, and incidence of common bile duct stones. End points were success of therapeutic strategy, morbidity, mortality, and length of hospitalization (preoperative, postprocedure, ICU, and total). Patients were divided into 2 groups according to age: group 1, younger than 65 years; and group 2, 65 years or older.

Results.—A total of 136 patients with BP were evaluated. There were 93 women and 43 men. The mean patient age was 59 years (range, 16–100 years). There were 68 group-1 patients (mean age, 42.2 years) and 68 group-2 patients (mean age, 76.6 years). Older patients had a significantly higher white blood cell count, compared with group-2 patients (10.27 10^6/L vs. 13.97 10^6/L). There were no between-group differences in serum amylase levels or any other relevant serum blood values. The initial numbers of Ranson criteria calculated from laboratory values indicated that older patients had significantly more severe illness. The overall rate of severe illness was low in this patient series.

The primary treatments were endoscopic retrograde cholangiography ($n = 36$) alone or with endoscopic sphincterotomy ($n = 27$); operative procedures, including cholecystectomy by laparoscopic ($n = 54$) or open ($n = 16$) approaches; and no definitive therapy ($n = 22$). Secondary treatments included laparoscopic transcystic bile duct exploration in 5 patients, open common bile duct exploration in 4, and postoperative endoscopic retrograde cholangiography in 10. The primary and secondary treatment strategies and outcomes were similar for both groups. There were no between-group differences in treatment approaches, morbidity, or recurrence among 30 patients (divided almost evenly between group 1 and 2) with deferred therapy. Length of ICU stay and overall hospital stay were similar for both groups and all treatment approaches.

Discussion/Conclusion.—Patients of all ages may be safely managed using a combined laparoendoscopic approach. Common bile duct stones are best managed in younger patients using laparoscopic transcystic duct exploration or open common bile duct exploration and older patients are best managed using laparoscopic transcystic duct exploration or postoperative endoscopic sphincterotomy. There is a substantial relapse rate for all patients for whom therapy is deferred.

▶ Older patients with their often more advanced gallstone biliary tract problems and associated medical problems can undergo a laparoscopic cholecystectomy with the safety of their younger counterparts. As expected, they have a higher incidence of stones within their bile ducts and a more advanced stage of pancreatitis as judged by Ranson's signs. But as is now known, age should not be included as a grave prognostic sign, which likely was done in this study. The resiliency of older patients never ceases to amaze me; however, there is no margin for therapeutic omission or error.

Medicare will have to be cautious as it attempts to improve its bottom line on its clients.

F.G. Moody, M.D.

Endoscopic Therapy for Organized Necrosis

Endoscopic Therapy for Organized Pancreatic Necrosis
Baron TH, Thaggard WG, Morgan DE, et al (Univ of Alabama, Birmingham)
Gastroenterology 111:755–764, 1996   7–4

Background.—There is debate regarding how to manage extensive pancreatic necrosis as a complication of severe acute pancreatitis. Some authorities suggest that surgical débridement is unnecessary unless infected necrosis is present, whereas others maintain that the necrotic areas should be débrided if the patient continues to be ill. The use of endoscopic drainage for patients with extensive, organized pancreatic necrosis was evaluated.

Methods.—Endoscopic drainage was attempted in 11 patients who had organized pancreatic necrosis after severe acute necrotizing pancreatitis. All patients were persistently ill and had persistent or progressive pancreatic collections on serial imaging studies (Table 1). The pancreatic necrosis was sterile in 8 cases and infected in 3. In all patients but 1, at least 50% of the pancreas was found to be necrotic on dynamic contrast-enhanced CT (Fig 1). The last 8 patients in the series were treated prospectively using a standardized protocol. This group had an intrapancreatic nasobiliary lavage catheter placed into the collection along with 10F stents.

Results.—The necrotic collections were drained successfully without surgery in 9 of the 11 patients. Five patients had procedure-related complications, including 4 with procedure-induced infected necrosis. In 1 patient, bleeding precluded entry into the pancreatic collection. The patients required a mean of 2.7 endoscopic procedures for the collections to resolve. The intrapancreatic nasobiliary lavage catheter was left in place for a mean of 19 days, and the nonoperatively treated patients were in the hospital for a mean of 9 days. The patients were followed up for a mean of 12 months. A pseudocyst developed in 1 patient, and was drained successfully.

Conclusions.—For some patients with organized pancreatic necrosis after an episode of acute pancreatic necrosis, endoscopic drainage may be a viable treatment option. The endoscopic approach is ideal for patients with necrosis in the accessible central area. Placement of an intrapancreatic lavage catheter is an important part of treatment. Further study of endoscopic therapy for organized pancreatic necrosis is needed before it is adopted for clinical use.

► This study provides evidence that endoscopic therapy may be a viable management option for a subset of patients who remain symptomatic after an episode of acute pancreatic necrosis in which the pancreas has become organized and partially liquefied (see Fig 1). The authors emphasize 2 points:

TABLE 1.—Results of Endoscopic Drainage for Organized Pancreatic Necrosis

Patient	Age (yr)	Sex	Etiology	Size (cm)	Indication	Timing (wk)	Necrosis (%)	CTSI	Drainage	Procedural complications	Nonsurgical resolution?	Hospital days	Follow-up (days)
1	21	F	Gallstone	18	Infection	7	>50	10	TG + TP	None	Yes	17	522
2	53	F	ERCP	20	Pain	7	>50	9	TG	Infection, G. perf.	No	58	545
3	15	M	Idiopathic	18	Pain	6	50	8	TG + lavage	Infection, pneumonia	Yes	19	527
4	64	M	Gallstone	15	Infection/ sepsis	6	50	8	TG + lavage	None	Yes	19	511
5	44	F	ERCP	10	Pain	6	50	8	TG + lavage	None	Yes	6	445
6	84	M	Idiopathic	10	Infection	9	>50	10	Tp + lavage	None	Yes	15	341
7	25	M	Alcohol	11	Pain/ GOO	4	50	8	TG + lavage	Infection	Yes	26	278
8	75	F	Pancreas divisum	8	Pain	10	50	7	TD + lavage	None	Yes	4	229
9	64	F	Gallstone	17	Pain/ GOO	7	>50	10	TG + lavage	Infection	Yes	34	231
10	45	M	Drug: Imuran	23	Pain/ GOO	11	30	6	TG (failed entry)	Bleeding	No	16	259
11	42	M	Idiopathic	12	Pain	6	50	7	TD + lavage	None	Yes	2	111

Note: Listed in chronological order.

Abbreviations: Timing, interval between onset of pancreatitis and drainage; *CTSI*, CT severity index; *TD*, transduodenal; *TG*, transgastric; *TP*, transpapillary; *G. perf*, gastric perforation; *ERCP*, endoscopic retrogade cholangiopancreatography; *GOO*, gastric outlet obstruction.

(Courtesy of Baron TH, Thaggard WG, Morgan DE, et al: Endoscopic therapy for organized pancreatic necrosis. *Gastroenterology* 111:755–764, 1996.)

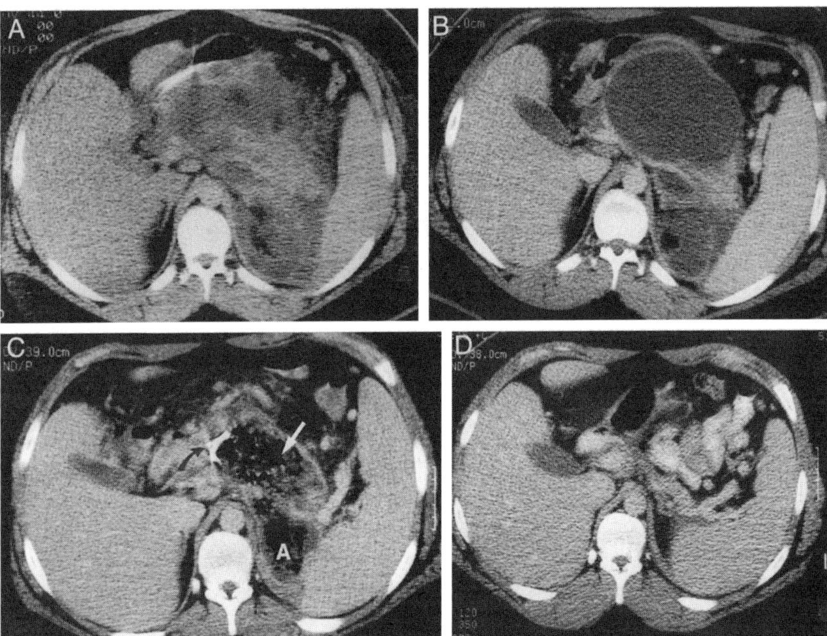

FIGURE 1.—A, acute pancreatitis with extensive necrosis. Contrast-enhanced CT shows large amounts of heterogeneous, inflammatory fluid surrounding the pancreas tail, extending into the left anterior pararenal space. Only the tail and uncinate portions of the pancreas enhance. CT severity index = 8. **B,** organized sterile pancreatic necrosis. Contrast-enhanced CT 6 weeks later shows evolution of the complex pancreatic collection. The attenuation of the collection is homogeneously low, with a well-formed wall and several septations. Except for the tail and uncinate, the pancreas is replaced by this large collection. **C,** 1 week after transgastric (TG) endoscopic drainage without lavage. The liquefied portion of the pancreatic collection has been drained. Solid, secondarily infected necrotic debris seen interspersed with gas is observed in the pancreatic bed (*white arrow*), and in the left anterior pararenal space (*A*). A TG pigtail stent is seen (*curved black arrow*). **D,** complete nonsurgical resolution of extensive infected organized pancreatic necrosis using intrapancreatic lavage. Contrast-enhanced CT 6 months after endoscopic drainage shows atrophy of most of the pancreatic head, neck, and body. (Courtesy of Baron TH, Thaggard WG, Morgan DE, et al: Endoscopic therapy for organized pancreatic necrosis. *Gastroenterology* 111:755–764, 1996.)

(1) the importance of accurately identifying pancreatic necrosis and differentiating this type of process from acute fluid collections, pseudocysts, and pancreatic abscesses; and (2) that these results apply to a specific group of patients with persistent symptoms attributable to well-defined, organized, and partially liquefied collections occurring 4–11 weeks (mean, 7 weeks) after the episode of acute pancreatitis.

N.J. Greenberger, M.D.

54 Chronic Pancreatitis

Natural History of Alcoholic Chronic Pancreatitis

Course of Alcoholic Chronic Pancreatitis: A Prospective Clinicomorphological Long-term Study

Ammann RW, Heitz PU, Klöppel G (Univ Hosp, Zurich, Switzerland; Univ of Kiel, Germany)
Gastroenterology 111:224–231,1996

7–5

Background.—Alcoholic chronic pancreatitis (ACP) appears to evolve from severe acute pancreatitis. Clinical findings were correlated with pancreatic histopathologic findings at early and advanced stages of disease.

Methods.—Seventy-three patients who progressed from clinically acute to chronic pancreatitis during a mean 12 years of follow-up were included in the analysis. Thirty-seven surgical and 46 postmortem pancreatic speci-

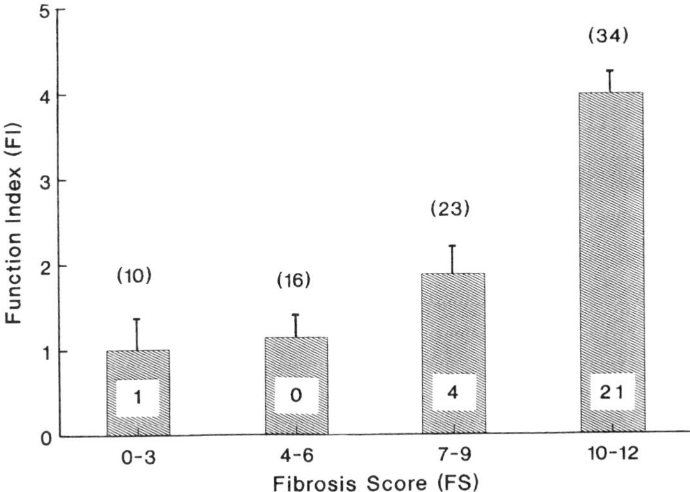

FIGURE 4.—Relationship between degree of fibrosis and pancreatic dysfunction in alcoholic chronic pancreatitis (FI; mean ± SEM). Numbers in parentheses at the top of bars are the number of patients; numbers inside bars are the number of patients with diabetes. The correlation of the 2 variables (fibrosis score and function index) is statistically significant ($P = 0.001$). (Courtesy of Ammann RW, Heitz PU, Klöppel G: Course of Alcoholic chronic pancreatitis: A prospective clinicomorphological long-term study. *Gastroenterology* 111:224–231, 1996.)

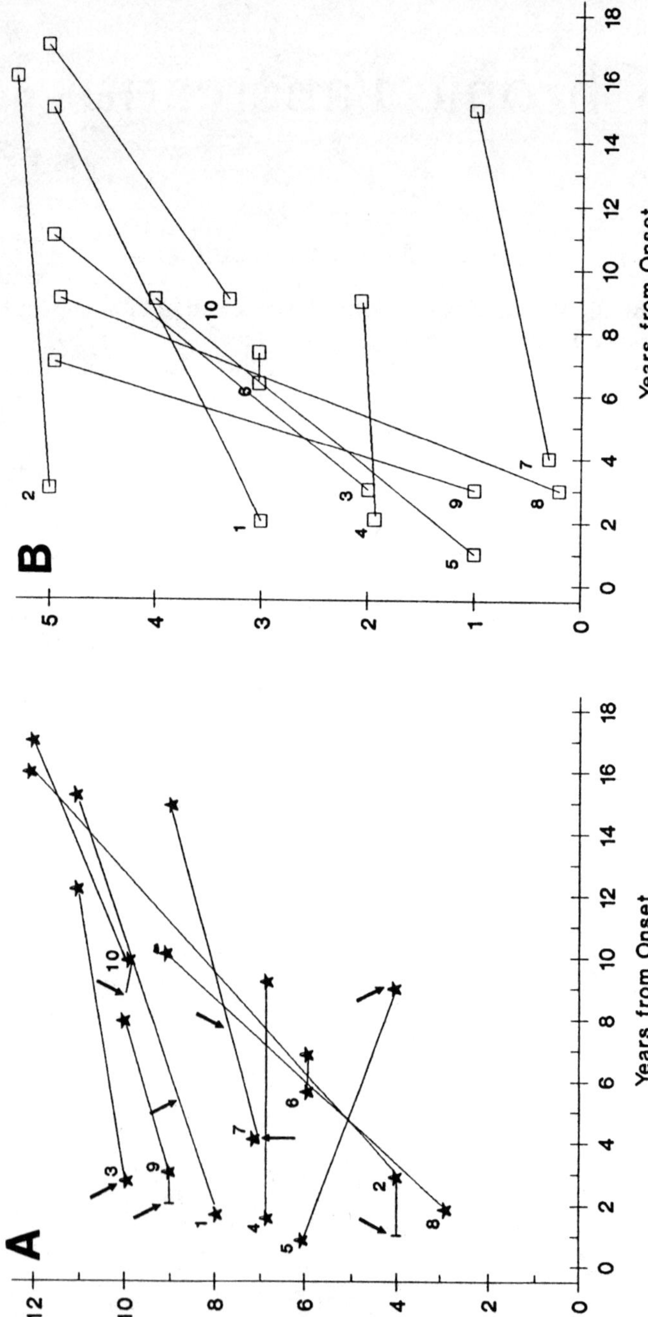

FIGURE 5.—Findings in the subgroup of 10 patients with 2 histologic studies. Evolution from onset of alcoholic chronic pancreatitis (time 0) to biopsy (*first symbol*) and to necropsy (*second symbol*) regarding fibrosis (fibrosis score, 0–12) (A) and dysfunction (function index, 0–5) (B). A, the onset of pancreatic calcification is indicated by an *arrow*; it preceded the surgical biopsy in 3 of 8 patients with calcific chronic pancreatitis (*line ahead of the asterisk*). The differences of the mean values of fibrosis score and function index (first vs. final) are statistically significant ($P < 0.01$). (Courtesy of Ammann RW, Heitz PU, Klöppel G: Course of alcoholic chronic pancreatitis: A prospective clinicomorphological long-term study. *Gastroenterology* 111:224–231, 1996.)

mens were assessed for morphologic changes, such as pseudocysts, auto-digestive necrosis, calcification, and perilobular and intralobular fibrosis. Pancreatic function had been monitored annually.

Findings.—Surgery was performed at a mean 4.1 years after onset. In the histologic assessment, focal necrosis predominated in 49% of the specimens and mild perilobular fibrosis in 54%. Eighty-eight percent of the specimens showed pseudocysts, mostly postnecrotic, within 6 years of disease onset. Eighty-five percent of the autopsy specimens, studied at a mean 12 years from onset, showed severe perilobular and intralobular fibrosis. Seventy-four percent showed calcifications. Only 4%, however, were necrotic. Fibrosis was associated with progressive pancreatic dysfunction, especially in the 10 patients with 2 histologic assessments (Figs 4 and 5).

Conclusions.—This study provided an analysis of the morphologic changes in the pancreas in the early stages of disease and the subsequent evolution of disease, terminating in ACP. The most important changes observed in the first 6 years after disease onset were frequent necrosis and pseudocysts and the scarcity of calculi (and protein plugs) in patients with mild fibrosis.

▶ This study provides further insights into the pathogenesis of ACP and supports the concept that chronic pancreatitis evolves as a direct result of severe alcoholic acute pancreatitis. Three mechanisms have been postulated to explain the relationship between alcohol and pancreatitis: (1) alcohol has direct toxic and metabolic effects on the pancreas; (2) episodes of acute alcoholic-induced pancreatitis occur in a setting of *pre-existent* chronic pancreatitis; and (3) ACP results from repeated episodes of necrotizing pancreatitis. The latter concept challenges the current notion that acute pancreatitis and chronic pancreatitis are separate disorders. Accumulating evidence suggests that this is not the case with alcohol-associated pancreatic disease. The authors have summarized the features common to both acute pancreatitis and chronic pancreatitis. First, alcohol abuse is the most common cause of both diseases. Second, ACP usually starts with acute episodes of pancreatitis that are indistinguishable from acute pancreatitis. In this regard, if patients with their first episode of alcohol-induced acute pancreatitis are studied and evaluated, 2–3 months later approximately 50% will be found to have impaired pancreatic exocrine function, suggesting that chronic pancreatitis is already established. Third, pseudocysts, which are common to both acute and chronic pancreatitis, present identical histologic features in the 2 conditions.

That alcohol is indeed toxic to the pancreas is further evident from studies by Gullo[1] who demonstrated that discontinuation of alcohol in patients with alcohol-induced chronic pancreatitis resulted in a slower deterioration of pancreatic function compared to similar patients who continued to ingest alcohol. Thus progression of ACP is slower and less marked if alcohol use ceases.

N.J. Greenberger, M.D.

Reference

1. Gullo L, Barbara L, Labo G: Effect of cessation of alcohol use in the course of pancreatic dysfunction in alcoholic pancreatitis. *Gastroenterology*, 95:1063–1068, 1988.

Pain Relapses in the First 10 Years of Chronic Pancreatitis

Talamini G, Bassi C, Falconi M, et al (Univ of Verona, Italy)
Am J Surg 171:565–569, 1996

7–6

Introduction.—A patient's drinking habits have been associated with painful acute exacerbations of chronic pancreatitis. Pain relapses have been reduced by pancreaticojejunostomy among patients who are also more willing to control their alcohol intake after surgery. To determine whether the number of pain recurrences in the course of the first 10 years of chronic pancreatitis was related to alcohol intake, sex, type of pancreatitis, cigarette smoking, presence of pancreatic intraductal calcifications, duration of follow-up, and performance of pancreaticojejunostomy, an evaluation was conducted.

Methods.—A follow-up was conducted of 582 patients who had well-documented chronic pancreatitis or typical abdominal pain symptoms accompanied by a significant increase in serum amylase levels in the absence of acute peptic or biliary disease. Of these, 205 patients were selected for study, and recordings were taken of the number of cigarettes smoked, number of grams of alcohol consumed daily, presence or absence of calcifications in the main pancreatic duct, performance of pancreaticojejunostomy, body mass index, and number of annual pain relapses.

Results.—The annual number of pain relapses was significantly associated with drinking, smoking, calcifications, pancreaticojejunostomy, and length of follow-up. Of these patients, 93% drank more than 40 g of alcohol per day. Of these patients, 87% were smokers who smoked an average of 23.3 cigarettes per day. Physically, pancreaticojejunostomy was effective in reducing pain by removing the largest intraductal calcifications and obstructions through drainage of Wirsung's duct. Psychologically, this surgery helped patients cut down their postsurgical alcohol intake. There was no correlation between pain relapses and sex or age at onset of chronic pancreatitis.

Conclusions.—Patients should reduce their alcohol intake and cigarette smoking, regardless of whether they receive surgical treatment. Once calcifications have formed, pancreaticojejunostomy is the procedure of choice to alleviate the pain.

▶ The physicians and surgeons in Verona, Italy, have done us a great service by subjecting their patients (205) to multivariate analysis after at least a 10-year follow-up. Pancreaticojejunostomy with an emphasis on intraductal stone removal offers long-term pain relief if the patients stop drinking and smoking. The authors make a good point: the operation provides a bond between the patient and the medical team, providing a vehicle for follow-up and reinforcement regarding compliance.

I was fascinated by the demographics. Eighty-nine percent of the 205 patients who drank more than 40 g of alcohol per day for almost 2 decades were male. In only 2% cirrhosis developed. It is of interest that although about 50% of patients stopped drinking during the follow-up period, only 10% stopped smoking. It would have been interesting to know how many patients later had pancreatic cancer.

F.G. Moody, M.D.

Endoscopic Stenting

Long-term Results of Endoscopic Stenting and Surgical Drainage for Biliary Stricture Due to Chronic Pancreatitis

Smits ME, Rauws EAJ, van Gulik TM, et al (Univ of Amsterdam, The Netherlands)
Br J Surg 83:764–768, 1996   7–7

Background.—Jaundice from obstruction of the intrapancreatic segment of the common bile duct reportedly occurs in 3% to 46% of patients with chronic pancreatitis. Authorities continue to disagree on whether endoscopic treatment or surgical drainage is the best long-term treatment. The long-term outcomes of polyethylene biliary stenting were investigated in 1 group of patients with benign biliary stricture from chronic pancreatitis.

Methods and Outcomes.—Fifty-eight patients aged 19–76 years were treated and followed for a median of 49 months. Endoscopic stent insertion immediately relieved jaundice and cholestasis in all patients. Complications occurred in 9% of the patients after therapeutic endoscopic retrograde cholangiopancreatography. Sixty-four percent had late stent-related complications. None of the patients died. In 28% of the patients, biliary stricture regressed, and stents were removed permanently. In 42 patients, biliary stricture persisted. Twenty-six had continued stenting and 16 underwent surgery. Six of these 16 patients had early morbidity after surgery, but no one died. Fifteen of the 16 patients had relief of jaundice postoperatively (Fig 1).

Conclusion.—Endoscopic stenting and surgery are both effective for alleviating biliary stricture in patients with chronic pancreatitis. Endoscopic stenting provides definitive treatment in more than one fourth of the patients. Although fewer early complications occur with endoscopic stenting than with surgery, the occurrence of stent-related complications is a major limiting factor.

▶ How best to manage cholestasis from a distal biliary stricture in chronic pancreatitis is an unresolved problem. Surgeons and gastroenterologists at the Academic Medical Center of the University of Amsterdam provide some interesting clinical results regarding the efficacy and morbidity of endoscopic stenting and surgical bypass. The flow diagram in Figure 1 relates the outcome. Stents are associated with relief of jaundice and an early low

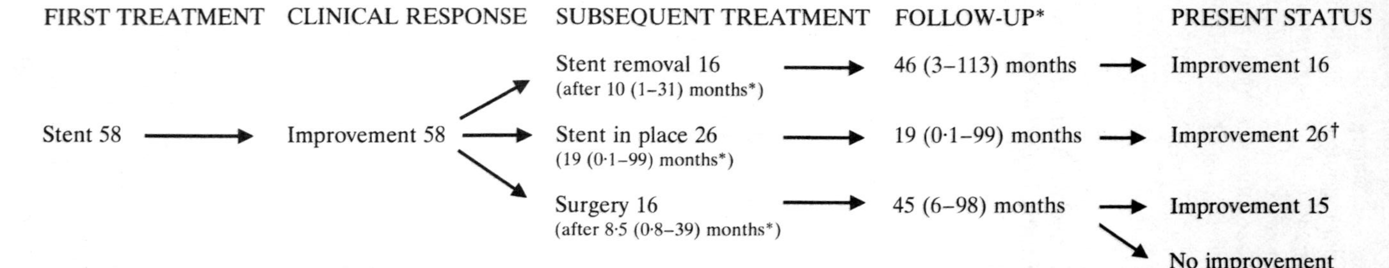

FIGURE 1.—Long-term results of endoscopic therapy and subsequent surgical drainage. *Asterisk* indicates that values are median (range); *dagger* indicates that 2 patients were lost to follow-up and 4 died. (Courtesy of Smits ME, Rauws EAJ, van Gulik TM, et al: Long-term results of endoscopic stenting and surgical drainage for biliary stricture due to chronic pancreatitis. *Br J Surg* 83:764–768, 1996. Publisher, Blackwell Science Ltd.)

morbidity, and almost one third of the patients had regression of their stricture and stent removal without recurrence. Sixty-four percent of those who required chronic stenting had a variety of complications related to stent migration or clogging in the majority. From this experience, the authors recommend stenting as an initial approach for up to 3 months. If the stricture persists, surgery is recommended for the young and fit and restenting for those at high risk. This sounds like good advice to me.

F.G. Moody, M.D.

Surgical Treatment Including Duodenum Preserving Resection

Duodenum Preserving Resection of the Head of the Pancreas in Painful Chronic Pancreatitis
Eddes EH, Masclee AAM, Lamers CBHW, et al (Univ Hosp, Leiden, The Netherlands)
Eur J Surg 162:545–549, 1996   7–8

Introduction.—Alcohol is one of the culprits of chronic pancreatitis, and damage to the gland is progressive and can end with endocrine and exocrine insufficiency. When pain is disabling, surgery may be necessary. Ideally, the surgery would combine low morbidity and mortality with effectiveness. The duodenum-preserving resection of the head of the pancreas removes only the diseased head, leaving the proximal gastrointestinal tract intact. Fifteen patients with painful chronic pancreatitis received this surgery.

Methods.—The retrospective study included 15 patients with painful chronic pancreatitis who had duodenum-preserving resection. For 11 patients, the cause was alcohol consumption, and for 4 patients the cause was unknown. The patients had a median age of 42 years, and there were 14 men and 1 woman. All patients were taking analgesics: 7 were taking opiates and 8 were taking non-opiates. Mortality, morbidity, pain relief, and endocrine and exocrine function were measured.

Results.—In all patients, surgery was successful. The hospital stay was a median of 24 days, ranging from 15 to 40 days. After a mean follow-up of 37 months, 11 of 15 patients were pain free after the operation, whereas 2 showed significant improvement. There was a small-bowel leak in 1 patient, obstructive ileus in 1 patient, and peri-anastomotic abscess in 2 patients. After resection, neither endocrine or exocrine function deteriorated significantly. After the operation, 7 of 9 patients who were not taking exocrine supplements previously needed them; however, they had no significant difference in mean urine paraaminobenzoic acid recovery.

Conclusions.—In patients with disabling pain caused by chronic pancreatitis with an inflammatory mass in the head of the pancreas, duodenum-preserving resection is an effective operation. Particularly in patients not taking opiate-like analgesics before the operation, pain relief is impressive after surgery.

▶ The surgical and medical gastroenterologists in Leiden report a high level of success for pain relief by using a duodenum-preserving resection of the pancreatic head. Although no deaths occurred in the 15 patients so treated, the operation was not without significant morbidity and a prolonged hospital stay.

A major question relates to the population of patients treated. The authors mention in the discussion that pain relief was especially effective in patients not receiving narcotic analgesics before operation. Most patients (if not all) referred to me for surgical therapy are already addicted to narcotics. This practice and attitude on my part does not detract from the appropriateness of their therapeutic decision to operate on patients early in the course of their painful experience with their disease, but one must weigh the risk, cost, and gain of such an approach. Obviously, the initial approach to the nonaddicted alcoholics with pain from chronic pancreatitis is to get them to stop drinking.

F.G. Moody, M.D.

Long-term Results of Pylorus-preserving Pancreatoduodenectomy for Chronic Pancreatitis

Martin RF, Rossi RL, Leslie KA (Lahey Clinic Med Ctr, Burlington, Mass; Harvard Med School, Boston)
Arch Surg 131:247–252, 1996   7–9

Background.—The treatment of chronic pancreatitis is challenging. Pancreatic head resection procedures appear to yield comparable pain relief outcomes. Authorities disagree, however, about which procedures have less deleterious adverse effects. The results of pylorus-preserving pancreatoduodenectomy (PPPD) in one series of patients with chronic pancreatitis were reported.

Methods.—The records of 45 patients who underwent PPPD for disabling chronic pancreatitis were reviewed. Follow-up ranged from 1 month to 13.7 years. Surviving patients were interviewed by telephone.

Findings.—The mean duration of pain before surgery was 50 months. Seventy percent of the patients needed daily narcotics. Portal vein resection was required in one patient. Another patient died within 30 days of surgery. Ninety-two percent of the patients reported improvement in pain 5 years postoperatively. On a scale of 0 to 10, the mean pain score was 9.2 before surgery, compared with 1.5 at 6 months, 0.8 at 1 year, 1.1 at 2 years, and 1.1 at 5 years. Seventy-four percent of the patients gained weight postoperatively to a mean of 92% of their pre-illness weight. Fourteen percent of the patients had new-onset diabetes by 6 months and 46% by 5 years. One patient, who underwent a total pancreatectomy, died from hypoglycemia. Four deaths were unrelated to PPPD. Ten percent of the patients had marginal ulcers. Nine patients needed late surgery.

Conclusions.—Pancreatic head resection produces long-term pain improvement in more than 90% of selected patients. Although the early development of diabetes mellitus is not common, the prevalence of diabetes after PPPD over time is similar to that of patients who did not undergo resection. Weight gain in the patients who underwent PPPD was superior to that previously reported for patients who underwent a standard Whipple procedure for chronic pancreatitis.

▶ In this report the surgeons at the Lahey Clinic establish the effectiveness of the pylorus-sparing Whipple procedure in relieving the addictive pain of chronic pancreatitis. They substantiate the value of the pylorus-sparing reconstruction by the fact that almost three quarters of the patients regained close to their pre-illness weight. I imagine that they are probably right; preserving the pylorus improves gastrointestinal function. *Warshaw*, in his lengthy discussion of the presentation of this work at the 76th Annual Meeting of the New England Surgical Society, pointed out potential shortcomings of the pylorus-sparing procedure, the major ones related to the high incidence of delayed gastric emptying and peptic ulcer disease. In fact, patients in this series required surgery at a later date for these problems.

F.G. Moody, M.D.

Laparoscopic Distal 70% Pancreatectomy and Splenectomy for Chronic Pancreatitis
Cuschieri A, Jakimowicz JJ, van Spreeuwel J (Univ of Dundee, Scotland; Catharina Hosp, Eindoven, The Netherlands)
Ann Surg 223:280–285, 1996   7–10

Background.—Resection can provide good pain relief in patients with chronic pancreatitis. However, a common localization of the bulk of the pathologic process in the head of the pancreas in many patients has inspired the possibility of localized resection. The technique of laparoscopic distal resections was described and the results reported.

Methods.—Five carefully selected patients with gross pathologic lesions confined to the left hemipancreas underwent laparoscopic distal pancreatectomy. All the patients had good nutritional health and no serious comorbidity. The 4 patients with alcohol habits stopped drinking.

Surgical Technique.—With the use of general endotracheal anesthesia, 5 port sites were used (Fig 1). The lesser omentum was divided without ligature of the left and right gastric vessels, and the lesser sac was entered through the gastrocolic omentum. The greater curvature was separated completely, with the division of any adhesions to the stomach. The common splenic artery was identified either by dissection or contact ultrasound scanning and was dissected from the pancreas. The pancreas was mobilized with careful dissection around to its posterior aspect until the main portal vein was identified and cleared. Then the splenic vein was doubly ligated and divided to allow complete mobilization of the pancreas. The pancreas was transected between the divided ends of the splenic vein and the pancreatic/splenic block was detached from

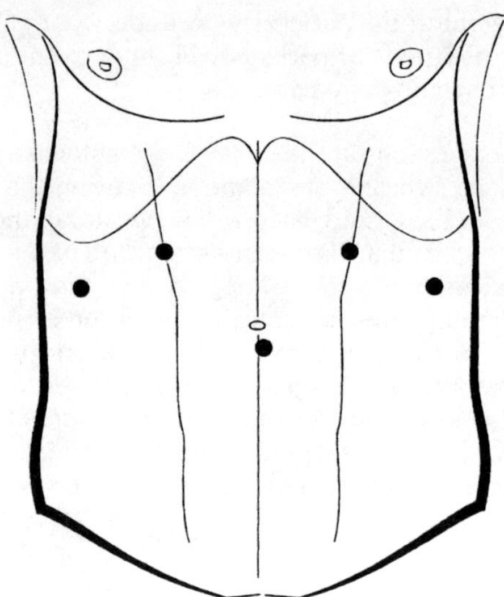

FIGURE 1.—Diagram of the port sites used for laparoscopic distal pancreatectomy. (Courtesy of Cuschieri A, Jakimowicz JJ, van Spreeuwel J: Laparoscopic distal 70% pancreatectomy and splenectomy for chronic pancreatitis. *Ann Surg* 223:280–285, 1996.)

right to left and removed. After irrigation and the placement of a drain adjacent to the transected pancreas, the port wounds were closed.

Results.—The surgery was performed in 4–6 hours. There were 2 postoperative complications: a minor, spontaneously resolving pancreatic leak in 1 patient and prolonged ileus in 1 patient. Hospital discharge occurred 6–7 days after surgery. All patients had substantial pain relief, and 2 patients had complete pain relief.

Conclusions.—A distal 70% pancreatectomy can be performed laparoscopically safely with good results. This approach accelerates postoperative progress and reduces postoperative hospital stay.

▶ This report by Cuschieri, Jakimowicz, and van Spreeuwel is more than just a show and tell of what can be done laparoscopically. It represents an important forward step in pancreatic surgery. But we must remind ourselves that these patients were treated by the combined efforts of the world's leaders in advanced laparoscopic technology. This procedure is not for the highly skilled and experienced laparoscopic surgeon. The question of whether this procedure was beneficial to these patients with chronic pain, of course, is another matter. The issue of patient selection and efficacy will have to be answered before this approach enters the mainstream of treating patients with the debilitating pain of chronic pancreatitis.

F.G. Moody, M.D.

55 Hereditary Pancreatitis

A Gene for Hereditary Pancreatitis Maps to Chromosome 7q35
Whitcomb DC, Preston RA, Aston CE, et al (Univ of Pittsburgh, Pa; Pittsburgh Veterans Affairs Med Ctr, Pa; Childrens Hosp of Pittsburgh, Pa; et al)
Gastroenterology 110:1975–1980, 1996   7–11

Background.—Hereditary pancreatitis (HP), an inherited disorder that encompasses clinical features of both acute and chronic pancreatitis, appears to result from a single genetic defect. The cause of HP, however, has not been determined. Investigators used the approach of genetic linkage technology to identify the HP gene.

Methods.—A comprehensive family tree was constructed for a 500-member pedigree centered in eastern Kentucky and western Virginia. Diagnosis of HP required characteristic pain with elevated amylase levels, CT or US findings consistent with pancreatitis, surgical findings, and repeated episodes of epigastric pain that started in childhood and were usually associated with vomiting. A detailed questionnaire was administered to ascertain the phenotype of all participants. In a 36-member subset of the family, a genome-wide search strategy was used to determine the genetic locus for HP. The search was began on chromosome 1 and proceeded through chromosome 7, with microsatellite markers spaced at 20-cM intervals.

Results.—The study participants were 103 family members who were interviewed, completed questionnaires, and gave blood. Linkage in the family subset was established between the HP phenotype and chromosome 7q. Modeled as an autosomal dominant disorder with 80% penetrance, a maximal multipoint logarithm of the odds score of 4.3 was obtained by using a 4-point analysis consisting of the markers D7S684, D7S661, and D7S505 and the HP locus. The centromeric limit for the location of the HP locus was defined by a recombination between HP and D7S684 located 8 cM centromeric to D7S661. The telomeric limit was defined by an obligate recombination between HP and D7S483 located 5 cM telomeric to D7S505. Thus the HP locus, as defined by this family subset, includes a 19-cM region on chromosome 7q. A break in the high-risk haplotype between D7S684 and D7S661 detected by using members from the extended pedigree suggests that an additional 8 cM may be excluded from the HP locus.

Discussion.—The onset of HP usually occurs between the ages of 5 and 10 years, and the disorder is one of the most common causes of chronic or recurrent pancreatitis in childhood. Symptoms of an acute attack of HP are similar to acute attack symptoms of pancreatitis from other causes. With the development of chronic pancreatitis in HP, patients experience chronic abdominal pain, weight loss, and diarrhea, and diabetes mellitus may be diagnosed. By linking the HP gene to a limited region, the molecular mechanism causing the disease may be defined and strategies developed to prevent or control its clinical manifestations.

▶ Hereditary pancreatitis is a chronic idiopathic inflammatory disorder affecting multiple family members over 2 or more generations. Hereditary pancreatitis is an autosomal dominant disorder with variable expression. This suggests that HP results from a single genetic defect that disrupts a critical mechanism protecting nonaffected individuals from pancreatitis. The pathogenesis of HP remains poorly understood. This elegant study by Whitcomb and colleagues links HP to the 7q35 region of chromosome 7q. Linking the HP disease gene to a limited region is a major step in defining the molecular mechanism causing HP. As Whitcomb et al. point out in their discussion, the observation focuses attention on new candidate genes within this area such as the T-cell receptor, carboxypeptidase A, and serine proteases.

N.J. Greenberger, M.D.

56 Shwachman Syndrome

Shwachman Syndrome: Exocrine Pancreatic Dysfunction and Variable Phenotypic Expression
Mack DR, Forstner GG, Wilschanski M, et al (Hosp for Sick Children, Toronto; Univ of Toronto)
Gastroenterology 111:1593–1602, 1996   7–12

Background.—Shwachman syndrome, first identified in 1964, is characterized by short stature, exocrine pancreatic hypoplasia, bone marrow dysfunction, and other features. The medical charts of 29 patients were reviewed to determine the clinical course and pathological findings of this inherited condition.

Methods.—All patients were monitored at The Hospital for Sick Children, Toronto. The mean age at diagnosis was 1.5 years; 17 patients were male. Diagnosis was established on the basis of exocrine pancreatic dysfunction and the presence of 1 or more of the clinical features typical of Shwachman syndrome (Fig 1). Quantitative tests of exocrine pancreatic function were performed in 24 patients, and 21 patients had measurements of serum cationic trypsinogen. All patients had fecal fat balance studies and radiologic skeletal studies at the time of diagnosis. The median follow-up was 5 years.

Results.—The mean birth weight of patients with Shwachman syndrome, both boys and girls, was within the lower limits of normal range. Growth velocity was subnormal for height and weight during the first 6 months of life but subsequently returned to normal. Skeletal abnormalities were present in 76% of the cases (Table 1), and liver abnormalities were also common. Severe fat maldigestion resulting from pancreatic insufficiency was present early in life. Despite persistent deficits of enzyme secretion, 45% of the patients demonstrated moderate improvements leading to pancreatic insufficiency as they grew older. The most common hematologic abnormality was neutropenia, which affected 88% of the patients. Eleven patients had abnormalities affecting all 3 cell lines, and the 5 deaths occurred in this group of patients. Two died of sepsis while severely neutropenic, and 5 died of acute myelogenous leukemia. Patients with severe neutropenia were prone to a variety of infectious organisms.

Discussion.—This is the largest group of patients with Shwachman syndrome described to date. Universal features in these patients were exocrine pancreatic dysfunction and an abnormality of 1 or more of the

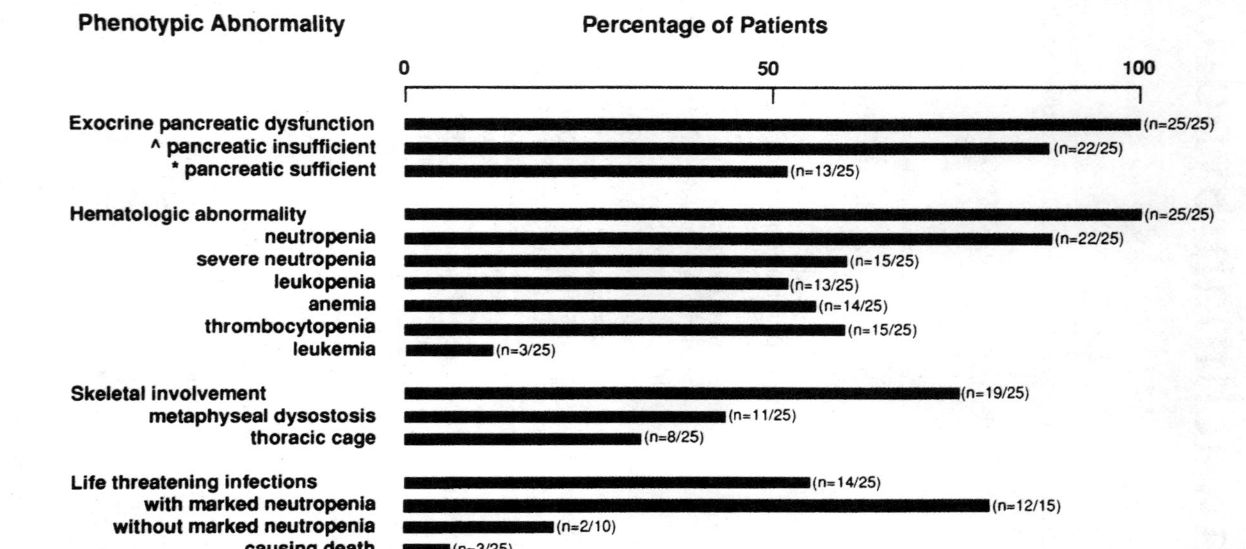

FIGURE 1.—Synopsis of the frequency of each clinical phenotype. ^At diagnosis; *at diagnosis or converted to pancreatic sufficiency after diagnosis. (Courtesy of Mack DR, Forstner GG, Wilschanski M, et al: Shwachman syndrome: Exocrine pancreatic dysfunction and variable phenotypic expression. *Gastroenterology* 111:1593–1602, 1996.)

TABLE 1.—Clinical Features

Patient No.	Sex	Clinical Findings	Age at Diagnosis (yr)	Pancreas Status	Hematology	Skeletal	Outcome
1	M	Thoracic, dystrophy	0.1	Pl-PS	A, NVL, W, P	CC, TD, RF, O	Death (AML)
2	M	PG, neutropenia, recurrent infections	0.25	Pl	A, NVL, W, P	MD	Death (AML)
3	M	PG, pancytopenia	16	Pl	A, NVL, W, P		Death (AML)
4	M	PG, pancytopenia	1.1	Pl	A, NVL, W, P	O	Death (sepsis)
5	F	PG, neutropenia, recurrent infections	1.5	Pl	A, NVL, P	O	Death (sepsis)
6	M	PG, recurrent infections	2.7	Pl-PS	A, NVL, W, P	MD, O	Unknown†
7	F	PG	0.4	Pl	A, NVL, W, P	MD	Unknown†
8	F	PG, neutropenia, recurrent infections hepatomegaly	2.25	Pl-PS	A, NVL, W, P	MD	
9	M	PG, recurrent infections	1.6	Pl-PS	A, NVL, W, P	MD	Death*
10	M	PG, neutropenia, recurrent infections	1	Pl	A, NVL, P	MD, CC, RF, O	
11	F	PG	0.25	Pl-PS	A, NVL, P	CC, TD, RF	
12	M	PG	6	Pl-PS	NL		Unknown†
13	M	Recurrent infections, neutropenia	9	PS	NVL, W	MD	Unknown†
14	M	PG, recurrent infections	10	Pl-PS	A, NVL, W	MD, O	Unknown†
15	F	PG, neutropenia	0.9	Pl-PS	NVL		
16	M	PG, neutropenia, recurrent infections	0.75	Pl	NVL, P	CC	
17	F	PG	0.3	Pl	A	CC, O	
18	F	PG, recurrent infections	0.6	Pl	A	O	Unknown†
19	M	PG	13.9	Pl	P	O	Unknown†
20	M	PG, skeletal abnormalities	3	Pl-PS	NL, W, P	MD, CC, RF, TD, O	Unknown†
21	M	PG	13	PS	NL, W, P	MD	
22	M	PG	1.5	Pl-PS	NL, W	MD, CC	
23	F	PG	29.5	PS	NL		
24	M	PG	3.75	Pl	NL		
25	M	Hepatomegaly	2.25	Pl	NL		

*Death unrelated to medical condition.

†Not currently monitored.

Abbreviations: PG, growth of less than the 5th percentile; *PI*, pancreatic insufficiency; *PL-PS*, pancreatic sufficiency developed during follow-up; *PS*, pancreatic sufficient at the time of diagnosis; *A*, fetal hemoglobin level greater than 2% or anemia (hemoglobin level of less than 12 g/dL for ages older than 6 years); *NVL*, neutrophil count of less than 500×10^6/L; *NL*, neutrophil count of less than 1500 $\times 10^6$/L; *W*, total white blood count of less than 4000×10^6/L; *P*, platelet count of less than 150×10^6/L; *MD*, metaphyseal dysostosis; *RF*, rib flaring; *TD*, thoracic dystrophy; *CC*, costochondral thickening; *O*, other. (Courtesy of Mack DR, Forstner GG, Wilschanski M, et al: Shwachman syndrome: Exocrine pancreatic dysfunction and variable phenotype expression. *Gastroenterology* 111:1593–1602, 1996.)

bone marrow cellular elements. Other phenotypic abnormalities varied widely in frequency. The prognosis is guarded for patients with severe bone marrow involvement.

▶ This study describes the largest group of patients with Shwachman syndrome ever reported and as such provides a wealth of information on the clinical features and natural history of this interesting disorder. The hallmarks of this condition include pancreatic exocrine insufficiency, skeletal abnormalities, short stature, hematologic abnormalities (especially neutropenia but also anemia and thrombocytopenia), and severe infections that are often life-threatening. The variable phenotypic expression is evident from Figure 1 and Table 1. Classically, Shwachman syndrome includes a triad of findings: (1) pancreatic insufficiency, (2) neutropenia, and (3) short stature. However, as pointed out in this report, exocrine pancreatic dysfunction and an abnormality of 1 or more bone marrow cellular products were the early features found in all 25 patients.

Two features of the pancreatic dysfunction bear emphasis. First, it is not generally appreciated that Shwachman syndrome is the second most common cause of exocrine pancreatic dysfunction. Second, pancreatic function may improve with age; 45% of the patients in this study showed gradual improvement leading to pancreatic sufficiency. Finally, note that in 5 patients Shwachman syndrome was first diagnosed after 10 years of age, i.e., at 10, 13, 13.9, 16, and 29.5 years.

N.J. Greenberger, M.D.

57 Pancreatic Neoplasms

Intraductal Papillary Mucinous Tumors and Other Intraductal Tumors

Intraductal Papillary-mucinous Tumors of the Pancreas: Clinicopathologic Features, Outcome, and Nomenclature

Loftus EV Jr, Olivares-Pakzad BA, Batts KP, et al (Mayo Clinic, Rochester, Minn)
Gastroenterology 110:1909–1918, 1996　　　　　　　　　　　　7–13

Background.—More and more cases of intraductal papillary-mucinous tumor (IPMT) of the pancreatic ducts are being reported. These tumors are dysplastic, frequently diffuse lesions that are associated with copious mucin production and duct dilatation and can cause episodes of pancreatic-like pain. Treatment is difficult because of inability to predict the presence

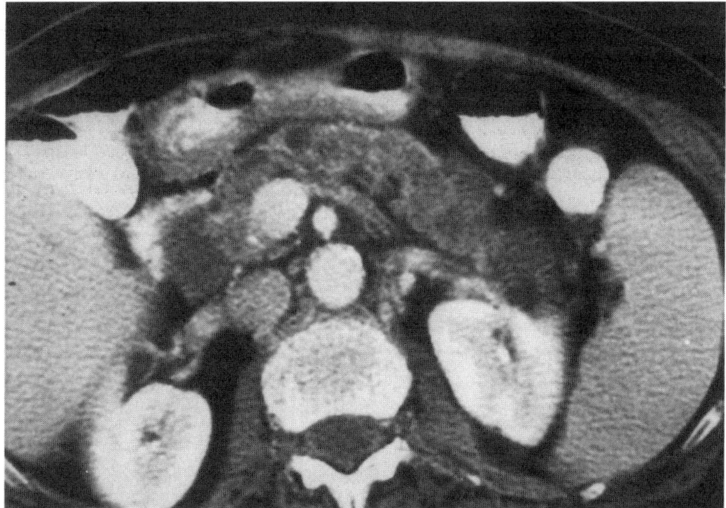

FIGURE 1.—Representative CT scan (patient 5) with dilatation of the main pancreatic duct, thinning of the pancreatic parenchyma, and numerous cystic structures throughout the gland. (Courtesy of Loftus EV Jr, Olivares-Pakzad BA, Batts KP, et al: Intraductal papillary-mucinous tumors of the pancreas: Clinicopathologic features, outcome, and nomenclature. *Gastroenterology* 110:1909–1918, 1996.)

of cancer and lack of knowledge about the natural history of disease. A series of 15 patients with IPMT was analyzed.

Methods.—The patients were 11 men and 4 women, with a median age of 68 years. Four patients had diabetes mellitus, and 9 had a previous diagnosis of chronic pancreatitis. All medical records, radiographs, and pathologic specimens were analyzed to see whether the clinical, imaging, or histologic features could predict disease outcome. In addition, an attempt was made to arrive at a reasonable treatment algorithm and to clarify the relations among IPMT, mucinous cystic neoplasms (MCNs) of the pancreas, and chronic pancreatitis.

Findings.—The results of CT scanning were abnormal in 93% of patients studied (Fig 1), and the results of endoscopic retrograde cholangiopancreatography (ERCP) were abnormal in 10 of 10 patients studied (Fig 2). One patient had hepatic metastases at the time of diagnosis. The remaining 14 patients underwent surgery: 6 had distal pancreatectomy, 4 had total pancreatectomy, and 4 had pancreaticoduodenectomy. At surgery, all patients were found to have chronic pancreatitis with dysplasia of the intraductal epithelium. Three had invasive adenocarcinoma in addition. At a median follow-up of 25 months, 10 patients were alive, including 9 of 11 patients with benign disease and 1 of 4 with cancer. None of

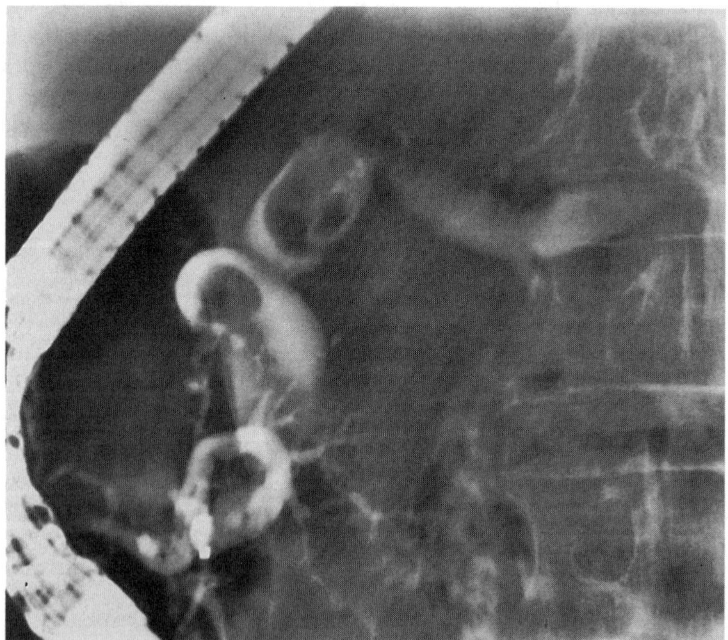

FIGURE 2.—Representative endoscopic retrograde cholangiopancreatography (patient 5) with diffuse dilatation of the main duct with numerous intraluminal filling defects. (Courtesy of Loftus EV Jr, Olivares-Pakzad BA, Batts KP, et al: Intraductal papillary-mucinous tumors of the pancreas: Clinicopathologic features, outcome, and nomenclature. *Gastroenterology* 110:1909–1918, 1996.)

TABLE 1.—Clinical Features and Outcome of 15 Patients With Intraductal Papillary-Mucinous Tumor of the Pancreas

Patient no.	Age (yr)	Sex	History of tobacco use	Symptoms	Duration	Previous diagnosis of chronic pancreatitis?	Abdominal mass	US/CT findings	ERCP findings	Operation	Outcome
1	78	M	Yes	Recurrent epigastric pain, elevated amylase levels	17 yr	Yes	No	MPD dilatation in body. ? cyst in tail	Segmental dilatation of MPD in tail	DP	Alive, 35 mo
2	71	M	Yes	Recurrent right-sided abdominal pain, diabetes mellitus	2 mo (DM, 11 yr)	No	No	MPD diffusely dilated	Prominent papilla, dilated MPD and one BD in uncinate, filling defects	DP	Alive, 27 mo
3	54	F	Yes	Recurrent back pain, elevated amylase levels, 17-kg weight loss	2 yr	Yes	No	Normal	Mild diffuse MPD dilatation	DP, then TP 7 mo later	Alive, 28 mo
4	53	M	Yes	Recurrent acute pancreatitis	3 yr	Yes	No	MPD dilatation in tail, cyst in tail	MPD dilatation, marked in tail, mild in head, stringy filling defects	DP	Alive, 27 mo
5	90	F	No	Hemosuccus pancreaticus	3 wk	No	No	Marked MPD dilatation, multiple cysts	Diffuse MPD and BD dilatation, filling defects	DP	Died of other cause, 18 mo
6	76	M	Yes	Steatorrhea, 9-kg weight loss, diabetes mellitus, jaundice	8 mo (DM, 31 yr)	Yes	No	Multicystic mass in head, uncinate; diffuse dilatation of MPD, biliary tree	Not done	TP	Alive, 25 mo
7	73	M	Yes	Recurrent epigastric pain, elevated amylase levels	15 yr	Yes	Yes	Cystic mass with mural nodules in head, dilated MPD in tail	Not done	WP	Died of cancer, 63 mo
8	66	F	No	Steatorrhea, 10-kg weight loss	1 yr	No	Yes	Diffusely dilated MPD, multiple small cysts	Dilated MPD in head, filling defects	TP	Died of cancer, 23 mo
9	59	F	No	Recurrent abdominal pain, elevated amylase levels, 9-kg weight loss	2 yr	Yes	No	Multicystic mass in body	Not done	DP	Alive, 66 mo

(*Continued*)

TABLE (cont.)

Patient no.	Age (yr)	Sex	History of tobacco use	Symptoms	Duration	Previous diagnosis of chronic pancreatitis?	Abdominal mass	US/CT findings	ERCP findings	Operation	Outcome
10	71	M	Yes	Abdominal pain, weight loss, diarrhea, diabetes mellitus	1 yr (DM, 2 yr)	No	No	Diffusely dilated MPD, local invasion	Diffusely dilated MPD, filling defects	No resection (history of hepatic metastasis)	Died of cancer, 6 mo
11	68	M	Yes	Constant periumbilical pain, 2-kg weight loss, diabetes mellitus	5 mo (DM, 13 yr)	Yes	No	Diffusely dilated MPD, multiple cysts	Prominent papilla, two focal dilatations BD in head, filling defects	DP	Alive, 53 mo
12	74	M	Yes	Incidental finding on magnetic resonance imaging for staging of bladder cancer	None	No	No	Cystic mass in head, MPD BD dilated	Not done	PPWP	Died postoperative, 4 mo
13	53	M	Yes	Recurrent acute pancreatitis	9 mo	No	No	Marked MPD dilatation	Dilated MPD body tail, filling defects mucin oozed from papilla after contrast injection	TP	Alive, 10 mo
14	54	M	Yes	Epigastric pain, elevated amylase, weight loss, steatorrhea	18 yr	Yes	No	Cystic mass in head, MPD dilated	Not done	PPWP	Alive, 14 mo
15	65	M	Yes	Epigastric pain, remote history of pseudocyst	10 yr	Yes	No	Complex cystic mass in head	Mucin oozed from major and minor papilla, diffusely dilated MPD and BD	PPWP	Alive, 11 mo

Abbreviations: BD, branch duct; DM, diabetes mellitus; ERCP, endoscopic retrograde cholangiopancreatography; MPD, main pancreatic duct; PPWP, pylorus-preserving Whipple pancreaticoduodenectomy; TP, total pancreatectomy; WP, Whipple pancreaticoduodenectomy.
(Courtesy of Loftus EV Jr, Olivares-Pakzad BA, Batts KP, et al: Intraductal papillary-mucinous tumors of the pancreas: Clinicopathologic features, outcome, and nomenclature. *Gastroenterology* 110:1909–1918, 1996.)

the patients with cancer had received a previous diagnosis of chronic pancreatitis (Table 1).

Conclusions.—Intraductal papillary-mucinous tumor of the pancreas may be considered a dysplastic, precancerous lesion, analogous to adenomatous polyps of the colon. It is distinct from MCN. There is no way to differentiate between patients with invasive noninvasive disease without surgery. The treatment of choice, therefore, is complete surgical excision with frozen section control of margins.

▶ This study provides important information on the clinical, imaging, and histologic features of IPMT of the pancreas. This disorder frequently masquerades as chronic pancreatitis, and most patients have had symptoms for many years (see Table 1). The diagnosis should be suspected on reviewing abdominal CT scan and ERCP findings. Virtually all patients will have both abnormal CT scan and ERCP examinations. The characteristic radiographic feature is the demonstration of a dilated main pancreatic duct that is either diffuse or segmental, along with intraluminal filling defects.

Intraductal papillary-mucinous tumor of the pancreas should be considered a dysplastic, precancerous lesion, but it is not possible to distinguish preoperatively patients with overt invasive carcinoma from those with dysplastic intraductal epithelium alone. However, the outcome of patients can be predicted by determining the histopathology at surgery. In the above series, 4 of 15 patients had overt cancer and 3 have died. By comparison, only 2 of 11 patients without cancer have died. The authors recommended a total pancreatectomy for patients with IPMT and diffuse dilatation. For elderly patients with co-morbid conditions, a subtotal resection or bilateral pancreatectomy is an acceptable alternative if they have dysplasia but no invasive carcinoma.

N.J. Greenberger, M.D.

Variant of Intraductal Carcinoma (With Scant Mucin Production) Is of Main Pancreatic Duct Origin: A Clinicopathological Study of Four Patients
Suda K, Hirai S, Matsumoto Y, et al (Juntendo Univ, Tokyo; Yamanashi Med Univ, Tokyo; Yamanashi Central Hosp, Tokyo; et al)
Am J Gastroenterol 91:798–800, 1996   7–14

Introduction.—Although ductal adenocarcinomas of the pancreas have a high malignant potential, intraductal tumors are associated with a favorable prognosis. Intraductal tumors typically derive from papillary structures and produce substantial amounts of mucin or demonstrate primarily ductal distention. Four patients were seen with "nodular" intraductal pancreatic tumors, which appear to be variants of intraductal carcinoma.

Methods.—Intraductal nodular carcinoma of the main pancreatic duct was discovered during pancreatoduodenectomy in 3 patients and at autopsy in 1 patient who died of cerebral hemorrhage. Each tumor was examined histologically and immunohistochemically. For comparison, 10 common ductal adenocarcinomas of the pancreas were examined immunohistochemically.

Results.—All 4 patients had a thickened, nodular, hard pancreas head, and 3 patients had metastasis to the regional lymph nodes. The tumors were very large in all cases, ranging from 3 to 7 cm in diameter. Histologic examination revealed a uniform pattern of well-differentiated tubular or papillotubular adenocarcinoma, demonstrating intraductal spreading and partial periductal invasion. The tumor cells typically did not produce mucus and had a columnar, rather than goblet cell-like or mucinous appearance. They did not stain for anti-CEA, and only stained on the luminar surface for anti-CA19-9, in contrast with the common ductal adenocarcinoma cells, which stained strongly for both. All 3 living patients had a favorable course, with 2 patients still alive 4 years after surgery, while 1 died 5 years after surgery.

Conclusions.—The nodular intraductal pancreatic tumor is a variant of intraductal carcinoma, characterized by minimal mucin production, slow progression, and a favorable prognosis.

▶ I wish that someone would refer more of this type of pancreatic ductal cancer my way. Possibly the few long-term survivors that I have in my many years of performing radical pancreaticoduodenectomies relates more to that the patients had intraductal nodular tumors rather than to my surgical skill. It is for this reason that I usually try to remove even relatively large tumors in otherwise healthy people if there is no evidence of distal spread. Note that 3 of the patients with long-term survival had a single lymph node involved.

F.G. Moody, M.D.

Intraductal Oncocytic Papillary Neoplasms of the Pancreas
Adsay NV, Adair CF, Heffess CS, et al (Mem Sloan-Kettering Cancer Ctr, New York; Armed Forces Inst of Pathology, Washington, DC)
Am J Surg Pathol 20:980–994, 1996   7–15

Introduction.—Traditionally referred to as pseudocysts, most cystic lesions of the pancreas are non-neoplastic. Recently, reports have been made of intraductal tumors with some histologic features that are similar to mucinous cystic neoplasms of the pancreas. These tumors have been given several names, such as mucin-producing tumor, mucinous duct ectasia, or ductectatic mucinous cystadenoma, but all of them are related histologically and biologically and represent variants of a single clinicopathologic entity. The clinical and pathologic features of 11 patients (6 men and 5 women) with a distinctive cystic intraductal tumor with oncocytic features and mucin production are described; they seem to represent a previously unrecognized tumor. The term intraductal oncocytic papillary neoplasm is suggested for these types of tumors.

Methods.—The files of 11 patients were reviewed. The clinical information was obtained by contacting the referring pathologists or clinicians and by reviewing the charts of the patients. Ultrastructural examination was done on the tissues.

Results.—Most of the pancreatic tumors were in the head, and the average tumor size was 6 cm. The tumors had mucin-filled cysts with nodular papillary projections. In some instances, there were dilated cuts communicating with the main tumor. In 10 of the 11 patients, the designation of intraductal oncocytic papillary carcinoma was justified because of the complexity of the architecture, even though the degree of cytologic atypia was not generally severe. The tumor was entirely intraductal in 9 patients. There was positive staining of the oncocytic cells with phosphotungstic acid hematoxylin and Novelli stains. Many of the cells were packed with mitochondria, as was noted ultrastructurally, and there was identification of mucin.

From 1 month to 3 months after resection, 7 patients were alive and free of tumor. Two died after resection and the other 2 died at 2.5 and 5 years, with no evidence of disease. The differential diagnosis of intraductal oncocytic papillary neoplasms when compared with mucinous cystic neoplasms and intraductal papillary mucinous neoplasms is that the intraductal oncocytic papillary neoplasms prominently show localized cystic dilation. Their complex architecture of the papillae and intraepithelial mucin-containing lumina and cribriforming are the hallmarks of this type of tumor (Table 4).

TABLE 4.—Differential Diagnosis of Intraductal Oncocytic Papillary Neoplasms With Similar Tumors

Findings	MCN	IPMN	IOPN
Gross features			
Multilocular cysts	++	+/−	++
Intraductal growth	−	++	++
Ductal dilatation	−	++	+
Mucin secretion	++	+	+
Extension outside the pancreas	+	+/−	+
Papillary growths	+/−	+	++
Microscopic features			
Arborizing complex papillae	−	+	++
Intraepithelial lumina	−	+/−	++
Goblet-like cells	+/−	+/−	++
Oncocytic change	−	−	++
Invasion	+	+	+/−
Ovarian type stroma	++	−	−

Abbreviations: MCN, mucinous cystic neoplasms; *IOPN,* intraductal oncocytic papillary neoplasms; *IPMN,* intraductal papillary mucinous neoplasms; −, not present, +/−, can be present/not prominent; +, present often; ++, very common/very prominent.

(Courtesy of Adsay NV, Adair CF, Heffess CS, et al: Intraductal oncocytic papillary neoplasms of the pancreas. *Am J Surg Pathol* 20:980–994, 1996.)

Conclusion.—Intraductal oncocytic papillary neoplasm is usually intraductal and is a distinctive pancreatic tumor. It may develop into invasive carcinoma, and complete resection should be the treatment.

▶ Pathologists at the Memorial Sloan-Kettering Cancer Center and the Armed Forces Institute of Pathology have teamed up to describe a unique pancreatic neoplasm characterized by an intraductal papillary mucus-producing epithelium. As is true of most cystic neoplasms, most appear to be benign but can recur locally if not adequately resected. Unfortunately, 2 of the patients died in the postoperative period, 1 after a total pancreatectomy and another after a distal pancreatectomy. One patient with a recurrence at the margin of resection at 2 years was successfully re-resected for cure.

The authors provide a comprehensive discussion of the features that distinguish these intraductal oncocytic papillary neoplasms from mucinous cystic neoplasms and intraductal papillary-mucinous neoplasms. As can be seen in Table 4, this is not a play on words. The distinguishing feature is the presence of oncocytes, unique cells that contain an abundant acidophilic cytoplasm made up primarily of mitochondria. The authors suggest that further identification and study of such lesions might lead to a better understanding of invasive pancreatic cancer. At the very least, these lesions should be treated with a great deal of therapeutic respect. All cystic lesions of the pancreas other than inflammatory pseudocysts should be removed if the clinical situation is not prohibitive.

F.G. Moody, M.D.

Pancreatic Carcinoma—Clinical, Immunocytochemical, and Molecular Studies

National Patterns of Care for Pancreatic Cancer: Results of a Survey by the Commission on Cancer
Janes RH Jr, Niederhuber JE, Chmiel JS, et al (Univ of Arkansas, Little Rock; Holt Krock Clinic, Ft Smith, Ark; Stanford Univ, Calif; et al)
Ann Surg 223:261–272, 1995   7–16

Background.—Although the prognosis of adenocarcinoma of the pancreas continues to be poor, the safety of the extensive surgery performed for an attempted cure has apparently improved. Cancer registries in the United States were surveyed to document the current methods of diagnosis, choice of treatment, morbidity and mortality associated with treatment, and patient survival over time.

Methods.—The 160-item survey was completed by 978 United States institutions for two time periods. A total of 8,917 cases were reported between 1983 and 1985, and 8,025 were reported for 1990.

Findings.—The male-to-female patient ratio was 1:1. Abdominal pain was the most common initial symptom. Surgical multimodality treatment patterns were influenced by patient age, ethnicity, neighborhood income, and type of insurance coverage, and by hospital annual caseload and facility type. The current patients had a higher reported history of smoking than United States population averages. Over time, increases were observed in the frequency of abdominal CT scans, endoscopic retrograde cholangiopancreatography, carcinoembryonic antigen, and CA 19-9 during assessment. There were time trends toward reduced surgical mortality and the greater use of extirpative surgery. There was also a slightly higher survival rate over time for patients who underwent surgical resection.

Conclusions.—Operative mortality in patients with pancreatic cancer has improved slightly with time. For carefully selected patients, cancer-directed surgery allows a chance for cure with excellent operative mortality and acceptable complication rates, particularly at centers with caseloads of 20 or greater per year.

▶ This survey of the outcome of 16,942 patients with pancreatic cancer who were studied for 2 periods with about equal numbers in each (1983 through 1985 and 1990) provides insight into trends in the natural history and management of this disease. The textbook notion of how pancreatic cancer presents should be modified because abdominal pain was the most common complaint. Jaundice was present in less than half of the patients. Computed tomographic scans emerged as the test with the highest sensitivity. The article clearly establishes that pancreatic cancer is a disease of older individuals and that survival is closely linked to its stage at the time of discovery. Although resectability rates remained stable during the 2 periods, the operative mortality rate dropped from 9% to 6%. As might be expected, institutions with the most surgical experience had the lowest surgical mortality. So where does that leave us? Just about where we were, unfortunately, and it is unlikely that we will see much further change in these statistics until the cause of the disease is elucidated. The aging of our population may make matters worse, because the incidence will increase, while the enthusiasm for a major surgical approach will likely be tempered by the risk and the marginal results thus far reported for other than the early stages of the disease.

F.G. Moody, M.D.

Isolated Portal Vein Involvement in Pancreatic Adenocarcinoma: A Contraindication for Resection?
Harrison LE, Klimstra DS, Brennan MF (Mem Sloan-Kettering Cancer Ctr, New York)
Ann Surg 224:342–349, 1996   7–17

Purpose.—In patients with pancreatic adenocarcinoma, even locally advanced disease may preclude curative resection. Sometimes the obstacle to resection is inability to separate the pancreas from the portal vein or local invasion of the portal vein. With modern techniques of portal vein resection (PVR), locally advanced disease need not be a contraindication to surgery. An 11-year experience with PVR in patients undergoing adenocarcinoma of the pancreas is evaluated.

Methods.—The analysis included 332 patients undergoing pancreatic resection for adenocarcinoma between 1983 and 1995. The patients were identified by review of the prospective pancreatic database at the study cancer center. Fifty-eight of the patients had isolated clinical involvement of the portal vein, and their pancreatic resection included PVR. Their morbidity, mortality, and overall survival were compared with those of patients undergoing curative pancreatic resection without PVR.

Results.—The in-hospital mortality was 5% for patients with PVR, similar to the 3% rate in patients who did not undergo PVR. The median survival was similar as well: 13 months for the PVR group and 17 months for the non-PVR group. Three of 11 5-year survivors were from the PVR group. Resection with PVR involved a longer operation, more blood loss, more transfusions, and a longer hospital stay.

Conclusions.—In patients with pancreatic adenocarcinoma, suspected isolated portal vein involvement should not be regarded as a contraindication to pancreatic resection. Portal vein resection can be done safely and with a low perioperative mortality. Survival is similar to that of patients undergoing pancreatic resection without PVR.

▶ The surgeons at the Memorial Sloan-Kettering Cancer Center add further credence to the concept that portal vein involvement by ductal adenocarcinoma of the pancreas is not a contraindication to a Whipple resection. They observed that the operative morbidity and mortality was similar for this procedure whether the portal vein was resected or left intact. The only difference was that the operation took longer and required more blood when PVR was performed. The overall survival rate was comparable, even though the patients who underwent PVR had larger lesions. I have not encountered a patient yet whereby the portal vein was invaded, and it was not obvious by preoperative assessment or at exploration that removal of the lesion would not effect a cure. For some reason, I remain skeptical as regards the advisability of a Whipple procedure for palliation except in highly selected cases.

F.G. Moody, M.D.

A Phase II Trial of Gemcitabine in Patients With 5-FU–Refractory Pancreas Cancer

Rothenberg ML, Moore MJ, Cripps MC, et al (Univ of Texas Health Science Ctr, San Antonio; Cancer Therapy and Research Ctr, San Antonio, Tex; Princess Margaret Hosp, Toronto; et al)
Ann Oncol 7:347–353, 1996   7–18

Background.—Survival remains poor for patients with pancreatic cancer. There have been no major treatment advances in more than 3 decades, since the introduction of 5-fluorouracil (5-FU). There are few treatment options for patients with locally advanced or metastatic pancreatic cancer. No treatment has been able to improve survival or reduce symptoms in patients with progressive disease. The new nucleoside analogue gemcitabine hydrochloride was evaluated for use in patients with progressive disease despite 5-FU therapy.

Methods.—The multicenter trial included 74 patients with inoperable pancreatic adenocarcinoma that had progressed despite a single course of treatment with 5-FU. All patients underwent a 2- to 7-day pain stabilization period to ensure that their baseline pain values were stable and reliable. Sixty-three went on to receive gemcitabine treatment with doses up to 1,250 mg/m^2, depending on toxicity. The study end point was reduction of cancer-related symptoms. Patients with at least a 50% reduction in visual analogue scale pain intensity, at least a 50% reduction in daily analgesic consumption, or a sustained improvement in Karnofsky performance status of at least 20 points were considered to have a Clinical Benefit Response.

Results.—Twenty-seven percent of patients achieved a Clinical Benefit Response. Fourteen patients had an improvement in pain. The responses lasted for a median of 14 weeks. Median survival for all gemcitabine-treated patients was 4 months, 7 months for patients with a Clinical Benefit Response. The treatment was fairly well tolerated, with few episodes of grade 2 or 4 toxicity.

Conclusions.—Gemcitabine appears to be useful in the treatment of advanced pancreatic cancer. It has significant clinical benefit in a group of patients who otherwise have no therapeutic options. The results are supported by a simultaneous trial showing that gemcitabine is superior to 5-FU in patients with newly diagnosed, inoperable pancreatic cancer.

▶ Current therapeutic options for patients with locally advanced metastatic pancreatic adenocarcinoma are limited. Patients who receive systemic chemotherapy usually are given 5-FU or a 5-FU–based regimen. When advanced disease develops, no agents have been demonstrated to improve survival or alleviate symptoms. Although this report is preliminary (a phase 2 trial), I selected it because it describes what appears to be a promising agent for the palliation of advanced pancreatic cancer. About 27% of patients with advanced pancreatic cancer attained a Clinical Benefit Response. Importantly, the therapy was generally well tolerated, with a low incidence of serious toxicities.

Another interesting agent being evaluated for the treatment of pancreatic cancer is sandostatin, the rationale being the inhibition of pancreatic acinar cell function. The performance of the agent in multiple drug regimens will be awaited with interest.

N.J. Greenberger, M.D.

Preoperative Staging of Cancer of the Pancreas: Value of MR Angiography Versus Conventional Angiography in Detecting Portal Venous Invasion

McFarland EG, Kaufman JA, Saini S, et al (Massachusetts Gen Hosp, Boston; Mallinckrodt Inst of Radiology, St Louis; Univ of California, Los Angeles)
AJR 166:37–43, 1996   7–19

Introduction.—Few published reports describe the role of MR angiography in pancreatic cancer. Conventional and MR angiography were prospectively compared in the detection of portal venous invasion in the preoperative stage of pancreatic carcinoma. Surgical findings were used as the reference standard.

Methods.—Twenty patients with pancreatic carcinoma underwent both conventional and MR angiography with a mean of 1.7 days between procedures. Data from the 2 studies were analyzed by blinded expert vascular radiologists. The main portal vein, splenoportal confluence, splenic vein, and superior mesenteric vein were evaluated in each imaging technique. Interpretations of both procedures were compared with each other and with surgical findings of the vascular involvement.

Results.—A curative pancreaticoduodenectomy was performed in 11 patients. Nine patients received a palliative bypass because of nonresectable tumor. The vascular status was concordant between studies in 13 of the 20 patients (7 resectable, 4 nonresectable, 2 false-negatives). The MR angiography studies correctly detected 11 of 11 resectable tumors, 5 of 9 nonresectable tumors, and had 4 false-negatives. Conventional angiography accurately found 7 of 11 resectable tumors, 6 of 9 nonresectable tumors, and had 4 false-positives and 3 false-negatives. A comparison of anatomical sites showed 100% concordance in the portal vein (14 of 14), 83% in the confluence (10 of 12), 66% in the superior mesenteric vein (12 of 18), and 92% in the splenic vein (11 of 12). The total concordance was 84% (47 of 56) for portal venous structures.

Conclusion.—These preliminary findings of MR angiography indicate that it has promise as a noninvasive technique for detecting resectability in tumors that involve the portal venous system in patients with pancreatic carcinoma. The presence of false-negatives with MR angiography demonstrates that the procedure does not fully eliminate unnecessary laparotomies. The lack of false-positives indicates that no patients with potentially resectable tumors would have been denied surgery in this cohort.

▶ Magnetic resonance imaging provides a useful screen for determining the resectability of pancreatic cases, but the relatively high rate of false negatives suggests that the approach with intent to resect will have to be modified relatively frequently at the time of exploration. I have found the spiral CT scan to be helpful in assessing the potential for resectability, and have become more aggressive towards exploring patients with this intent, because a bypass by a biliary-enteric anastomosis gives better, more worry-free palliation than sequential restenting transendoscopically. For reasons that are not entirely clear, we seem to be able to accomplish these procedures with a much lower morbidity and length of stay than in the past, even in the elderly.

F.G. Moody, M.D.

Immunocytochemical Detection of p53 Protein From Pancreatic Duct Brushings in Patients With Pancreatic Carcinoma

Ishimaru S, Itoh M, Hanada K, et al (Hiroshima Univ, Japan)
Cancer 77:2233–2239, 1996

7–20

Background.—Often imaging techniques cannot distinguish between pancreatic carcinoma and chronic pancreatitis. Cytologic examination, using material obtained by endoscopic retrograde pancreatic duct brushing (ERPDB), has had a wide range of sensitivities. Mutations of the p53 tumor suppressor gene have been found in 40% to 70% of the patients with pancreatic carcinomas, but not in patients with benign pancreatic disease. The utility of measuring p53 protein overexpression in brushing samples obtained with ERPDB was compared with that of conventional cytologic examination in the differentiation of malignant and benign pancreatic lesions.

Methods.—Twenty-eight patients with narrowed or obstructed main pancreatic ducts, including 20 with duct cell carcinoma and 8 with chronic pancreatitis, were studied. Brushing samples obtained with ERPDB were analyzed with cytologic examination, using the Papanicolaou technique, and with p53 immunocytochemistry. The ability of each technique to differentiate malignant from benign pancreatic lesions was compared.

Results.—Papanicolaou staining cytologic examination had a sensitivity of 60% and a specificity of 100% in the diagnosis of carcinoma, whereas p53 immunocytochemistry had a sensitivity of 90% and a specificity of 100%. The overall accuracy was 93% with p53 staining, 71% with cytology, and 95% with a combination of both.

Conclusions.—The technique of p53 immunocytochemistry, used in conjunction with conventional cytologic examination, can improve the accuracy of differentiation between ductal cell carcinoma and chronic pancreatitis preoperatively.

▶ How accurate is pancreatic duct brushing in detecting pancreatic ductal cancer? If you add p53 immunocytochemistry to your cytologic analysis, the sensitivity is 90%, the specificity, 100%, and the accuracy, 93%. These sound like great numbers to me since the diagnosis of an early pancreatic cancer is an unresolved challenge in our center, especially in patients with chronic pancreatitis.

F.G. Moody, M.D.

Molecular Diagnosis of Exocrine Pancreatic Cancer Using a Percutaneous Technique

Evans DB, Frazier ML, Charnsangavej C, et al (Univ of Texas, Houston)
Ann Surg Oncol 3:241–246, 1996   7–21

Background.—The diagnosis of pancreatic adenocarcinoma is commonly established by the cytologic findings of CT-guided percutaneous fine-needle aspiration (FNA) of the pancreas. However, false negative FNA results are common. Most patients with exocrine pancreatic cancer have the K-*ras* oncogene, which is characterized by point mutations at codon 12. The feasibility of detecting the K-*ras* mutation by extracting DNA from the FNA material discarded during preparation of the cytologic slide was investigated.

Methods.—Twenty-five patients with a pancreatic mass who underwent CT-guided FNA and in whom pancreatic adenocarcinoma was cytologically or histologically diagnosed were included. The FNA sample was centrifuged, and the DNA was extracted from the supernatant. The DNA was amplified with 15 cycles of polymerase chain reaction (PCR) by using primers K-*ras* 5' and K-*ras* 3', then digested with BstNI to remove the wild-type K-*ras* codon 12, which has a BstNI restriction site not found on mutant K-*ras* codon 12. The PCR and digestion steps were repeated, then subjected to gel electrophoresis.

Results.—Each specimen yielded a median of 3.33 µg of DNA. Mutant K-*ras* DNA was detected in 21 of 25 samples, including the samples from 6 of 8 patients who had potentially resectable disease and from 15 of 17 patients who had locally advanced or metastatic disease. All these patients had positive cytology results.

Conclusion.—The extraction of DNA for PCR analysis from the material usually discarded from FNA samples is feasible and does not interfere with FNA preparation for cytologic analysis. This technique provides objective data, which can be used as an adjunct to cytologic analyses of FNA specimens. Molecular analysis may be useful at institutions that do not have cytopathologists experienced in the interpretation of pancreatic FNA specimens.

▶ It is heartening to learn that molecular biological techniques are now creeping into clinical diagnoses. The K-*ras* oncogene is in the forefront of this important growing point of technology. I am sure that others will follow if our hospital-based pathology services can keep up. The M.D. Anderson Hospital, where this work was done, happens to be highly specialized in gene analysis technology. Fortunately, PCR technology is commonplace and easily mastered by medical technologists. The diagnosis of pancreatic cancer needs all the help that it can get.

F.G. Moody, M.D.

An Aggressive Therapeutic Approach to Carcinoma of the Body and Tail of the Pancreas
Ozaki H, Kinoshita T, Kosuge T, et al (Natl Cancer Ctr Hosp, Tokyo; Natl Cancer Ctr Research Inst, Tokyo)
Cancer 77:2240–2245, 1996

7–22

Background.—Patients with adenocarcinoma of the pancreatic body and tail have a dismal prognosis after conventional simple distal pancreatectomy. The results of more aggressive therapy with extended radical surgery and adjuvant radiochemotherapy were assessed.

Methods.—A total of 101 patients with carcinoma of the body and tail of the pancreas were treated between 1962 and 1990. Thirty-two of the patients underwent distal pancreatectomy. The 10 patients, including 3 with distant metastasis, treated between 1962 and 1979, underwent simple distal pancreatectomy with dissection limited to the lymph nodes adjacent to the pancreas. Between 1980 and 1990, 24 patients, including 7 with distant metastases, underwent distal pancreatectomy with dissection extended into the lymph nodes and other adjacent structures, particularly the retropancreatic space. After 1984, intraoperative radiation and adjuvant chemotherapy with mitomycin C were also used in 7 patients without distant metastasis.

Results.—The 10 patients treated between 1962 and 1979 all died within 20 months postoperatively. Twenty-two patients treated between 1980 and 1990 with the more aggressive approach survived longer, with a median survival of 10.1 months and survival rates of 34% at 1 year, 24% at 3 years, and 20% at 5 years. However, all 7 patients in this group with distant metastasis died within 10 months postoperatively. Extrapancreatic invasion was common, with lymph node metastasis in 91%, retropancreatic soft-tissue invasion in 95%, perineural space invasion in 94%, extrapancreatic nerve plexus invasion in 79%, left adrenal gland invasion in 23%, stomach invasion in 23%, and duodenal invasion in 14%. After extended dissection of the retropancreatic structures was implemented, invasion to the posterior margin was reduced to 36%.

Conclusions.—Extended resection plus intensive radiochemotherapy improves the outcome of patients with advanced carcinoma of the body and tail of the pancreas.

▶ These aggressive Japanese surgeons have taken on a difficult task, that of curing an incurable lesion. There are few reported 5-year survivors with proven carcinoma of the body and tail of the pancreas. They report 4 patients who lived 5 or more years, 3 of whom were still alive at the time of this report. Two patients had lymph nodes involved; three had involvement of retroperitoneal structures. A resection, intraoperative irradiation, and mitomycin (chemotherapy) were components of the therapeutic protocol that seemed to lead to this unique outcome. This article is worth tucking away in your reprint file.

F.G. Moody, M.D.

Surgery for Left-sided Pancreatic Cancer

Fabre JM, Houry S, Manderscheid JC, et al (Hôpital Saint Eloi, Montpellier, France; Hôpital Tenon, Paris)
Br J Surg 83:1065–1070, 1996   7–23

Introduction.—Although the 5-year survival rate for pancreatic cancer after resection is poor, surgery remains the treatment of choice for this malignancy. For small tumors, with no lymph node or vascular involvement, the 5-year survival rate has been reported to be about 37%. However, when the tumor occurs in the body or tail of the pancreas, the survival rate is only about 10%. Patients with pancreatic cancer were studied retrospectively to determine the factors associated with a poor surgical outcome and to identify the indications for surgery.

Methods.—The medical records of patients with pancreatic cancer were reviewed for a 7-year period. Patients with cancer located in the body or tail of the pancreas were identified. The type of procedure performed, factors associated with prognosis, and postoperative morbidity and mortality were determined.

Results.—A total of 590 patients with body and tail pancreatic cancer were identified. One hundred and twenty-eight patients underwent pancreatic resection (group 1); 12 had a total pancreatectomy and 116 had a left pancreatectomy. Palliative bypass was performed in 164 patients (group 2) and laparotomy in 293 (group 3). The procedure was not identified for 5 patients. Metastases were present in 61% of patients. In group 1, metastases were found in 28% of patients; in group 2, 66%; and in group 3, 73%. Among patients who underwent resection, significantly more tumors (29%) were smaller than 4 cm as compared with the other 2 groups. Reasons for not performing a resection included the presence of metastases (50%), vascular involvement (34%), age or health status (17%), and lymph node involvement (7%). For 49% of patients, the resection was considered to be curative, whereas in 51%, it was palliative. For all procedures, the postoperative mortality rate was 12%, with the highest mortality rate in group 2 (19%). When combined, age older than 70 years and failure of 1 or more organs were associated with mortality rates of 40% and 45% in groups 1 and 2, respectively. The overall rate of postoperative morbidity was 22%, with a significantly higher rate in group 1 among patients who were younger than 70 years (31%) and did not have organ failure (33%). Morbidity was also significantly higher among patients in group 1 who had metastases (42%), as compared with patients undergoing the other procedures. Overall, a 5-year survival rate of 1% was found, with a median survival of 4.5 months. The median survival for patients with metastases was 3.4 months and did not differ significantly between the groups. Patients in group 1 who did not have metastases or lymph node involvement had a median survival of 9.2 months and a 3-year survival rate of 12%. As compared to pancreatic cancer of the head and isthmus, median survival after resection for cancer of the body and tail was significantly lower. Factors that were found to be significant prognostic determinants included adjacent organ involvement, lymph node involvement, metastasis, and primary tumor size.

Conclusion.—Only a small number of patients, with small tumor size and no lymph node involvement, were found to benefit from resection. However, only a small percentage of patients are suitable for surgery. For most patients, pancreatic resection should be considered palliative, with no effect on survival.

▶ Adenocarcinoma of the body and tail of the pancreas is a uniformly fatal disease. This large series adds statistical validity to this somber fact. The authors provide wise and informed advice. Palliative surgery should be reserved for digestive bypass purposes, and nonsurgical palliation should be the primary treatment objective. However, be on the lookout for the small lesion whose removal may offer prolonged survival.

F.G. Moody, M.D.

Intraoperative Fine Needle Aspiration Cytology of Pancreatic Lesions
Sáez A, Català I, Brossa R, et al (Ciutat Sanitaria i Universitaria de Bellvitge, Barcelona)
Acta Cytol 39:485–488, 1995   7–24

Objective.—Intraoperative biopsy of pancreatic lesions often fails to detect cancer and may result in serious complications. This issue prompted a study of intraoperative fine needle aspiration cytology (FNAC).

Method.—A total of 109 studies were done in 90 consecutive patients, 60 of whom had a final diagnosis of malignant disease of the pancreas.

Results.—The cytologic findings were reported as positive for carcinoma in 42 of 60 cases, and suspicious in 4 others. Seven patients with benign findings and 7 with unsatisfactory studies were later shown to have malignant disease. The cytologic findings were benign in 26 of 30 patients without cancer; 4 had unsatisfactory studies. Intraoperative FNAC was 80% sensitive and 100% specific, with positive and negative predictive values of 100% and 70%, respectively. No complications were ascribed directly to aspiration biopsy.

Conclusions.—Intraoperative FNAC is a very reliable way to distinguish malignant from benign pancreatic lesions. It can be performed rapidly and is a safe procedure.

▶ Fine needle aspiration cytology has come of age as a way to establish the benign or malignant nature of pancreatic mass lesions either before or at the time of exploratory laparotomy. The sensitivity of only 80% is problematic if you are of the school that requires a positive histologic diagnosis of cancer before performing a radical pancreaticoduodenectomy (Whipple's procedure). I have moved towards the other side and now resect lesions that obstruct the bile duct and are highly suspect for malignancy. The problem arises when a lesion cannot be resected for whatever reason, and this is where FNAC offers a relatively risk-free way to obtain a histologic diagnosis.

F.G. Moody, M.D.

Pancreaticoduodenectomy: Does It Have a Role in the Palliation of Pancreatic Cancer?

Lillemoe KD, Cameron JL, Yeo CJ, et al (Johns Hopkins Med Insts, Baltimore, Md)
Ann Surg 223:718–728, 1996   7–25

Objective.—Recent data indicate that patients with pancreatic carcinoma have improved survival after pancreaticoduodenectomy, even with lymph node involvement and positive margins. Unresectable pancreatic carcinoma usually is treated palliatively with biliary and gastric bypass. Perioperative complications and overall survival were compared in patients undergoing pancreaticoduodenectomy and patients undergoing standard surgical palliation.

Methods.—Prospective data were collected regarding 64 patients (aged 37–85 years) who underwent palliative pancreaticoduodenectomy and had positive margins between 1986 and 1994 and 62 patients (aged 41–82) who underwent standard surgical palliation because of local invasion with no evidence of metastatic disease between 1986 and 1991. Of the

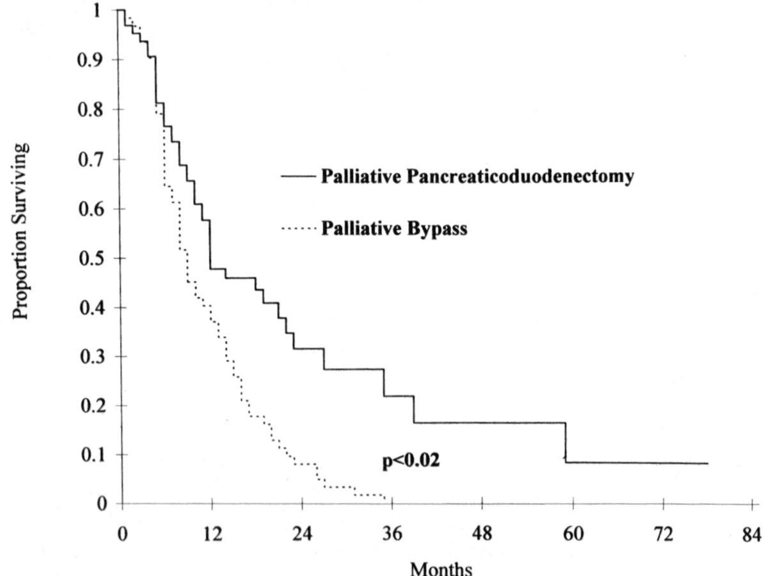

FIGURE 1.—The actuarial survival curves (Kaplan-Meier) for patients undergoing palliative pancreaticoduodenectomy (*n* = 64) and palliative bypass (*n* = 62). (Courtesy of Lillemoe KD, Cameron JL, Yeo CJ, et al: Pancreaticoduodenectomy: Does it have a role in the palliation of pancreatic cancer? *Ann Surg* 223:718–728, 1996.)

patients who did not undergo resection, 87% received combined biliary and gastric bypass. Survival was analyzed statistically.

Results.—Hospital mortality rates and complications were similar between the 2 groups, but the pancreaticoduodenectomy group had a significantly longer hospital stay. Postoperative chemotherapy and radiation therapy were administered to 48% of the unresected group and 78% of the pancreaticoduodenectomy group. Overall survival was significantly improved for the pancreaticoduodenectomy group II (Fig 1). Postoperative adjuvent therapy improved survival significantly.

Conclusion.—For patients with pancreatic cancer, pancreaticoduodenectomy improves survival significantly over standard palliative surgery without increasing perioperative morbidity and mortality.

▶ Lillimoe and his associates at Johns Hopkins provide a retrospective analysis of morbidity and survival of patients with advanced pancreatic cancer, with 1 group undergoing pancreaticoduodenectomy, and a second, biliary and gastric bypass. Adjuvant therapy was employed in a nonrandomized manner in some patients in both groups. The operative mortality rate (1.6%) was comparable and sufficiently low to justify a radical surgical approach in patients with incurable lesions. The mean tumor diameter in the resected cases was 3.6 cm, and 78% had positive nodes. All had positive margins. These patients lived longer and had a higher quality of life. The question remains, was this because their lesions, though advanced, were not as far along as those of their counterparts who had the bypass, or did they have a better response to chemoradiation because of a reduced tumor burden? Lest the reader assume that I am a skeptic, I will state that I also resect lesions that on final analysis are more advanced than I originally thought. And I also am surprised at how well such patients do and how long they survive, even without adjuvant therapy, which I often do not recommend in patients who are frail or elderly. I must confess that I do not knowingly embark on a pancreaticoduodenectomy suspecting that I will find a node distal from the tumor or cancer at a resected margin, and even with the excellent protocols for adjuvant therapy available to my patients at the M.D. Anderson Cancer Center, I do not believe that I will until a controlled trial establishes the efficacy of such an approach.

F.G. Moody, M.D.

The Use of Somatostatin Receptor Scintigraphy in the Differential Diagnosis of Pancreatic Duct Cancers and Islet Cell Tumors

van Eijck CHJ, Lamberts SWJ, Lemaire LCJM, et al (Univ Hosp, Rotterdam, The Netherlands; Univ of Berne, Switzerland)
Ann Surg 224:119–124, 1996
7–26

Introduction.—A variety of tumors, such as carcinoids, paragangliomas, brain tumors, and meningiomas, have somatostatin receptors. It is important to differentiate between pancreatic duct carcinomas and islet cell tumors to determine proper treatment and palliative surgery. In the workup of patients with pancreatic endocrine and exocrine tumors, the diagnostic value of somatostatin receptor scintigraphy, a new nuclear medical technique, was determined. With this new technique, somatostatin receptor-positive tumors could be visualized in vivo after the administration of a radionuclide-labeled somatostatin analogue. The results of the in vivo technique were compared with the results of in vitro receptor autoradiographic studies in the tumor specimen.

Methods.—The study included 48 patients with islet cell tumors and 26 patients with suspected primary pancreatic duct cancers. Using the radionuclide-labeled somatostatin analogue indium-111 octreotide, the somatostatin receptor scintigraphy technique was done. This technique also was used on another group of 12 patients who were still alive more than 3 years after pancreaticoduodenectomy for pancreatic duct adenocarcinomas.

Results.—The primary pancreatic islet cell tumor and metastases could be visualized in 31 of 48 patients (65%). There was no visualization of the 26 pancreatic adenocarcinomas or their metastases. Metastatic lesions were visualized with the new technique in 5 of 12 patients who were alive more than 3 years after pancreaticoduodenectomy. These patients were operated on for "nonfunctioning" islet cell tumors rather than for adenocarcinomas, as was noted retrospectively.

Conclusions.—In the preoperative differential diagnosis of islet cell tumors and pancreatic duct cancers, as well as in the follow-up, somatostatin receptor scintigraphy has a place, particularly in those patients in which no tumor histologic analysis was obtained, or when the pathologic examination of the tumor tissue did not include special staining procedures for neuroendocrine characteristics. If no histologic analysis and staining for neuroendocrine characteristics was done, the evaluation of the results of investigations on the role of surgery or radiation therapy and chemotherapy or both in pancreatic duct cancer have to be interpreted with caution.

▶ Somatostatic receptor scintigraphy as reported here sounds like a remarkable advance in our ability to distinguish endocrine from exocrine tumors of the pancreas. This is an important issue, as was well discussed by the authors; endocrine tumors should be resected whenever possible, even when distal sites are involved, because debulking enhances subsequent therapy. This is not the case to date for ductal adenocarcinoma of the pancreas.

F.G. Moody, M.D.

Prognostic Factors After Resection of Ampullary Carcinoma: Multivariate Survival Analysis in Comparison With Ductal Cancer of the Pancreatic Head
Klempnauer J, Ridder GJ, Pichlmayr R (Hanover Med School, Germany)
Br J Surg 82:1686–1691, 1995   7–27

Background.—In contrast to ductal cancer of the pancreatic head, the prognosis of ampullary cancer in relation to the tumor node metastasis (TNM) classification has not been widely studied. Identifying prognostic factors is important for predicting survival probability and for making treatment decisions. The outcomes of resection for ampullary carcinoma were analyzed and prognostic factors were determined in a comparison study of patients with ampullary carcinoma and ductal cancer of the pancreatic head.

Methods and Findings.—Eighty-five patients with ampullary and 150 patients with ductal pancreatic head carcinoma underwent resection. Ninety-eight percent in the former group and 87% in the latter group were cured. Five-year survival rates were 38% and 16%, respectively, excluding hospital deaths. In a multivariate analysis, residual tumor stage and tumor size and grading independently predicted the prognosis in patients with pancreatic carcinoma. For patients with ampullary carcinoma, however, only the tumor size was a prognostic indicator. In univariate analysis only, lymph node metastasis adversely affected prognosis. The *Union Internacional Contra la Cancrum* classification system did not reliably predict prognosis in patients with ampullary carcinoma after resection.

Conclusions.—The prognosis of ampullary cancer appears to be intrinsically better than that of pancreatic head tumors. This is not simply because patients with ampullary cancer are initially seen at an earlier disease stage. Furthermore, a differential importance of the various survival variables does not adequately explain the difference in prognoses.

▶ The authors conducted a retrospective review of their surgical experience with periampullary neoplasms to find out why patients with lesions arising in the ampulla of Vater have a better prognosis than those whose neoplasms arose in the pancreatic duct. Their study reveals several interesting points, the most striking being the high resectability rate (98%) for ampullary cancers compared with those arising in the pancreas (46%). The favorable 5-year survival rate of 38% for ampullary carcinoma was related to tumor size rather than to the presence or absence of lymph node metastases. The relatively high (16%) 5-year survival rate for patients with pancreatic cancer who survived resection is also interesting. Apparently, the TNM staging criteria are not applicable to prognosis following resection of ampullary cancer.

F.G. Moody, M.D.

58 Pancreatic Trauma

Is Octreotide Beneficial Following Pancreatic Injury?
Nwariaku FE, Terracina A, Mileski WJ, et al (Univ of Texas, Dallas)
Am J Surg 170:582–585, 1995   7–28

Introduction.—Injury to the pancreas poses a therapeutic challenge and is a cause of significant morbidity in patients with trauma. Octreotide has been reported to reduce morbidity and enhance closure of pancreatic fistulae after major elective pancreatic resections for cancer and chronic pancreatitis in a large prospective series. The influence of octreotide on the incidence and severity of abdominal complications after pancreatic injury was reviewed retrospectively in 96 patients.

Methods.—Patient records were reviewed for the presence of intra-abdominal and pancreatic abscesses, pseudocyst, pancreatitis, and pancreatic fistula. Patients who received octreotide were compared with those who did not receive octreotide for fistula incidence, duration, amylase output, and length of hospital stay.

Results.—Mean patient age of the 68 males and 28 females was 29 years. Fifty patients had penetrating injuries and 26 had blunt injuries. Thirty-eight patients had gunshot wounds. Sixteen patients died within 48 hours and 1 patient died after 48 hours. Of the remaining 80 patients, 21 received octreotide and 55 did not receive octreotide. Forty-one percent of patients experienced pancreatic fistula complications postoperatively. In patients with minor pancreatic injury (grades I and II), the octreotide-treated group had a fistula rate of 46%, compared to 35% in the group that was not treated. In patients with more severe pancreatic injury (grades III, IV, and V), the fistula rates for the octreotide-treated and non-treated groups were 50% and 56% (not a significant difference), respectively. Regardless of the severity of injury, the duration of pancreatic fistula drainage and peripancreatic drain amylase levels were higher in treated than non-treated patients. There was no significant difference between treated and non-treated patients with an injury severity scale score greater than or equal to 25 in length of stay, pancreatitis, pseudocyst, or mortality rates.

Conclusion.—The use of octreotide for the reduction of pancreatic complications after pancreatic injury was not determined to benefit patients in this series. Biased patient selection may have affected the complication rate in patients who receive octreotide. Controlled, prospective investigation is needed.

▶ The trauma team at the University of Texas Southwestern in Dallas reports that octreotide adjunctive therapy does not reduce the morbidity associated with pancreatic injury. In fact, the incidence of fistula formation was higher in those who received the normal treatment. Keep in mind that this was a retrospective review, not a controlled trial. I suspect that the results, however, would have been the same even in a controlled trial. As you can gather, I am not a fan of octreotide administration in the treatment of pancreatic disease.

F.G. Moody, M.D.

Operative Strategies in Pancreatic Trauma

Farrell RJ, Krige JEJ, Bornman PC, et al (Univ of Cape Town, South Africa; Groote Schuur Hosp, Cape Town, South Africa)
Br J Surg 83:934–937, 1996   7–29

Introduction.—Injuries to the pancreas are primarily associated with major trauma in other organs, which account for most deaths in those with pancreatic trauma. Because of changes in the proportion of blunt vs. penetrating trauma injuries, advances in prehospital care and transportation of patients with trauma, and improved management of associated injuries, previous institutional series may not be relevant to the current management of pancreatic trauma. A review was conducted of pancreatic trauma, and the significance of the mechanism of injury along with its influence on operative management.

Methods.—Fifty-one patients who had operations for pancreatic trauma were reviewed: 21 had stab wounds, 17 had gunshot wounds, and 13 had blunt trauma. Recordings were taken of demographic data, mechanism of injury and operative findings, postoperative course, and complications. The severity of pancreatic injury was graded using the Lucas classification system, with a class 1 injury having a contusion or peripheral laceration with minimal parenchymal damage, and a class 4 injury having combined pancreaticoduodenal injury.

Results.—There were 17 injuries in the pancreatic head, 15 in the body, and 19 in the tail. There were associated injuries of surrounding organs in most patients. There were 7 pancreatoduodenectomy operations, 7 distal pancreatectomy operations, and 35 external drainages. Five (10%) of the 51 patients died, 2 of multiple-organ failure, 2 of hemorrhage, and 1 of acute subdural hematoma. Among the 46 survivors, their hospital stay ranged from 4 to 47 days, with a median of 10 days. The hospital stays were longer from blunt trauma and gunshot wounds than for stab wounds. Pancreatic fistula developed in 10 (20%) of the patients. Four of these patients had pancreatic fistula develop after gunshot wounds, 4 after blunt trauma, and 2 with stab wounds. Drainage procedures were conducted on all but 1 of these patients. A low incidence of duct injury was associated with stab wounds, and external drainage was satisfactory in most cases. Patients with a higher grade of pancreatic injury tended to have more postoperative complications.

Conclusions.—It is essential that an experienced surgeon conduct careful exploration because duct injuries were common and easily missed after blunt trauma and gunshot wounds. Pancreatic resection can be done with good results in appropriately selected patients. External drainage should be used to manage minor contusions, lacerations, or gunshot wounds. Distal pancreatectomy should be used to manage major contusions and lacerations of the body/tail of the pancreas, gunshot wounds in the region of the pancreatic duct in the body/tail and stab wounds of the body/tail with visible duct involvement.

▶ The surgeons at the Groote Schuur Hospital in Capetown, South Africa, offer a sensible approach to pancreatic injuries. Distal resections should be done for major lacerations or contusions of the body and tail of the gland. The indications for extirpation become more stringent for injuries to the head. In this instance, they reserve pancreaticoduodenectomy for devitalizing injuries, such as what gunshot wounds and massive blunt trauma do to the area. Only 7 of 51 pancreatic injuries required a pancreaticoduodenectomy. Of interest is that less than 4% of the injured patients who required exploration had evidence of pancreatic injury, and of the 5 patients with pancreatic injury who died, none did so as a consequence of their pancreatic injury. I guess that this relative immunity relates to the pancreas' favorable location within the depths of the retroperitoneum.

F.G. Moody, M.D.

59 Pancreatic Transplantation

Solitary Pancreas Transplantation: Experience With 50 Consecutive Cases
Stratta RJ, Taylor RJ, Sudan D, et al (Univ of Nebraska, Omaha)
Transplant Proc 27:3022–3023, 1995

7–30

Introduction.—Pancreas transplantation (PT) is generally accepted when performed concomitantly with kidney transplant. Because of its inferior results, solitary PT is considered controversial. The experience of 50 consecutive solitary PTs is reported in 45 patients with diabetes mellitus (DM).

Methods.—Thirty-one patients with DM underwent 35 solitary PTs, and 14 patients with DM with well-functioning kidney transplants underwent 15 sequential pancreas-after-kidney transplants. Mean patient age was 35 years. Mean duration of DM was 27 years. Indications for solitary PT included the presence of 2 or more overt diabetic complications and/or glucose hyperlability with hypoglycemic unawareness and impaired quality of life, and adequate renal functional reserve. A minimum of a 2-antigen match was required for transplantation.

Results.—The mean time to wait for transplantation was 2.3 months. The mean initial hospital length of stay was 16.7 days. The mean hospital bill was $100,664. The incidence of rejection was 70%. The complication rate was 44%. Fifty-seven percent of patients had major infection. The cause of 22 graft losses were 5 thrombosis, 11 rejection, and 6 infection. There were 12 resultant pancreatectomies. Four patients died: 1 cardiac arrest, 1 pulmonary embolism, and 2 sepsis. Two-year patient survival was 90%. Two-year graft survival was 63%. At a mean follow-up of 22 months, all patients with functioning grafts had excellent metabolic control and had achieved good rehabilitation without major cardiovascular, renal, or progressive diabetic problems.

Conclusion.—Compared to combined pancreas-kidney transplantation, solitary PT is associated with an increased risk of thrombosis and rejection. Despite the increase in morbidity, insulin independence and improved quality of life was achieved in over 60% of patients. Long-term results are needed to document the role of solitary PT in the treatment of DM and its potential in the prevention or arrest of secondary diabetic complications.

▶ Stratta and his associates at the University of Nebraska Medical Center pack a considerable amount of information into this 2-page article. They share the experience of their use of PT performed either prior to or at some point after renal transplantation. Their experience reflects an extraordinary effort to stave off the ravages of diabetes. Just imagine the amount of "blood, sweat, and tears" associated with a rejection rate of 70%, a surgical complication rate of 44%, and an infection rate (major) of 57%. Four of the 45 patients treated died in the course of the study, and the hospital charges alone were $100,000. This clearly has to be considered a heroic application of a technology that, even when done simultaneously with renal transplantation, still appears to be in its evaluative phase in terms of cost benefit and effectiveness.

F.G. Moody, M.D.

PART EIGHT

ACQUIRED IMMUNODEFICIENCY DISEASE AND RELATED TOPICS

Introduction

The following four articles describe some interesting aspects of gastrointestinal problems in patients with HIV infections.

Norton J. Greenberger, M.D.

60 Complications

Fluconazole Compared With Endoscopy for Human Immunodeficiency Virus–infected Patients With Esophageal Symptoms
Wilcox CM, Alexander LN, Clark WS, et al (Emory Univ, Atlanta, Ga; Grady Mem Hosp, Atlanta, Ga)
Gastroenterology 110:1803–1809, 1996   8–1

Introduction.—A common complication of HIV infection is esophageal disease, and *Candida* esophagitis is the most common cause of esophageal disease. The first line of treatment is antifungal treatment, and if this fails, endoscopy is the next step. Because of the potential multiplicity of causes and prognostic value of endoscopic findings, some favor pretreatment endoscopy. Fluconazole treatment was compared with endoscopy for HIV-infected patients with new-onset esophageal symptoms. The cost-effectiveness, safety, and efficacy were evaluated.

Methods.—One hundred thirty-four patients infected with HIV who had esophageal symptoms were randomly assigned to receive either fluconazole treatment or endoscopy. The fluconazole group received 200 mg orally at the time of evaluation and then 100 mg for 2 weeks. Endoscopy was

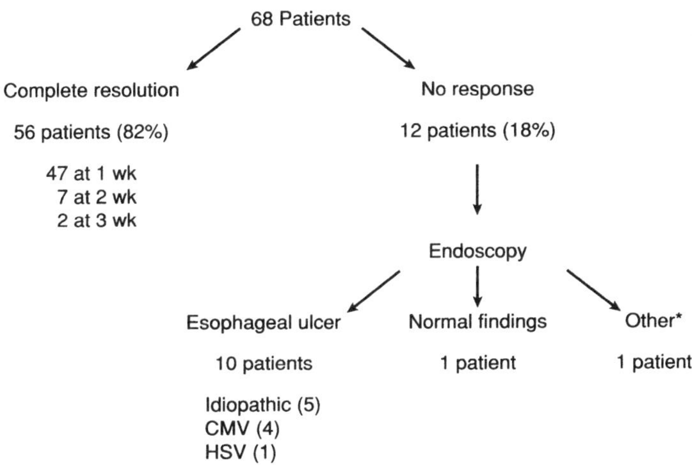

FIGURE 1.—Outcome of patients randomized to the empirical fluconazole group. *Hypopharyngeal edema, otherwise normal endoscopic findings. *Abbreviations: CMV,* cytomegalovirus; *HSV,* herpes simplex virus. (Courtesy of Wilcox CM, Alexander LN, Clark WS, et al: Fluconazole compared with endoscopy for human immunodeficiency virus–infected patients with esophageal symptoms *Gastroenterology* 110:1803–1809, 1996.)

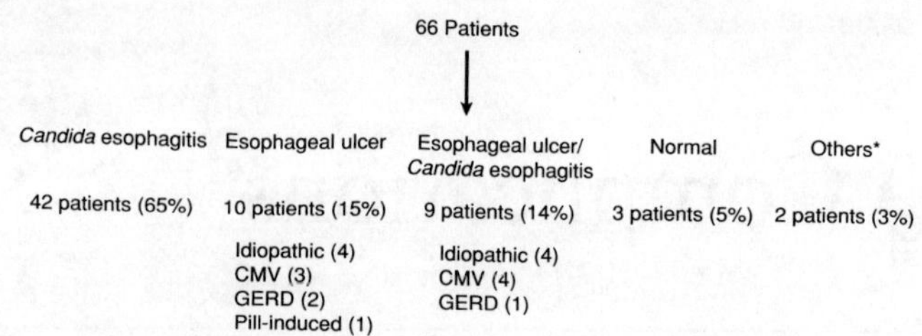

FIGURE 2.—Outcome of patients randomized to the endoscopy group. *One patient failed to return for endoscopy, and 1 patient had herpes simplex virus stomatitis. *Abbreviations: CMV,* cytomegalovirus; *GERD,* gastroesophageal reflux disease. (Courtesy of Wilcox CM, Alexander LN, Clark WS, et al: Fluconazole compared with endoscopy for human immunodeficiency virus–infected patients with esophageal symptoms. *Gastroenterology* 110:1803–1809, 1996).

recommended if symptoms worsened. An endoscopy procedure was performed with meperidine, midazolam, and droperidol used for conscious sedation. Biopsy specimens were evaluated.

Results.—Fifty-six of the 68 patients in the fluconazole group (82%) had a complete symptomatic response, usually within 1 week (Fig 1). *Candida* esophagitis was found in 42 of 66 patients (64%) in the endoscopy group, and ulcerative esophagitis was found in 10 patients (15%) (Fig 2). Severe symptoms were less likely to develop among patients who had *Candida* esophagitis alone at endoscopy or who responded to empirical antifungal therapy. Nonresponders usually had odynophagia as the only symptom, or they had odynophagia and dysphagia. Nonresponders also had thrush. The most cost-effective treatment was empirical fluconazole, which saved $738.16 per patient. The average patient in the endoscopy group paid $977.77 for treatment, whereas the average patient in the fluconazole group paid $239.61.

Conclusion.—For HIV-infected patients with new-onset esophageal symptoms, empirical oral antifungal therapy with fluconazole is highly efficacious, cost-effective, and safe. Endoscopy should be reserved for patients whose symptoms worsen or do not improve after 1 week of fluconazole therapy.

▶ This study supports the concept that most HIV-infected patients with new onset of esophageal symptoms may safely undergo empirical fluconazole therapy. Endoscopy can be reserved for patients whose symptoms worsen or are unchanged at 1 week or in whom an apparent complication develops. Such a strategy could substantially reduce the cost of care without apparent ill effects to the patient.

N.J. Greenberger, M.D.

Etiology, Evaluation, and Outcome of Jaundice in Patients With Acquired Immunodeficiency Syndrome
Chalasani N, Wilcox CM (Emory Univ, Atlanta, Ga; Grady Mem Hosp, Atlanta, Ga)
Hepatology 23:728–733, 1996   8–2

Purpose.—Many patients with AIDS have abnormal results on liver tests, which may result from a variety of causes. Although abnormal results of biochemical tests are common, jaundice appears to be uncommon. The prevalence, causes, diagnostic evaluation, and outcomes of jaundice in AIDS patients were studied prospectively.

Methods.—All HIV-infected patients with abnormal liver test results at 1 large inner-city U.S. hospital were studied during a 4-year period. Patients whose serum bilirubin concentration was 3 mg/dL or greater were considered to have jaundice, the cause of which was assessed by biochemical tests, radiographic studies, liver biopsy, clinical follow-up, and autopsy.

Results.—Of 541 patients with HIV infection investigated for liver disease during the study period, 7% had jaundice. Jaundice was most commonly caused by drug-induced hepatitis (31% of cases) and alcoholic liver disease (13% of cases) (Table 2). Antimycobacterial therapy, especially isoniazid, was responsible for most of the drug-induced cases. The liver test abnormalities cleared up after the offending medication was stopped or the dose reduced. The patients with alcohol-related jaundice were clinically similar to non–HIV-infected patients with alcoholic liver disease. Some cases of jaundice were caused by opportunistic infections or tumors; some patients had several potential causes. Ultrasound and CT helped in assessing the underlying cause of jaundice. Of 16 patients who died in the hospital or within 6 months after evaluation, 7 died of liver disease.

Conclusions.—There are several different potential causes of jaundice in HIV-infected patients, drug-induced hepatitis being the most common. The diagnostic approach is similar to that used in non–HIV-infected patients. A complete diagnostic evaluation may identify the cause, which is

TABLE 2.—Causes of Jaundice

Intrahepatic (n = 23)	Extrahepatic (n = 5)	Cholangiopathy (n = 3)	Unknown (n = 5)
Drugs (11)	Neoplasms (3)	Cholangiography + papillary stenosis (2)	No work-up (3)
Alcohol (5)	Lymphoma (2)		No diagnosis (2)
Lymphoma (2)	KS (1)	Papillary stenosis (1)	
KS (1)	Tuberculosis (1)		
MAC (1)	Ductal stone (1)		
Multifactorial (3)			

(Courtesy of Chalasani N, Wilcox CM: Etiology, evaluation, and outcome of jaundice in patients with acquired immunodeficiency syndrome. *Hepatology* 23:728–733, 1996.)

TABLE 5.—Suggested Approach for the Evaluation of Jaundice in AIDS Patients

1. Discontinue all potentially hepatotoxic medications.
2. Hepatic imaging studies for the evaluation of biliary ductal dilation, hepatic mass lesions, or associated intraabdominal diseases: Abdominal CT is preferred in most patients, although US may be reasonable in the patient with mild jaundice and right upper quadrant pain where gallstone disease or papillary stenosis is strongly suspected.
3. Liver biopsy of identified hepatic mass lesions: In patients without focal liver lesions, percutaneous liver biopsy should be individualized, given the overall low yield for disorders requiring specific management.
4. ERCP is appropriate for a definitive diagnosis and potential endoscopic therapy in patients with biliary ductal dilation by abdominal imaging.

(Courtesy of Chalasani N, Wilcox CM: Etiology, evaluation, and outcome of jaundice in patients with acquired immunodeficiency syndrome. *Hepatology* 23:728–733, 1996.)

---

often potentially treatable (Table 5). However, overall survival is poor, even for patients with drug-induced hepatitis.

▶ This paper provides useful information on the prevalence, causes, and outcome of jaundice in patients with AIDS. Jaundice was defined as a serum bilirubin concentration of 3.0 mg/dL or greater. I would like to emphasize the key findings:

• Jaundice is infrequent in patients with AIDS and occurred in only 36 of 511 cases (7%) in this large series.

• Drug-induced hepatitis was the most common cause of jaundice and was identified in 11 of 36 cases (31%). The most common single drug implicated was isoniazid and not other antiretroviral drugs. Discontinuation of the putative drug often resulted in normalization of liver tests.

• Alcoholic liver disease was the second most frequent cause of jaundice.

• Infrequent causes included neoplasm, cholangiopathy, and gallstones.

• The short-term mortality is high, overall survival is poor, and drug-induced hepatitis may result in a lethal outcome.

The authors provide a very useful approach to the evaluation of jaundice in patients with AIDS (Table 5).

N.J. Greenberger, M.D.

Biliary Cryptosporidiosis in HIV-Infected People After the Waterborne Outbreak of Cryptosporidiosis in Milwaukee

Vakil NB, Schwartz SM, Buggy BP, et al (Univ of Wisconsin, Milwaukee; Med College of Wisconsin, Milwaukee)
N Engl J Med 334:19–23, 1996   8–3

Introduction.—An outbreak of cryptosporidiosis occurred in Milwaukee in 1993. The impact of this outbreak on individuals infected with HIV was examined retrospectively.

Methods.—A retrospective study was performed on the clinical presentation, CD4 count, and survival of a group of 82 patients with HIV who had cryptosporidiosis develop during the outbreak. Stool samples were used to confirm infection. Follow up continued for 1 year after the outbreak.

Results.—After the water contamination, a dramatic increase occurred in the number of HIV-infected patients who had cryptosporidiosis develop. Of the 24 patients with biliary symptoms, 4 were alive at the 1 year follow-up. Of the 58 patients without biliary symptoms, 30 were alive at the 1 year follow-up. Eighty-eight percent of patients with biliary symptoms had CD4 counts of no more than $50/mL^3$, whereas only 63% of patients without biliary symptoms had CD4 counts that low. During the 1-year study period, 72% of patients with low CD4 counts died, whereas only 25% of those with higher CD4 counts died. Lower CD4 counts, associated with older age and the presence of nausea and vomiting, were independent predictors of death in this patient group.

Conclusions.—When HIV-infected patients were exposed to waterborne cryptosporidium during the Milwaukee outbreak, those with CD4 counts of no more than $50/mL^3$ were at increased risk of biliary symptoms and death within 1 year of infection. National surveillance for infections with cryptosporidium does not occur.

▶ Waterborne outbreaks of cryptosporidiosis have been described in the United States and other countries, and the outbreak in Milwaukee was devastating in that it affected more than 400,000 individuals. Not surprising, immunocompromised patients were found to be much more susceptible to biliary infections with *Cryptosporidium*. In particular, HIV-infected patients with CD4 counts of less than 50 per cubic millimeter were found to be at greatly increased risk of biliary symptoms and of death within 1 year after the infection. Finally, it is important to note that *Cryptosporidium* is not a reportable disease in most states. Apparently there are no national standards for surveillance for infection with this organism.

N.J. Greenberger, M.D.

Long-term Follow-up of Endoscopic Retrograde Cholangiopancreatography Sphincterotomy for Patients With Acquired Immune Deficiency Syndrome Papillary Stenosis
Cello JP, Chan MF (Univ of California, San Francisco; San Francisco Gen Hosp)
Am J Med 99:600–603, 1995   8–4

Introduction.—Reports of AIDS-related cholangiopathy have appeared with increasing frequency. Patients have been given short-term relief of pain with endoscopic sphincterotomy. The effect of endoscopic retrograde cholangiopancreatography (ERCP) sphincterotomy in 25 patients with AIDS and stenosis of the ampulla of Vater are reported.

Methods.—All patients experienced moderate-to-severe right upper quadrant and/or mid-epigastric abdominal pain that was either persistent or initiated by food intake. All patients had common bile ducts greater than 8 mm in diameter, 5- to 10-mm long tapered narrowing of the distal common bile duct with no distal intraductal or duodenal mass lesions, and normal pancreatograms. All patients had elevated levels of serum alkaline phosphatase and/or alanine aminotransferase and/or bilirubin. Patients underwent standard ERCP sphincterotomy. Pain scores were rated on a scale of 0 to 4. Patients were followed weekly or bimonthly by their primary care physician in an AIDS clinic.

Results.—Patients had been diagnosed with AIDS at a mean of 13.3 months before they underwent ERCP evaluation. All patients had a variety of underlying opportunistic infections and malignancies at the time of initial ERCP. Six patients had cutaneous Kaposi's sarcoma. Three patients had immediate postoperative complications. Patients were followed for a mean of 9.4 months. Six patients were alive at the time of their final evaluation. Mean pain score went from 3.88 on the day of the procedure to 1.33 at 1-month follow-up, a significant difference. Pain scores were significantly lower from months 1 to 11, compared to pre-procedure scores. Pain scores of 8 of 25 patients still alive at 12 months or longer after the sphincterotomy were not significantly different from those recorded on the day of the procedure. Twelve patients underwent repeat ERCP evaluation at a mean of 4.1 months after ERCP sphincterotomy because of continued abdominal pain and/or marked elevations of serum alkaline phosphate levels. There was no significant difference between pre- and post-procedure serum phosphatase levels.

Conclusion.—Patients with AIDS-associated papillary stenosis received long-term relief of biliary-type pain after ERCP sphincterotomy was performed. The procedure did not affect mean serum alkaline phosphatase levels.

▶ The AIDS-related stenosing papillitis is more than a curiosity in this complication-plagued disease. It represents a pain-producing entity that responds to the relatively safe and simple procedure of endoscopic papillotomy. Apparently, the pain is from distal obstruction, since its relief is not associated with a decrease in alkaline phosphatase, a finding apparently related to more proximal strictures within the biliary tree. The etiology of these unique lesions remains unknown but, as this article alludes, it could be related to the unique organisms that populate the afflicted host.

F.G. Moody, M.D.

Capsules and Comments

The Esophagus

Mechanisms of Oral-Pharyngeal Dysphagia in Patients With Parkinson's Disease
Ali GN, Wallace KL, Schwartz R, et al.
Gastroenterology 110:383–392, 1996   9–1

▶ Dysphagia is a well-recognized manifestation of Parkinson's disease and is associated with considerable morbidity from nutritional and pulmonary sequelae. The authors studied 19 patients with Parkinson's disease, of whom 12 had oral-pharyngeal dysphagia and 7 had no symptoms, and 23 healthy control subjects using simultaneous video radiography and pharyngeal manometry. The clinical severity of Parkinson's disease predicted neither the presence nor the severity of dysphagia. The data obtained indicated that oral-pharyngeal dysphagia in Parkinson's disease is multifactorial and includes all the following abnormalities: (1) incomplete upper esophageal sphincter (UES) relaxation; (2) reduced UES diameter; (3) lower pharyngeal contraction pressures; and (4) abnormal pharyngeal wall motion. Most of the patients showed oral and pharyngeal dysfunction even before the clinical expression of dysphagia. Impaired pharyngeal bolus transport is the major determinant of dysphagia in patients with Parkinson's disease.

The Incidence of Adenocarcinoma in Barrett's Esophagus: A Prospective Study of 170 Patients Followed 4.8 Years
Drewitz DJ, Sampliner RE, Garewol HS
Am J Gastroenterol 92:212–221, 1997   9–2

▶ Barrett's esophagus is a complication of gastroesophageal reflux disease and is defined by intestinal metaplasia in the esophagus. Although Barrett's epithelium predisposes patients to the development of adenocarcinoma of the esophagus, past studies have demonstrated widely differing frequencies of adenocarcinoma. Drewitz and colleagues prospectively monitored 170 patients with Barrett's esophagus for a mean of 57 months, or 4.8 years (range 6–156 months). Adenocarcinoma developed in 4 patients, for an incidence of 1 per 208 patient-years of follow-up. It was concluded that surveillance of patients with Barrett's esophagus for dysplasia remains an appropriate clinical practice. In an accompanying editorial, Cameron[1] questioned the benefit of frequent surveillance and suggested that longer intervals, such as 2–5 years, may be more appropriate, provided there is no focal abnormality on endoscopy and no dysplasia on biopsy.

Reference

1. Cameron AJ: Barrett's esophagus: Does the incidence of adenocarcinoma matter? *Am J Gastroenterol* 92:193–194, 1997.

The Stomach and Duodenum

A Randomized Prospective Comparison of Percutaneous Endoscopic Gastrostomy and Nasogastric Tube Feeding After Acute Dysphagic Stroke

Norton B, Homer-Ward M, Donnelly MT, et al.
BMJ 312:6–13, 1996

9–3

▶ Thirty patients who had clinical evidence of severe stroke and dysphagia and who were unconscious at hospital admission were entered into a 6-week randomized trial to determine the effectiveness of percutaneous endoscopic gastrostomy compared with nasogastric tube feeding. Two weeks after hospital admission, 14 patients were allocated to feeding by nasogastric tube and 16 by percutaneous endoscopic gastrostomy tube. The key finding was a dramatic reduction in the 6-week mortality rate associated with gastrostomy feeding; 2 of 16 patients (12.5%) fed by gastrostomy tube had died compared with 8 of 14 patients (57%) fed by nasogastric tube. Patients fed by gastrostomy tube had an improved nutritional status, as evidenced by a mean increase of 0.27 g/dL in the serum albumin level compared with a mean decrease of 0.95 g/dL in patients fed by nasogastric tube. Feeding by percutaneous gastrostomy tube reduced mortality and improved nutritional status.

Sucralfate Suppresses *Helicobacter pylori* Infection and Reduces Gastric Acid Secretion by 50% in Patients With Duodenal Ulcer

Banerjee S, El-Omar E, Mowat A, et al.
Gastroenterology 110:717–724, 1996

9–4

▶ Sucralfate is an effective therapeutic agent in the treatment of duodenal ulcer. It also has been observed that the relapse rate after duodenal ulcer healing with sucralfate is lower than that after healing with histamine H_2 receptor antagonists. Although sucralfate has been classified in the cytoprotective category of ulcer healing drugs, the precise mechanism by which it heals duodenal ulcers remains incompletely defined. The effect of sucralfate on *Helicobacter pylori* infection and on the accompanying hypersecretion of gastric acid induced by this infection in patients with duodenal ulcer disease was studied. Plasma gastrin levels, basal acid output, gastric urease activity, and *H. pylori* density were studied in 10 patients with duodenal ulcer disease who tested positive for *H. pylori* before, during, and after 4 weeks of treatment with sucralfate at a dosage of 2 g twice daily. The density of *H. pylori* decreased by 70% during sucralfate treatment but returned to pretreatment levels after therapy was discontinued. The suppression of *H. pylori* infection was associated with approximately a 50% decrease in basal acid output and an 80% decrease in gastric urease activity; both returned to pretreatment levels after sucralfate treatment was discontinued. Sucralfate suppresses *H. pylori* infection and reduces gastric acid secretion in patients with duodenal ulcer disease. These effects may be important mechanisms by which the drug promotes duodenal ulcer healing.

Duodenal Bicarbonate Secretion: Eradication of *Helicobacter pylori* and Duodenal Structure and Function in Humans

Hogan D, Rapier R, Dreilinger A, et al.
Gastroenterology 110:705–716, 1996

9–5

▶ Basal and acid-stimulated proximal duodenal mucosal bicarbonate secretion are impaired in most patients with duodenal ulcer disease. The possible contribution of *Helicobacter pylori* infection to the diminished proximal duodenal mucosal bicarbonate secretion observed in patients with duodenal ulcers was investigated. Basal, peak, and total acid-stimulated proximal duodenal mucosal bicarbonate secretion was determined in 18 normal *H. pylori*–negative participants, 5 normal *H. pylori*–positive participants, 6 duodenal ulcer *H. pylori*–positive patients, and 6 duodenal ulcer *H. pylori*–negative patients. Duodenal mucosal bicarbonate secretion was measured before and after the eradication of *H. pylori,* and mucosal structure was characterized by duodenal bulb histopathology. Patients with duodenal ulcer and successful *H. pylori* eradication demonstrated normalized proximal duodenal mucosal bicarbonate secretion. The histologic examination of duodenal biopsy specimens was comparable in patients with duodenal ulcer and normal study participants, and there was no apparent relation between inflammation and duodenal mucosal bicarbonate secretion. The key finding is that eradication of *H. pylori* in patients with duodenal ulcer resulted in normalization of basal and acid-stimulated proximal duodenal mucosal bicarbonate secretion. Such normalization of duodenal bicarbonate secretion may be a factor in the markedly reduced rate of ulcer recurrence after the eradication of *H. pylori.*

Lymphocytic Gastritis and Gastric Permeability in Patients With Celiac Disease

Vogelsang H, Oberhuber G, Wyatt J
Gastroenterology 111:73–77, 1996   9–6

▶ Lymphocytic gastritis has been described in patients with celiac disease. The possibility that mucosal changes caused by celiac disease in the stomach and small bowel lead to functional changes (e.g., abnormal gastric and small-bowel permeability) was investigated. Of 28 patients with sprue who were not on a gluten-free diet, 3 showed reactive gastritis, 17 showed lymphocytic gastritis, and 8 showed *Helicobacter pylori* with lymphocytic gastritis. Of the 15 patients who were on a partially gluten-free diet, 4 showed reactive gastritis, 8 showed lymphocytic gastritis, and 3 showed *H. pylori* with lymphocytic gastritis. Gastric and intestinal permeability were measured by oral or duodenal administration of a triple sugar solution containing sucrose, lactulose, and mannitol. Gastric permeability was elevated in 60% of the patients with celiac disease and correlated with antral intraepithelial lymphocyte counts. Further, intestinal permeability also was elevated in 69% of these patients and correlated with duodenal antral epithelial counts. The prevalence of lymphocytic gastritis associated with increased gastric permeability in untreated celiac disease is high. Celiac disease appears to be a general disorder of the gastrointestinal tract associated with altered permeability.

The Colon

Identifying Patients with a High-risk of Relapse in Quiescent Crohn's Disease

Sahmoud T, Hoctin-Boes G, Modigliani R, et al.
Gut 37:811–818, 1995   9–7

▶ Crohn's disease is characterized by alternating phases of quiescent and unpredictable clinical activity. There currently is no reliable way to identify patients with quiescent Crohn's disease who have a high risk of relapse. The natural history of Crohn's disease in patients with quiescent, untreated disease was studied to determine which patients are at risk for relapse. A relapse was defined as either a Crohn's disease activity index (CDAI) of 200 or higher or a CDAI of at least 150 that exceeds the baseline value by more than 100 points. Using a Cox model, the following "bad" prognostic factors were identified: (1) age 25 years or younger at onset of disease; (2) interval since first symptoms 5 years or more; (3) interval since previous relapse 6 months or less; and (4) colonic involvement. The group at highest risk was composed of patients with at least 3 of the 4 bad prognostic factors. These data should permit the design of clinical trials in patients with quiescent Crohn's disease who have a high risk of relapse.

Colorectal Adenocarcinoma in Crohn's Disease

Ribeiro MB, Greenstein AJ, Sachar DB, et al.
Ann Surg 223:186–193, 1996

9–8

▶ Twenty-one patients with colorectal cancer were identified from among 1,695 with Crohn's disease who were admitted to Mt. Sinai Hospital between 1960 and 1989. An additional 9 patients were identified from discharge records up to December 1989. Their mean ages at the onset of Crohn's disease and at the diagnosis of cancer were 32 and 53 years, respectively. Four patients had cancer in the first decade of Crohn's disease, 10 in the second decade, 9 in the third decade, 6 in the fourth decade, and 1 in the fifth decade. Fifteen patients (50%) had ileocolitis, 8 (27%) had colitis, and 7 (23%) had ileitis only. The 5-year actuarial survival rate was 44% for the overall series. The incidence, characteristics, and prognosis of colorectal cancer complicating Crohn's disease were similar to the features of cancer in ulcerative colitis, and include young age, long duration of disease, and multiple neoplasms. Surveillance programs should be instituted for Crohn's disease of the colon similar to those used for ulcerative colitis of comparable duration and extent.

An Increased Risk of Crohn's Disease in Individuals Who Inherit the HLA Class II DRB3*0301 Allele

Forcione DG, Sands B, Isselbacher KJ, et al.
Proc Natl Acad Sci USA 93:5094–5098, 1996

9–9

▶ The pathogenesis of both forms of inflammatory bowel disease (i.e., ulcerative colitis and Crohn's disease) remains incompletely understood. Immune mechanisms play an important role in inflammatory bowel disease, and it has been suggested that a combination of genetic, especially immunogenetic, and environmental factors contributes to the development of these disorders. Further, the role of the inflammatory T cell in Crohn's disease suggests that inherited variations in major histocompatibility complex (MHC) class II genes may be of pathogenetic importance in inflammatory bowel disease. T-cell techniques were used to molecularly type individual alleles of all DRB1, DRB3, DRB4, and DRB5 loci to compare the frequency of the known alleles among ethnically matched populations that consisted of 40 patients with ulcerative colitis, 42 patients with Crohn's disease, and 93 healthy control subjects. A very strong association between HLA–DRB3*0301 and Crohn's disease was reported. A single allele of the infrequently typed HLA class II locus is strongly associated with Crohn's disease, and MHC class II molecules may be important in its pathogenesis.

Mesalazine Induced Exacerbation of Ulcerative Colitis
Kapur KC, Williams GT, Allison MC
Gut 47:838–839, 1996

9–10

▶ Watery diarrhea occurs in up to 15% of patients given 5-aminosalicylic acid (5-ASA) in the form of olsalazine and, to a lesser extent, in patients receiving other forms of 5-ASA analogues. A patient with ulcerative colitis was described in whom 3 different 5-ASA analogues—Asacol, Pentasa, and Salofalk—each seemed to exacerbate diarrhea and bleeding. Both endoscopic and histologic evidence of disease relapse developed after rectal challenge with mesalazine. In addition to the usual factors considered in patients with ulcerative colitis who experience relapse during treatment, the possibility of exacerbation of the disease by a 5-ASA analogue needs to be kept in mind.

Epidermoid Anal Cancer: Results From the UKCCCR Randomized Trial of Radiotherapy Alone Versus Radiotherapy, 5-Fluorouracil, and Mitomycin
UKCCCR Anal Cancer Trial Working Party
Lancet 348:1049–1054, 1996

9–11

▶ Epidermoid anal cancer is believed to be predominantly locoregional, but in surgical series, only approximately 50% of patients have survived for 5 years after radical or local excision. Nonsurgical management with radiation therapy alone or combined with chemotherapy in uncontrolled series has yielded survival rates comparable to those of surgery. Combined modality therapy (CMT) was compared with radiation therapy alone in patients with epidermoid anal cancer. Of 585 patients, 290 were randomly assigned to receive radiation therapy alone and 295 to receive 5-fluorouracil and mitomycin in addition to radiation therapy. After a median follow-up of 42 months, 164 of 279 patients (59%) receiving radiation therapy alone had local failure compared with 101 of 283 patients (36%) receiving CMT. Standard therapy for most patients with epidermoid anal cancer should be a combination of radiation therapy and infused 5-fluorouracil and mitomycin, with surgery reserved for those who fail to respond to CMT.

The Liver

Hepatitis C Virus Genotypes and Risk of Hepatocellular Carcinoma in Cirrhosis: A Case-Control Study
Silini E, Bottelli R, Asti M, et al.
Gastroenterology 111:199–205, 1996

9–12

▶ The possible role of hepatitis C virus (HCV) genotypes in patients with cirrhosis and primary liver cancer complicating hepatitis C was investigated. Three hundred eighty-five patients with cirrhosis with or without hepatocellular carcinoma were studied; 166 patients had hepatocellular carcinoma and cirrhosis, and 219 had cirrhosis alone. The frequency of HCV genotypes was analyzed in these 2 groups of patients to investigate whether the HCV genotype influenced clinical presentation and survival in patients with hepatocellular carcinoma, and to determine the cirrhosis-related risk of hepatocellular carcinoma in patients with different genotypes. Hepatitis C virus type 1b infection was more prevalent in patients with hepatocellular carcinoma compared with patients with cirrhosis but without hepatocellular carcinoma and chronic hepatitis. Age, male sex, and HCV type 1b significantly influenced the risk of cancer in patients with cirrhosis by univariate analysis. Hepatitis C virus type 1b significantly influenced the risk of hepatocellular carcinoma independent of age, sex, and Child's class.

Ciprofloxacin and Long-term Prevention of Spontaneous Bacterial Peritonitis: Results of a Prospective Controlled Trial

Rolachon A, Cordier L, Bacq Y, et al
Hepatology 22:1171–1174, 1995   9–13

▶ Spontaneous bacterial peritonitis (SBP) is a frequent complication in decompensated patients with cirrhosis who have ascites, and is especially likely to occur when ascitic fluid protein levels are less than 1.5 g/dL. Aerobic gram-negative bacilli account for more than two thirds of all cases of spontaneous bacterial peritonitis. Previous studies have demonstrated that daily treatment with antibiotics such as norfloxacin and Bactrim reduces the incidence of recurrent SBP in patients with cirrhosis. The efficacy of long-term antibiotic prophylaxis with ciprofloxacin for the prevention of SBP in 60 patients with cirrhosis and low ascitic fluid protein levels was evaluated. Twenty-eight patients received 750 mg of ciprofloxacin once weekly for 6 months and were compared with 32 placebo recipients who also were followed up for 6 months. Spontaneous bacterial peritonitis developed in only 1 of the 28 patients who received ciprofloxacin (3.6%) compared with 7 of the 32 placebo recipients (22%). Long-term antibiotic prophylaxis with ciprofloxacin at a dosage of 750 mg once weekly is effective in the prevention of SBP in patients with cirrhosis.

Spontaneous Bacterial Empyema in Cirrhotic Patients: A Prospective Study

Xiol X, Castellvi JM, Guardiola J, et al.
Hepatology 23:719–723, 1996   9–14

▶ Although spontaneous bacterial peritonitis (SBP) is a well-known entity with a reported incidence between 15% and 20% in hospitalized patients with cirrhosis and ascites, spontaneous bacterial empyema—the infection of a pre-existing hydrothorax—has been reported only rarely. To define better the incidence and primary characteristics of spontaneous bacterial empyema, hospitalized patients with cirrhosis and hydrothorax were studied. Sixteen of the 120 patients (13%) had 24 episodes of spontaneous bacterial empyema. In 10 of the 24 episodes (43%), spontaneous bacterial empyema was not associated with SBP. Because half the episodes of spontaneous bacterial empyema were not associated with SBP, thoracentesis should be performed in patients with cirrhosis, pleural effusion, and suspected infection. Culture of the pleural fluid should be performed by inoculating 10 mL into blood culture bottles at the bedside.

Evaluation of the Efficacy and Safety of Flumazenil in the Treatment of Severe Portal Systemic Encephalopathy: A Double-blind, Randomized, Placebo Controlled Multicenter Study

Gyr K, Meier R, Haussler J, et al.
Gut 39:319–324, 1996

9–15

▶ Flumazenil is a competitive benzodiazepine receptor antagonist that rapidly reverses the hypnotic sedative effects of benzodiazepines after IV administration. Anecdotal clinical observations suggest that flumazenil may be effective in ameliorating the symptoms of portal systemic encephalopathy (PSE) in patients with chronic liver disease. The efficacy of flumazenil in patients with non-comatose, mild to moderate PSE (stages I–III) caused by severe chronic liver disease was evaluated. Forty-nine patients were randomly assigned to receive either 3 sequential bolus injections of flumazenil or placebo at 1-minute intervals, followed by IV infusion of either flumazenil 1 mg/hr or placebo for 3 hours. A clinically relevant response was seen in 25% to 36% of the patients receiving flumazenil but in none of the patients receiving placebo, and the difference was statistically significant. This suggests that agonists of the benzodiazepine receptor may have a significant role in the pathogenesis of PSE and may be clinically useful in patients with PSE.

Ultrasonographic Determination of Ascitic Volume

Inadomi J, Cello JP, Koch J
Hepatology 24:549–551, 1996

9–16

▶ Physical examination often is inaccurate in the evaluation of ascites. Noninvasive imaging procedures such as CT scanning and US are sensitive and specific for the detection of ascites but have not been developed further to determine the volume of ascitic fluid. A method was described by which ascitic fluid volume could be calculated using transcorporeal US. This method was validated by comparing it with the volume of distribution of a radiolabeled tracer. Ultrasonic measurements were obtained along the ventral surface of the abdomen, and the greatest vertical depth of ascitic fluid was recorded along with the abdominal circumference measured from this point. The median volume of ascites as measured by an indicator dilution technique using [99mTc]-labeled macroalbumin was 11.2 L, with a range of 1.5–17.0 L. The median volume calculated by the US method was 10.3 L (range, 1.2–18 L). Ultrasonic measurements appear to be a useful technique for accurately determining the volume of ascitic fluid.

Management and Follow-up of 78 Giant Haemangiomas of the Liver
Pietrabissa A, Giulianotti P, Campatelli A, et al.
Br J Surg 83:915–918, 1996   9–17

▶ With an ever-increasing number of patients undergoing imaging of the upper abdomen for a variety of indications, the incidental finding of liver hemangiomas has increased considerably. This has led to the term "incidentaloma," which refers to the incidental finding of mass lesions in the liver. Most often, these lesions turn out to be hemangiomas. However, the natural history and appropriate treatment of giant liver hemangiomas remain poorly defined. Seventy-eight patients with giant hemangiomas of the liver were described, 16 of whom underwent resection and 62 of whom had asymptomatic hemangiomas that were managed conservatively; the latter group was monitored for a mean of 55 months. Among those who underwent resection, surgery permanently relieved their symptoms and their hemangiomas did not recur. Of those who received treatment, 6 have died of unrelated diseases and 20 were living in distant areas and could not participate in the US follow-up protocol. Of the 36 unresected lesions monitored according to the protocol, 32 remained stable in size and only 4 showed minor changes. None ruptured or became symptomatic. Asymptomatic large hemangiomas can be managed safely by observation. Resection should be considered only for symptomatic patients and rapidly growing lesions.

The Pancreas

Urinary Trypsinogen-2 Test Strip for Acute Pancreatitis
Hedstrom J, Korvuo A, Kenkimaki P, et al.
Lancet 347:729–731, 1996   9–18

▶ Proteolytic enzymes appear to have a role in the pathophysiology of pancreatitis, and the concentration of trypsinogen in serum reflects pancreatic damage. Serum concentrations of trypsinogen-2 are increased in patients with acute pancreatitis. A trypsinogen-2 test strip was evaluated in patients with clinically suspected acute pancreatitis. In 57 patients with acute pancreatitis, there were 52 positive and 5 negative test results. By contrast, in 40 control subjects with abdominal pain from extrapancreatic causes, there were 36 negative and 4 false positive test results. These findings should be confirmed in larger, randomized, blinded, and appropriately controlled trials.

Serum Antibodies to Carbonic Anhydrase I and II in Patients with Idiopathic Chronic Pancreatitis and Sjögren's Syndrome
Kino-Ohsaki J, Nishimori I, Morita M, et al.
Gastroenterology 110:1579–1586, 1996   9–19

▶ Approximately 30% of patients with chronic pancreatitis have no apparent underlying cause of their disease. Various immunologic alterations have been described in patients with chronic pancreatitis, suggesting autoimmunity as a possible etiologic factor in idiopathic chronic pancreatitis. Chronic pancreatitis also has been observed as a complication in patients with Sjögren's syndrome. It recently has been demonstrated that patients with Sjögren's syndrome may have antibodies to carbonic anhydrase II. Serum from 51 patients with idiopathic chronic pancreatitis and Sjögren's syndrome was evaluated. Serum antibodies against carbonic anhydrase I and II were detected in 7 and 11 of 33 patients with idiopathic chronic pancreatitis, respectively, and in 8 and 13 of 21 patients with Sjögren's syndrome, respectively. Immune sensitization against carbonic anhydrase II or its derived peptide has occurred in some patients with idiopathic chronic pancreatitis and Sjögren's syndrome.

The Gallbladder

The Role of Gallbladder Emptying in Gallstone Formation During Diet-induced Rapid Weight Loss
Gebhard RL, Prigge WF, Ansel HJ, et al.
Hepatology 24:544–548, 1996   9–20

▶ Rapid weight loss in obese individuals has been reported to result in cholesterol gallstones. In 1 series,[1] gallstones developed in 28% of obese individuals who rapidly lost weight on a liquid diet containing 520 kcal/day and less than 2 g of fat per day. Gebhard et al. evaluated and compared biliary physiology in individuals given 2 different low-calorie liquid diets: a 520-kcal diet with less than 2 g of fat per day and a 900-kcal diet with 30 g of fat per day. Both diets produced comparable weight loss of 22%. Gallbladder emptying was significantly faster in the individuals given the 900-kcal diet, which included 1 meal containing 10 g of fat to stimulate maximal gallbladder emptying, than in the individuals given the 520-kcal diet. Gallstones developed in 4 of 6 individuals who received the 520-kcal/day diet. By contrast, none of 7 individuals who received the 900-kcal/day diet had gallstones. This suggests that gallstone risk during rapid weight loss may be reduced by maintenance of gallbladder emptying with a small amount of dietary fat.

Reference

1. Shiffman ML, Kaplan GD, Brunkafan-Kaplan V, et al: Prophylaxis against gallstone formation with ureodeoxycholic acid in patients participating in a very low calorie diet program. *Ann Intern Med* 122:899–905, 1996.

Miscellaneous

Clinical Implications of Endoscopic Ultrasound: The American Endosonography Club Study

Nickl NJ, Bhutani M, Catalano M, et al.
Gastrointest Endosc 44:371–377, 1996   9–21

▶ Four hundred twenty-eight patients were enrolled in a prospective, multicenter study to evaluate the clinical outcomes of endoscopic US (EUS). The specific aim of the study was to determine whether the results of EUS led to changes in treatment and management plans. Endoscopic US findings led to treatment plan changes in 74% of patients, and to management changes of major importance in 31% of patients. The latter included decisions regarding surgery (62 patients), nonsurgical invasive management (36 patients), and further follow-up (22 patients). Importantly, the changes in management were directed toward less costly, lower-risk invasive management in 55% of patients and toward more costly, risky, or invasive procedures in 37%. The most common organ-specific indications for EUS examination were to stage a known esophageal cancer, stage a known anorectal cancer, evaluate upper gastrointestinal submucosal lesions, evaluate a known pancreatic mass, identify or confirm pancreatitis, or differentiate pancreatitis vs. a pancreatic mass. Changes in management plans may occur in most patients based on the results of EUS, and are more likely to be in the direction of less costly, risky, or invasive management options.

Subject Index*

A

C

M

W

Author Index